BONE TUMORS

BONE TUMORS

General Aspects and

Data on 3,987 Cases

(Second Edition, Third Printing)

by

DAVID C. DAHLIN, M.D.

Consultant

Section of Surgical Pathology, Mayo Clinic

Professor of Pathology

Mayo Graduate School of Medicine

University of Minnesota

Rochester, Minnesota

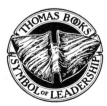

CHARLES C THOMAS · PUBLISHER
Springfield · Illinois · U.S.A.

Published and Distributed Throughout the World by
CHARLES C THOMAS · PUBLISHER
Bannerstone House
301-327 East Lawrence Avenue, Springfield, Illinois, U.S.A.

© *1957 and 1967, by* CHARLES C THOMAS · PUBLISHER
ISBN-0-398-00386-6
Library of Congress Catalog Card Number: 66-27430

First Edition, 1957
Second Edition, First Printing, 1967
Second Edition, Second Printing, 1970
Second Edition, Third Printing, 1973

With THOMAS BOOKS *careful attention is given to all details of manufacturing and design. It is the Publisher's desire to present books that are satisfactory as to their physical qualities and artistic possibilities and appropriate for their particular use.* THOMAS BOOKS *will be true to those laws of quality that assure a good name and good will.*

Printed in the United States of America
B-7

Preface to Second Edition

THE BASIC CLASSIFICATION (modified from Lichtenstein's) employed in the first edition, with tumors comprising histologically distinctive types that have significant clinical and therapeutic implications, has stood the test of time and has gained wide acceptance. Nevertheless, some minor but useful modifications and additions have been developed and are incorporated in this volume. A few of the tumors in the earlier series have been reclassified in the light of recent knowledge.

The 9 years ending December 31, 1964, have provided more than 1,700 additional tumors, all in patients who consulted the Mayo Clinic and all studied pathologically, to augment the original series. These new cases have been incorporated into the total. The combined material has been reviewed pathologically and clinically in continuing studies in collaboration with my colleagues in the Section of Orthopedics and the Section of Diagnostic Roentgenology. It has provided significantly more follow-up information, which is critical to advancement of knowledge concerning each type of tumor. The continuing cooperation of our Section of Medical Statistics, Epidemiology, and Population Genetics has provided us with follow-up data on from 97 to 100% of the various categories of malignant bone tumor. The only group I have not studied in detail is the series of 1,044 myelomas that have been diagnosed on material obtained by aspiration of bone marrow. Patients in this group are examined and treated in the Special Hematology Laboratory, the Section of Therapeutic Radiology, and the Section of Clinical Oncology.

The new data have necessitated amplification of most of the chapters. Illustrations have been increased in order to document many of the concepts gained from study of our own material and of material sent in from elsewhere on some 1,200 problem cases in the past few years. Notable additions include comments on desmoplastic fibroma, mesenchymal chondrosarcoma, postirradiation sarcomas, and sarcomas secondary to chondromatosis and to multiple exostoses. A new chapter deals with odontogenic tumors. The bibliography for each chapter has been increased. Many of the articles that cover general aspects of diagnosis and treatment of bone tumors, and several of the more comprehensive texts available, are listed at the end of Chapter 1.

Members of the Section of Publications, the Section of Photography, and the Section of Medical Illustrations and Scientific Exhibits have made indispensable contributions to this work.

D. C. Dahlin, M.D.

Preface to First Edition

Many of the major advances in present-day understanding of neoplastic and nonneoplastic diseases of bone have been made in the last two decades. In the light of current concepts, I have reviewed systematically all the bone tumors in the files of the Mayo Clinic prior to 1956. I began this review 9 years ago, and have had the help of several of my colleagues who have collaborated in the study of various facets of the over-all problem, as is indicated in the bibliography. The study has embraced more than 2,000 consecutive, unselected bone tumors. Correlation of the clinical features with the gross and microscopic features has been possible because both the case records and the gross and microscopic specimens have been available for study. Complete follow-up studies were available in almost 100% of cases largely because of the work of Dr. Henry W. Meyerding, emeritus member, Section of Orthopedic Surgery, Mayo Clinic, and emeritus professor of orthopedic surgery, Mayo Foundation, Graduate School, University of Minnesota, whose active interest in bone tumors covered a span of nearly 40 years.

Data derived from this study were first presented in the form of an exhibit at the annual meeting of the American Medical Association held in Chicago in June, 1956. Information on skeletal localization and on age and sex distribution, as well as roentgenograms, photomicrographs, and illustrative moulages of gross specimens, was included. As a result of this exhibit, a number of orthopedic surgeons, roentgenologists and pathologists asked me to make the accumulated data available for reference. This I have attempted to do in this small volume, which is an amplification of the material presented in the exhibit.

Because proper understanding of the neoplasms of bone demands correlation of their roentgenologic, gross and microscopic features, these features are liberally illustrated. Textual material has been kept to a minimum and theoretical considerations have been almost completely avoided. The bibliography has been restricted to a few of the pertinent contributions on each subject.

In the final chapter I have discussed briefly several nonneoplastic diseases of bone because they are among those that may be confused clinically and roentgenologically with neoplasms of bone. Odontogenic tumors, because of the special problems they pose, have not been included in the series.

I am indebted to Dr. David G. Pugh, of the Section of Roentgenology of the Mayo Clinic, for his review of the illustrative roentgenograms and of the comments on the roentgenologic features of bone tumors. From Dr. Einer W. Johnson, Jr., and Dr. William H. Bickel of the Section of Orthopedic Surgery, I have received invaluable aid in preparation of the comments on therapy. I am also indebted to the entire staff of the Section of Orthopedic Surgery for their co-operation in this project. To Dr. Carl M. Gambill, of the Section of Publications, and to the Section of Photography, the Section of Biometry and Medical Statistics and the Art Studio I am grateful for their contributions to this book. Dr. Arthur H. Bulbulian, of the Mayo Foundation Museum of Hygiene and Medicine, did much of the work on the original exhibit of bone tumors.

D. C. D.

Contents

CHAPTER 1 3
    Introduction and Scope of Study. Practical Approach to Rapid Histologic Diagnosis, Literature, Classification. Hematopoietic Tumors. Chondrogenic Tumors. Osteogenic Tumors. Tumors of Unknown Origin. Fibrogenic Tumors. Notochordal Tumors. Tumors of Vascular Origin. Lipogenic Tumors. Neurogenic Tumors. Unclassified Tumors. Skeletal and Age Distribution.

CHAPTER 2 18
    Osteochondroma (Osteocartilaginous Exostosis)

CHAPTER 3 28
    Chondroma

CHAPTER 4 38
    Benign Chondroblastoma

CHAPTER 5 48
    Chondromyxoid Fibroma

CHAPTER 6 58
    Osteoma

CHAPTER 7 62
    Osteoid Osteoma

CHAPTER 8 70
    Benign Osteoblastoma (Giant Osteoid Osteoma)

CHAPTER 9 78
    Giant Cell Tumor (Osteoclastoma)

CHAPTER 10 90
    Fibroma (Nonosteogenic Fibroma of Bone, Metaphyseal Fibrous Defect, Fibrous Cortical Defect) and "Xanthoma"

CHAPTER 11 100
    Vascular Tumors

CHAPTER 12 110
    Lipoma and Liposarcoma

CHAPTER 13 114
    Neurilemmoma and Related Tumors

CHAPTER 14 116
    Myeloma

CHAPTER 15 126
    Malignant Lymphoma of Bone (Reticulum Cell Sarcoma)

CHAPTER 16 138
    Chondrosarcoma (Primary, Secondary, and Mesenchymal)

CHAPTER 17 156
    Osteogenic Sarcoma

CHAPTER 18 176
    Parosteal Osteogenic Sarcoma (Juxtacortical Osteogenic Sarcoma)

CHAPTER 19 186
    Ewing's Tumor

CHAPTER 20 196
    Malignant Giant Cell Tumor

CHAPTER 21 204
    "Adamantinoma" of Long Bones

CHAPTER 22 212
    Fibrosarcoma and Desmoplastic Fibroma

CHAPTER 23 222
    Chordoma

CHAPTER 24 234
    Conditions That Commonly Simulate Primary Tumors of Bone. Metastatic Carcinoma. Fibrous Dysplasia. Aneurysmal Bone Cyst. Heterotopic Ossification. Exuberant Callus. Simple Cyst. Epidermoid Cyst. "Cysts" Associated with Diseases of Joints. Osteomyelitis. Histiocytosis X (Reticuloendotheliosis). Giant Cell Reparative Granuloma. Paget's Disease. Hyperparathyroidism. Synovial Chondromatosis and Para-Articular Chondromas. Bone Infarcts

CHAPTER 25 268
    Odontogenic Tumors

INDEX 281

BONE TUMORS

Chapter 1

Introduction and Scope of Study

THE TABULATED STATISTICS included in this book are those of an unselected series of bone tumors except for the following factors. A case was included only if a complete surgical specimen or adequate material for biopsy had been obtained. No case was included in which histologic verification of the diagnosis according to modern pathologic concepts was impossible. The pathologic features were currently reviewed in every case. The patients had all come to the Mayo Clinic for care, thus introducing a possible selection factor of questionable significance.

Accurate analysis of many of the tumors from the earlier years embraced by this study would have been impossible but for the fact that the entire gross specimen, preserved in 10% formalin solution, was available for review in practically every case. A sufficient number of new microscopic sections were made to assure that the various gross features of each lesion could be studied histologically. Such new sections were essential for the correct interpretation of certain lesions. In the average aneurysmal bone cyst, for example, the microscopic section on file was often from a nonspecific solid portion, and it was necessary to embed the curetted fragments from the specimen bottle in paraffin to obtain a preparation that reconstructed the true pathologic appearance to a degree sufficient for correct diagnosis.

Roentgenograms or the interpretation of them were correlated with the gross and histopathologic features. Although x-ray shadows do not supplant microscopic sections in final diagnosis, they frequently afford practically conclusive evidence of the malignant or benign nature of bony lesions and often indicate the histologic type. The roentgenogram may be considered part of the gross pathologic picture, delimiting as it does the part of the bone affected and, in large measure, the extent of the disease. The pathologist responsible for the diagnosis of osseous lesions handicaps himself immeasurably if he ignores their roentgenographic features. These features provide a useful guide for proper biopsy. Anyone can determine, for instance, the inadequacy of an inconclusive needle biopsy specimen or a gram of necrotic tissue excised from a tumor that gives the roentgenologic appearance of having destroyed half of a femur. A recognized limitation is that rather gross destruction, especially of cancellous bone, is necessary for a lesion to be reflected in the roentgenogram. This is well illustrated in Figures 11-13 and 11-14.

INTRODUCTION

In the case of most bone tumors the patient's local symptoms and the results of physical examination are relatively nonspecific. The usual symptoms, pain or swelling or both of these, serve mainly as a guide to the correct site for roentgenographic studies and for biopsy. Accordingly, clinical features of bone tumors have been relegated to a relatively minor place in the discussions to follow. Occasionally, however, as with osteoid osteoma that may give referred pain at a site well away from the lesion, clinical judgment is all-important.

Laboratory studies are of little aid in the diagnosis of the average bone tumor. Myeloma, with its sometimes practically pathognomonic alteration of proteins in serum or urine, is a notable exception. Alkaline phosphatase levels may be elevated in osteoid-producing neoplasms, either primary or metastatic. Elevated levels of acid phosphatase point to metastatic prostatic carcinoma. The ominous nature of rapidly growing sarcomas such as Ewing's tumor may be suggested by systemic evidences that include fever, anemia, and rapid sedimentation rate of erythrocytes.

Physiologists, chemists, and electron microscopists are attempting to clarify some of the basic problems relative to the diagnosis and nature of neoplasms, including those in bone. Some day a simpler method may be found for indicating the biologic capability of each bone tumor that presents a problem. As of now, however, the diagnosis on which therapy must be predicated and prognosis estimated depends upon correct interpretation of material removed for biopsy and stained by techniques that have been known for decades, sometimes augmented significantly by gross pathologic alterations including those reflected in the roentgenogram.

In the interest of brevity a somewhat dogmatic stand will be presented in the chapters to follow. This will be based on the study of Mayo Clinic cases and a review of the literature. When significant differences of opinion exist, these will be indicated in the text or in the bibliography.

Practical Approach to Rapid Histologic Diagnosis

Successful therapy of malignant disease depends upon the institution of treatment before systemic dissemination has occurred. It is axiomatic, therefore, that when the treatment of choice is ablative surgery it should be instituted at the earliest practicable moment in an attempt to remove the tumor before the neoplastic embolization that leads to death of the patient has occurred.

In at least 90% of bone tumors there are soft portions that can be sectioned and examined for immediate diagnosis. In most cases these soft portions afford the best material for diagnosis. For example, in sclerosing osteogenic sarcoma there are almost invariably such noncalcified zones at the periphery of the tumor. Study of the roentgenogram will guide the surgeon to these zones from which to obtain biopsy specimens for early diagnosis. Protracted decalcification of densely sclerotic portions of the tumor or adjacent cortical bone add nothing but delay in the institution of therapy.

Fresh frozen sections allow an immediate, accurate, definitive diagnosis in more than 90%

of the cases of bone tumor. There should be no problem in recognizing the rare lesion too difficult or too ossified for rapid interpretation. As with fixed sections of various types, good histologic preparations and sound basic understanding of the pathologic features are requisites for successful interpretation of fresh frozen sections. Deficiency in either requisite will tend to make one deprecate this diagnostic medium. Actually it has several advantages over conventional permanent-section techniques. First, it allows immediate appraisal of the adequacy of the specimen for biopsy. Edematous tissue around the tumor, necrotic neoplastic tissue, or benign portions of the lesion with frankly malignant foci may otherwise be considered representative of the pathologic process. Second, if the lesion proves to be of an inflammatory nature, the pathologist is guided to proper bacteriologic techniques. Finally, and most important, in the case of those malignant tumors best treated by ablative surgery, definitive therapy can be carried out immediately. Dockerty, in 1953, detailed the technique that has been employed successfully in our laboratory, with minor variations, for more than 50 years.

The pathologist who is averse to making a definitive diagnosis on fresh frozen sections should have permanent sections ready for diagnosis in 24 hours in the case of most bone tumors, provided the surgeon has procured the most suitable tissue for biopsy. Pathologists are becoming increasingly aware that they can, after examination of the roentgenograms, give the surgeon valuable counsel regarding the biopsy procedure.

Use of permanent-staining techniques other than the ordinary technique with hematoxylin and eosin are rarely necessary because they are of insignificant value in most cases. On some occasions a stain for mucus helps in the differentiation of metastatic carcinoma from primary neoplasm of bone. A stain for reticulin in examples of reticulum cell sarcoma has questionable value because atypical tumors often show equivocal amounts of stainable reticulin. Even techniques for the demonstration of alkaline phosphatase in fresh material proved of no value to me in classification, this enzyme appearing in such cells as those of a pure chondrosarcoma and the endothelial cells intermixed in typical reticulum cell sarcoma.

The procurement of material for biopsy of bone tumors by aspiration through a needle or trochar has become increasingly favored. Positive results obtained by this technique are dependable and of value, and at the Mayo Clinic its greatest usefulness has been in lesions of the vertebrae where it can supplant an extensive operation for surgical removal of tissue. The use of this technique is limited, however, since a negative result has little value in the face of clinical and roentgenologic evidence of significant disease. Also, in some tumors such as low-grade, well-differentiated chondrosarcomas, a large sample may be necessary to provide adequate evidence of malignant disease.

When decalcification is necessary a number of satisfactory techniques are available. Detailed considerations of them were published by Morris and Benton in 1956. A good principle is to avoid the dense bone that requires severe measures for decalcification if at all possible.

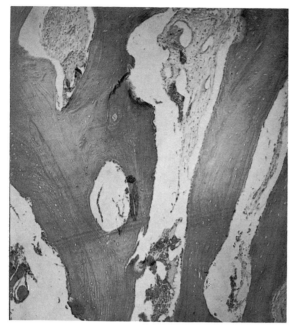

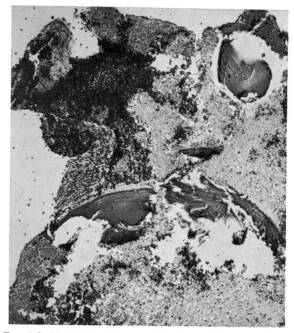

Fig. 1-1. Lymphoma permeating dense bone, a poor place for biopsy. Decalcification has ruined the cytologic features (×50).

Fig. 1-2. Nondiagnostic, necrotic tissue. Frozen sections could have provided guidance to adequate tissue (×75).

Literature

Numerous articles and books concerned with bone tumors have appeared in recent years. Most authors now recognize that a useful classification must comprise entities that are pathologically distinct and have significant clinical, therapeutic, and prognostic implications. Nearly everyone has accepted the several entities that have been clarified by the works and writings of Jaffe and Lichtenstein. There are still some differences of opinion regarding exact definitions of some tumors. Accordingly, at the end of this chapter, I have provided the interested reader with a bibliography which includes the major texts that have been written in English. The list also includes many of the classic articles related to diagnostic techniques and therapy as well as some of the comprehensive studies of bone tumors in general and of those in special locations.

Classification

The classification used in this book (Table 1) is similar to that advocated by Lichtenstein. One of the significant differences is that there has been little attempt to draw a relationship between the benign and the malignant tumors because so few of the latter take origin from the former. The classification is based on the cytology or the recognizable products of the proliferating cells. In most instances, the tumors apparently arise from the type of tissue they produce, but such an assumption cannot be proved correct. For example, most chondrosarcomas begin in portions of bone that normally contain no obvious benign cartilaginous zones. In any event, basing a classification on what is actually seen histologically allows reduplication of results on subsequent

6

analysis. Some of the lesions in the general classification are probably not neoplasms in the strict sense.

Myxomas of the jaws are probably of odontogenic derivation. Myxomas are practically never seen elsewhere in the skeleton. Chondrosarcomas, fibrosarcomas, chondromyxoid fibromas, and portions of foci of fibrous dysplasia may have prominently myxoid features.

Hematopoietic Tumors

The hematopoietic tumors, numbering 1,481, were the most prevalent tumors of bone in the files of the Mayo Clinic. These included 1,286 cases of myeloma. Malignant lymphomas of bone, which ordinarily contain a predominance of reticulum cells and are generally referred to as reticulum cell sarcomas, contributed 195 cases. Leukemic tumor nodules in bone, while commonly found in the terminal phases of leukemia, rarely masquerade clinically as primary malignant disease of bone, although osteoarticular symptoms and signs may be prominent in acute leukemia.

Chondrogenic Tumors

The second largest group consisted of chondrogenic tumors. The tumors in this group were placed there because their histologic appearance proved or suggested a relationship to hyaline cartilage. Nearly a fourth of the total series were in this group, and the osteochondromas (osteocartilaginous exostoses) constituted nearly half of the chondrogenic group. Osteochondromas result from growth of their cartilaginous caps, making them basically chondrogenic. Chondromas, whether they be centrally or subperiosteally located, are tumors of hyaline cartilage which may show variable amounts of calcification and ossification within their substance. Benign chondroblastomas have been separated from the "wastebasket" of giant cell tumors of bone because their proliferating cells produce foci of a matrix substance quite like that of hyaline cartilage. Although chondromyxoid fibromas have a variegated histologic appearance, large or small zones ordinarily bear a striking resemblance to hyaline cartilage. Both primary and secondary chondrosarcomas are obviously related to the chondrogenic neoplasms. Mesenchymal chondrosarcoma is a distinctive subtype.

Osteogenic Tumors

In the osteogenic group of tumors the 650 sarcomas dominated the picture. For a tumor to qualify for this group the malignant neoplastic cells of the given tumor must, in at least some portions, produce recognizable osteoid substance. With this basic qualification the osteogenic sarcomas logically fall into three classes, namely osteoblastic, chondroblastic, and fibroblastic, depending upon the dominant histologic picture. The basic biologic behaviors of these three

INTRODUCTION

tumor subtypes, however, are quite similar, as will be shown in the chapter devoted to osteogenic sarcoma.

The clinically indolent and pathologically slowly progressing low-grade tumors that have become generally known as parosteal or juxtacortical osteogenic sarcomas have been placed in a separate subdivision.

In the Mayo Clinic files there are 102 examples of ordinary osteoid osteoma. Without delving into the controversy as to whether this lesion represents a true neoplasm or some peculiar reaction in bone, we have arbitrarily classed it with the bone tumors. The 28 tumors that we previously called "giant osteoid osteomas" represent an unusually controversial group of cases. Lesions of this type have been called "osteogenic fibromas," "ossifying fibromas" and more recently "osteoblastomas." We employed the term "giant osteoid osteoma" because this tumor bears such a close histologic resemblance to ordinary osteoid osteoma. The prefix "giant" was meant to indicate a different biologic behavior, since tumors of this type do not share the strictly limited growth potential of the average osteoid osteoma. Benign osteoblastoma is now the generally accepted name for this tumor.

Tumors of Unknown Origin

The commonest tumor of unknown origin was Ewing's tumor, constituting 210 cases. Benign giant cell tumor, with 155 cases, was almost as prevalent. The giant cells of the benign giant cell tumor appear to arise from the stromal cells the exact origin of which is unknown. It has been suggested that they arise from undifferentiated mesenchymal cells of bone. It is impossible to substantiate the diagnosis of malignant giant cell tumor unless one can demonstrate typical zones of benign giant cell tumor in the current or previous tissue from the same case. We had only 14 bona fide malignant giant cell tumors. Adamantinoma of long bones is of unknown origin and only nine examples were present in this series.

Fibrogenic Tumors

The pathologic entity called "fibromas of bone," although quite likely not neoplastic, has been included among the bone tumors because of common usage. The files contained 50 examples. Only 100 pure fibrosarcomas of bone were encountered. It should be stressed, however, that multiple sections of all of the tumors were made, and osteoid production in any portion of a predominantly fibroblastic tumor relegated it to the osteogenic sarcoma group. The three desmoplastic fibromas encountered, although histologically benign, will be discussed in relation to fibrosarcomas.

Notochordal Tumors

This series included 122 chordomas. Although this tumor rarely metastasizes, it commonly produces death of its host by local recurrence and extension and hence it has been placed in the category of malignant tumors.

Tumors of Vascular Origin

Although the angiomatous tumors are relatively commonly manifested in roentgenograms, less that 1.5% of the histologically verified neoplasms in this series were in this group. Forty-seven of these were hemangiomas, four were hemangiopericytomas, and seven were malignant blood vascular tumors. The designation of hemangiopericytoma as benign in Table 1 is debatable.

Lipogenic Tumors

Four lipomas of bone were found. In no case did it seem possible to substantiate the unequivocal diagnosis of liposarcoma of bone. The occasional tumor with multinucleated malignant cells, possessing foamy cytoplasm and suggesting the possibility of an origin from adipose connective tissue, was classed with the osteogenic sarcomas. This decision was based on the observation that a similar histologic appearance was present in other tumors which contained zones of obvious osteogenic sarcoma.

Neurogenic Tumors

Four of the seven neurilemmomas of bone in the present series involved the mandible. No malignant neurogenic tumors originating in bone were recognized.

Unclassified Tumors

A few tumors had to be discarded from the total series because there was insufficient tissue for accurate classification. Another group, constituting approximately 1% of the total, did not fall into a niche in the classification. These neoplasms form a heterogeneous group that, for the time being, must be called "unclassified."

Skeletal and Age Distribution

Table 2 shows the skeletal distribution of the various types of tumors. It affords the reader a convenient guide for comparative incidence whether he is interested in a specific neoplasm or an affected bone. The knowledge that certain bones are practically immune to some tumors and have a marked predilection to be the site of development of other neoplasms often assists one in arriving at a correct diagnosis. It is noteworthy, for instance, that only 3 of 650 osteogenic sarcomas affected bones of the hands and wrists and that all but 1 of the 26 tumors of the sternum were malignant.

Some tumors have a decided predilection for patients in certain age groups. Knowledge of this predilection is often useful in arriving at a preoperative diagnosis. The succeeding chapters indicate, with bar graphs, the age distribution for each neoplasm. For specific figures the reader is referred to Table 3.

TABLE 1

CLASSIFICATION OF 3,987 PRIMARY TUMORS OF BONE*

Histologic type	Benign	Cases	Malignant	Cases
Hematopoietic 1,481 cases (37%)			Myeloma Reticulum cell sarcoma	1,286 195
Chondrogenic 969 cases (24%)	Osteochondroma Chondroma Chondroblastoma Chondromyxoid fibroma	464 117 24 20	Primary chondrosarcoma Secondary chondrosarcoma Mesenchymal chondrosarcoma	299 35 10
Osteogenic 805 cases (20%)	Osteoid osteoma Benign osteoblastoma	102 28	Osteogenic sarcoma Parosteal osteogenic sarcoma	650 25
Unknown origin 388 cases (10%)	Giant cell tumor	155	Ewing's tumor Malignant giant cell tumor Adamantinoma	210 14 9
Fibrogenic 153 cases (4%)	Fibroma Desmoplastic fibroma	50 3	Fibrosarcoma	100
Notochordal 122 cases (3%)			Chordoma	122
Vascular 58 cases (1.5%)	Hemangioma Hemangiopericytoma	47 4	Hemangioendothelioma	7
Lipogenic 4 cases	Lipoma	4		
Neurogenic 7 cases	Neurilemmoma	7		
	Total benign	1,025	Total malignant	2,962

* Classification based on that advocated by Lichtenstein, Louis: Classification of Primary Tumors of Bone. *Cancer* 4: 335–341, 1951.

INTRODUCTION

TABLE 2

LOCALIZATION DATA ON BONE TUMORS

(*Exclusive of 1,011 Patients with Multiple Myelomas, 50 with Multiple Exostoses, and 19 with Multiple Chondromas*)

	Femur	Tibia	Innominate	Humerus	Vertebra	Ribs	Sacrum	Hand	Scapula
Osteochondroma	148	64	33	81	11	13	1	7	23
Chondroma	15	1	3	15	3	3		44	2
Chondroblastoma	6	2	5	6	1	1			3
Chondromyxoid fibroma	5	7	2						
Osteoid osteoma	37	26	4	9	3			6	2
Benign osteoblastoma	3	4		2	9		2		
Giant cell tumor	51	38	8	7	3	2	14	1	
Fibroma	19	20		2					
Desmoplastic fibroma									
Hemangioma	3	1	1	1	8	1			
Hemangiopericytoma			1		1	1	1		
Lipoma	1								
Neurilemmoma	1					1			1
Total benign	289	163	57	123	39	22	18	58	31
Myeloma	8	4	30	9	90	35	11		4
Reticulum cell sarcoma	35	18	23	17	19	16	8		12
Primary chondrosarcoma	54	9	71	23	21	54	6	3	17
Secondary chondrosarcoma	2	4	14	3	3	1	1		3
Mesenchymal chondrosarcoma			1		1	2			1
Osteogenic sarcoma	274	116	55	64	10	12	4	3	11
Osteoblastic	177	51	16	39	7	3	1	2	4
Chondroblastic	43	31	25	10	3	6	2		2
Fibroblastic	54	34	14	15		3	1	1	5
Parosteal	20	4		1					
Ewing's tumor	54	20	34	19	7	15	9	1	12
Malignant giant cell tumor	8	2	1	2			1		
Adamantinoma		8							
Fibrosarcoma	27	19	12	5	4	1	7		5
Chordoma					20		62		
Hemangioendothelioma			3		3				
Total malignant	482	204	244	143	178	136	109	7	65
Total series	771	367	301	266	217	158	127	65	96

* Excludes 4 myelomas diagnosed on basis of lymph nodes, 1 on skin, 1 on pleural fluid, and 1,044 on marrow.

† Excludes 2 chondrosarcomas of hyoid and 1 of knee joint.

TABLE 2 (Continued)

Fibula	Skull	Mandible	Maxilla and nasal cavity	Clavicle	Radius	Ulna	Tarsals	Foot	Sternum	Carpals	Patella	Total
18				1	6	2	4	2				414
3					2			5		1	1	98
												24
					1	1	1	3				20
2		1			1	3	5	1		2		102
1	2	2						1		1	1	28
6	2				13	8	1		1			155
7					2							50
		1			1		1					3
1	24	3	3								1	47
												4
	2					1						4
		4										7
38	30	11	3	1	26	15	13	11	1	4	3	956
	2	6	18	11					8			236*
2	16	17			1	2	2		6		1	195
2	6	1	14	4	1		2	1	7			296†
3				1								35
	1		3					1				10
19	13	21	29	3	5	3	4	1	3			650
11	10	9	6		4		2	1				
2		8	15	3		1	2		2			
6	3	4	8		1	2			1			
												25
13	2	3		6	3	3	5	3	1			210
												14
1												9
1	4	10	2		2	1						100
	40											122
1												7
42	84	58	66	25	12	9	13	6	25		1	1,909
80	114	69	69	26	38	24	26	17	26	4	4	2,865

TABLE 3

DISTRIBUTION OF TUMORS BY HISTOLOGIC TYPE AND BY AGE OF PATIENTS

Histologic type	Age distribution by decades									Total patients
	1	2	3	4	5	6	7	8	9	
Benign										
Hematopoietic										None
Chondrogenic										
Osteochondroma	51	206	93	58	30	18	6	2		464
Chondroma	11	28	23	21	18	10	5	1		117
Chondroblastoma	1	14	4	1	1	3				24
Chondromyxoid fibroma	3	6	7	1	1	2				20
Osteogenic										
Osteoid osteoma	16	43	28	10	2	2	1			102
Benign osteoblastoma	2	12	9	3	1		1			28
Unknown origin										
Giant cell tumor		17	52	42	31	8	4	1		155
Fibrogenic										
Fibroma	11	33	6							50
Desmoplastic fibroma		1	2							3
Notochordal										None
Vascular										
Hemangioma	2	1	7	7	17	7	5	1		47
Hemangiopericytoma				1	2		1			4
Lipogenic										
Lipoma				1	2		1			4
Neurogenic										
Neurilemmoma		2	2		1		2			7
Total benign	97	363	233	145	106	50	26	5		1,025

TABLE 3 (*Continued*)

Histologic type	Age Distribution by Decades									Total patients
	1	2	3	4	5	6	7	8	9	
Malignant										
Hematopoietic										
Myeloma			4	14	59	76	64	25	0	242*
Reticulum cell sarcoma	10	17	25	21	32	55	28	7		195
Chondrogenic										
Chondrosarcoma										
Primary	1	7	25	58	66	88	39	13	2	299
Secondary		1	10	11	8	4		1		35
Mesenchymal chondrosarcoma			3	3	3	1				10
Osteogenic										
Osteogenic sarcoma	25	294	121	60	63	44	34	9		650
Osteoblastic	19	185	53	28	23	18	14	3		343
Chondroblastic	5	62	39	14	19	11	4	1		155
Fibroblastic	1	47	29	18	21	15	16	5		152
Parosteal osteogenic sarcoma		4	7	8	5	1				25
Unknown origin										
Ewing's tumor	45	103	41	13	6	2				210
Malignant giant cell tumor			1	6	2	4	1			14
Adamantinoma		3	4	1		1				9
Fibrogenic										
Fibrosarcoma	2	14	12	23	16	19	8	3	3	100
Notochordal										
Chordoma	1	1	10	21	28	33	22	4	2	122
Vascular										
Hemangioendothelioma	1	1		4		1				7
Lipogenic										None
Neurogenic										None
Total malignant	85	445	263	243	288	329	196	62	7	1,918

* Exclusive of 1,044 tumors diagnosed only by marrow aspiration.

INTRODUCTION

Bibliography

1948 Guri, J. P.: Tumors of the Vertebral Column. *Surg., Gynec., & Obst., 87*:583-598.

1948 Hatcher, C. H.: The Diagnosis of Bone Sarcoma. *Rocky Mountain M. J., 45*:968-978 (Nov.)

1948 Hatcher, C. H.: Treatment of Bone Sarcoma. *Rocky Mountain M. J., 45*:999-1009 (Nov.)

1949 Geschickter, C. F., and Copeland, M. M.: *Tumors of Bone.* Ed. 3, Philadelphia, J. B. Lippincott Co., 810 pp.

1950 Copeland, M. M.: Benign Tumors of Bone. *Surg., Gynec., & Obst., 90*:697-712.

1950 Prevo, S. B.: A Clinical Analysis of 205 Cases of Malignant Bone Tumor. *J. Bone & Joint Surg., 32A*:298-306.

1951 Pugh, D. G.: *Roentgenologic Diagnosis of Diseases of Bones.* Baltimore, The Williams and Wilkins Co., pp. 352-568.

1951 Lichtenstein, L.: Classification of Primary Tumors of Bone. *Cancer, 4*:335-341.

1953 Dockerty, M. B.: Rapid Frozen Sections—Technique of Their Preparation and Staining. *Surg., Gynec., & Obst., 97*:113-120.

1953 Haggart, G. E., and Copel, J. W.: Early Diagnosis of Primary Malignant Bone Tumors. *J.A.M.A., 152*:883-885.

1953 Johnson, L. C.: A General Theory of Bone Tumors. *Bull. New York Acad. Med., 29*:164-171.

1955 Ottolenghi, C. E.: Diagnosis of Orthopaedic Lesions by Aspiration Biopsy. Results of 1,061 Punctures. *J. Bone & Joint Surg., 37A*:443-464.

1955 Schajowicz, F.: Aspiration Biopsy in Bone Lesions. Cytological and Histological Techniques. *J. Bone & Joint Surg., 37A*:465-471.

1955 Lichtenstein, L.: Tumors of Periosteal Origin. *Cancer, 8*:1060-1069.

1955 Barrett, N. R.: Primary Tumours of Rib. *Brit. J. Surg., 43*:113-132.

1955 Thomson, A. D., and Turner-Warwick, R. T.: Skeletal Sarcomata and Giant-Cell Tumour. *J. Bone & Joint Surg., 37B*:266-303.

1956 Morris, R. E., Jr., and Benton, R. S.: Studies on Demineralization of Bone: I. The Basic Factors of Demineralization. II. The Effect of Electrolytic Technics in Demineralization. III. The Effect of Ion Exchange Resins and Versenate in Demineralization. IV. Evaluation of Morphology and Staining Characteristics of Tissues After Demineralization. *Am. J. Clin. Path., 26*:579-595, 596-603, 771-777, 882-898.

1956 Sirsat, M. V.: Sarcoma of Bone: Observations on 150 Cases, With Special Reference to Incidence, Location and Pathology. *Indian J. Surg., 18*:1-30.

1957 Schobinger, R., and Stoll, H. C.: The Arteriographic Picture of Benign Bone Lesions Containing Giant Cells. *J. Bone & Joint Surg., 39A*:953-960.

1957 Bickel, W. H., and Lewis, R. C., Jr.: Hemipelvectomy for Malignant Disease. *J.A.M.A., 165*:8-12.

1957 Tracey, J. F., Brindley, H. H., and Murray, R. A.: Primary Malignant Tumors of Bone. *J. Bone & Joint Surg., 39A*:554-560.

1958 Jaffe, H. L.: *Tumors and Tumorous Conditions of the Bones and Joints.* Philadelphia, Lea and Febiger, 629 pp.

1959 Bucalossi, P., Di Pietro, S., and Rock, T.: Tumori della gabbia toracica. *Tumori, 45*:695-750.

1959   Strickland, B.: The Value of Arteriography in the Diagnosis of Bone Tumours. *Brit. J. Radiol., 32*:705-713.

1962   Vittali, Horst-Peter: Zur Diagnose der bösartigen "zystischen" Knochentumoren. *München. med. Wchnschr., 104*:2494-2497; 2511-2512.

1962   Ackerman, L. V., and Spjut, H. J.: *Tumors of Bone and Cartilage.* Atlas of Tumor Pathology, Section II, Fascicle 4, Armed Forces Institute of Pathology, Washington, D.C., National Research Council, 347 pp.

1963   Gilmer, W. S., Higley, G. B., Jr., and Kilgore, W. E.: *Atlas of Bone Tumors: Including Tumorlike Lesions.* Saint Louis, The C. V. Mosby Co., 165 pp.

1963   Aegerter, E., and Kirkpatrick, J. A.: *Orthopedic Diseases.* Ed. 2. Philadelphia, W. B. Saunders Co., pp. 477-652.

1964   Gabrielsen, T. O., and Kingman, A. F., Jr.: Osteocartilaginous Tumors of the Base of the Skull. Report of a Unique Case and Review of the Literature. *Am. J. Roentgenol., 91*:1016-1023.

1964   Pack, G. T., and Ariel, I. M.: *Treatment of Cancer and Allied Diseases.* Vol. 8. Tumors of the Soft Somatic Tissues and Bone. New York, Harper and Row Co., 574 pp.

1964   Cohen, D. M., Dahlin, D. C., and MacCarty, C. S.: Apparently Solitary Tumors of the Vertebral Column. *Mayo Clin. Proc., 39*:509-528.

1965   Lichtenstein, L.: *Bone Tumors.* Ed. 3. Saint Louis, The C. V. Mosby Co., 411 pp.

Chapter 2

Osteochondroma (Osteocartilaginous Exostosis)

This most common of the benign bone tumors logically belongs in the chondrogenic group. Although the average osteochondroma is predominantly osseous, the bony mass is produced by progressive enchondral ossification of its growing cartilaginous cap. Growth of these tumors usually parallels that of the patient, and they often become quiescent when the epiphyses have closed.

One may question whether osteochondromas are correctly classed with the neoplasms of bone, but their clinical features and their rare malignant transformation make it reasonable to include them among the tumors. Their pathologic features make it apparent that the tumors are produced by growth of aberrant foci of cartilage on the surface of bone. Hence one could consider these tumors among the congenital anomalies.

Multiple Osteochondromas

A much smaller group of patients has numerous osteochondromas affecting many bones. In this condition, which has a strong familial tendency, each individual tumor has the characteristics that will be described for the solitary form. The incidence of development of secondary chondrosarcoma in patients with multiple osteochondromas is probably more than 10%. Osteochondromas result from a distinctive form of dysplasia that should not be confused with enchondromatosis.

Most patients with multiple exostoses have many, sometimes innumerable, lesions that may be grossly deforming. An occasional patient has only two or three.

Subungual Exostoses

These peculiar projections from the distal portion of a terminal phalanx, usually of the first toe, are almost certainly the result of trauma with or without superimposed infection. They are not included in the data on osteochondromas although they possess many of the roentgenologic and pathologic features of them.

Osteochondroma

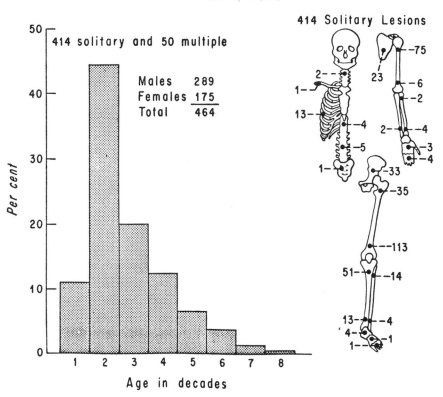

FIG. 2-1. Skeletal, age, and sex distribution of osteochondromas.

Incidence

Osteochondromas comprised 45% of the benign bone tumors and 12% of the total in this series. Many of these tumors are asymptomatic and never found, and many of those discovered are never excised, so their actual incidence is much greater than these figures for surgical cases indicate. Nearly 90% (414) of the patients had solitary lesions.

Sex

A trifle more than 60% of patients in both the solitary and multiple exostoses groups were males. The literature indicates little sex predilection.

Age

More than half the patients were less than 20 years of age at the time of excision of their osteochondromas, and 44.4% were in the second decade of life. The age at the time of first operation for those with multiple exostoses was used in the illustration above and paralleled closely the age of patients with single exostoses who required surgical treatment.

Localization

Osteochondromas may occur on any bone that develops by enchondral ossification. They usually occur in the metaphyseal region of the long bones of the limbs; rarely they are near or

OSTEOCHONDROMA

in the middle third of such bones. More than half in this series involved the femur and humerus. The ilium contributed 25 of the 33 arising from innominate bones.

Symptoms

The patient's complaints are related to the size of the tumor; the complaint of a hard swelling, usually of long duration, is the commonest. The presence of the mass may induce the patient, because of fear or vanity, to seek medical care. Pain may result from the tumor's impinging on neighboring structures or from weight bearing or other activity. Pain was due to fracture of the tumor's stalk in two patients in this series.

Physical Findings

Palpable mass is ordinarily the only finding. Secondary effects may occur, especially when the tumor infringes upon the spinal canal.

Roentgenologic Features

The characteristic appearance is that of a projection composed of a cortex continuous with that of the underlying bone and a spongiosa, similarly continuous. The adjacent cortex often flares to become the base of the tumor. The projection may have a broad base or be distinctly pedunculated. Irregular zones of calcification may be present, especially in the cartilaginous cap, but extensive calcification with consequent irregularities of the cap should arouse the suspicion of malignant change. Osteochondromas commonly arise at the site of tendon insertions and the direction of their growth is often along the line of the tendon's pull. The affected bone is often abnormally wide at the level of an osteochondroma owing to failure of normal tubulation. Such widening is especially apt to be seen in patients with multiple exostoses.

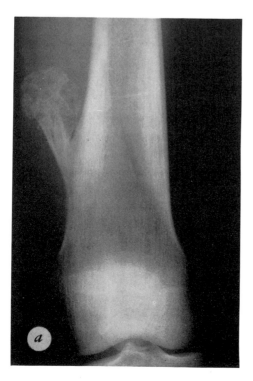

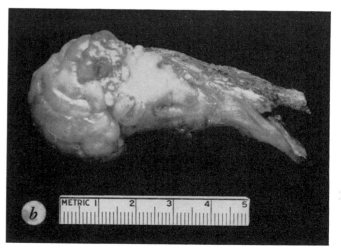

Fig. 2-2. *a*. Pedunculated osteochondroma of the medial aspect of the femur. *b*. Gross specimen in the same case showing a regular, smooth, cartilaginous cap.

Fig. 2-3. *Right*. Osteochondroma of 19 years' known duration in a 24-year-old woman. The mass had been partially excised at the age of 11. This roentgenogram shows the flaring of the bony cortex as it becomes the base of the tumor. *Below*. The excised tumor is composed chiefly of fatty, cancellous bone. The cortex is markedly attenuated where it covers the broad stalk of the tumor. Most of the cartilaginous cap has undergone involution. The excised segment of humerus was replaced by a bone graft. Similar block excisions were employed for two other humeral and one femoral osteochondroma because their size and roentgenographic appearances suggested the possibility of chondrosarcoma.

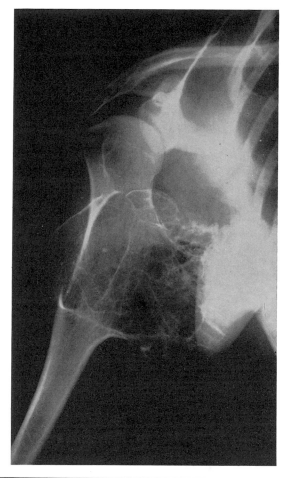

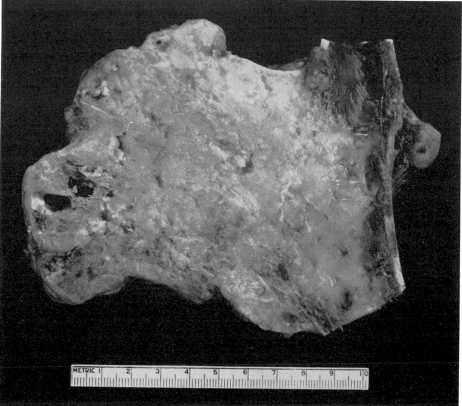

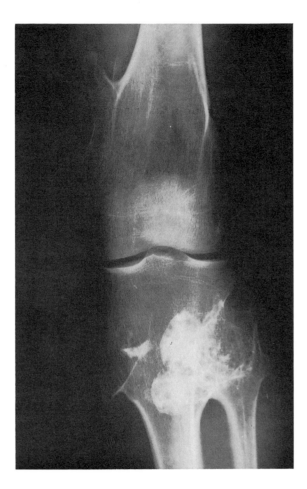

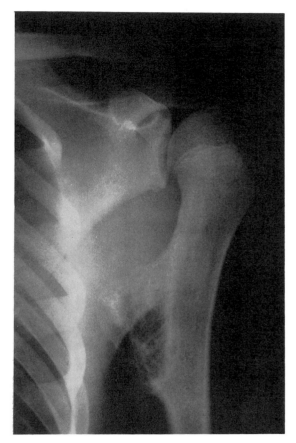

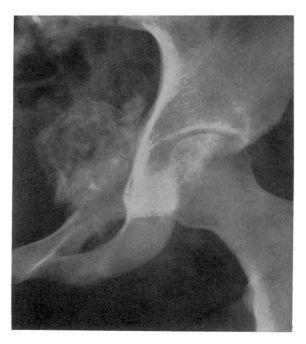

Fig. 2-4 *Above, left*. Hereditary multiple osteochondromas about the knee.

Fig. 2-5 *Above, right*. Sessile exostosis in one of the commoner sites. Gross specimen is shown in Figure 2-8.

Fig. 2-6 *Left*. Osteochondroma proved benign but with roentgenologic features suggestive of chondrosarcoma.

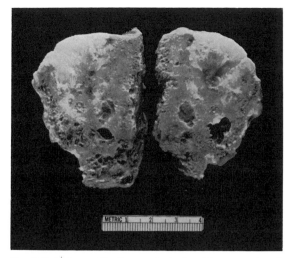

Fig. 2-7. Osteocartilaginous exostosis with a prominent, irregular cartilaginous cap. Such lesions require careful sampling to exclude secondary chondrosarcomatous change. Note cyst formation secondary to degeneration.

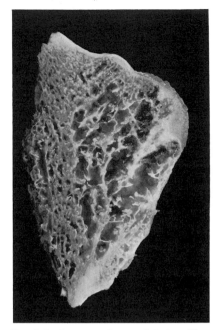

Fig. 2-8. Gross specimen of lesion illustrated in Figure 2-5. There is a prominent cancellous core and a thin cartilaginous cap.

Gross Pathology

The gross pathologic features confirm the roentgenologic picture. Sessile exostoses may be very flat, whereas pedunculated ones are sometimes very long and slender, and all gradations between these exist. Many are cauliflower-shaped with or without a stalk.

The tumor's cortex and its periosteal covering are continuous with those of the underlying bone. A bursa often develops over the exostosis. The marrow of the tumor may be fatty or hematopoietic often mirroring the status of the spongiosa of the underlying bone with which it merges.

The hyaline cartilage of the tumor's cap is ordinarily 2 to 3 mm thick. This cap may cover the entire external surface of a sessile tumor, whereas it covers only the rounded end of a stalked exostosis. The cartilage may be 1 cm or more thick in the actively growing benign exostosis of adolescence. Irregularity and thickening of the cap, especially when the patient is postpubertal, demand careful histologic study because of the likelihood of secondary chondrosarcoma. If the cartilaginous rim is thin and regular and the underlying spongiosa appears normal the tumor is always benign. In the case of arrested exostosis there may be practically no cartilaginous cap.

The bursa overlying an exostosis may be the site of ossified or calcified cartilaginous loose bodies. In this series there were three with numerous and one with single such loose bodies.

Histopathology

Microscopic study confirms the gross appearance of regular cortical and underlying medullary bone with its fatty or hematopoietic component. The chondrocytes of the cartilaginous cap are often arranged in clusters in parallel, oblong lacunar spaces, reminiscent of normal epiphyseal cartilage. This histologic orientation strongly suggests that the lesion is benign. The typical benign chondrocyte has a single small nucleus. During the age of active bone growth fairly frequent binucleate cartilage cells may be seen in benign exostoses. Malignant transformation of an exostosis is nearly always in the form of chondrosarcoma, the histologic features of which are described in a later chapter. Islands of cartilage are sometimes imbedded in the underlying cancellous bone, and these may undergo degeneration with irregular calcification, which is sometimes demonstrable on the roentgenograms. The exostosis is covered by periosteum which is continuous with that of the adjacent bone. As indicated by the gross appearance, the cartilaginous cap involutes after growth of the osteochondroma ceases, and it may even disappear entirely.

Trauma may produce fibroblastic proliferation and even new bone formation, especially in the peripheral portions of an osteochondroma. Those few osteochondromas of the hands and feet not in the subungual zones tended to have more admixed fibroblastic tissue and less regularity of their cartilaginous and bony components, suggesting that they may have resulted from prior trauma.

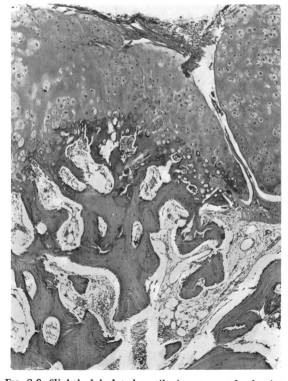

FIG. 2-9. Slightly lobulated cartilaginous cap of a benign osteochondroma. Enchondral ossification is producing regular bony trabeculae separated by fatty marrow. A strip of periosteum overlies the tumor (×30).

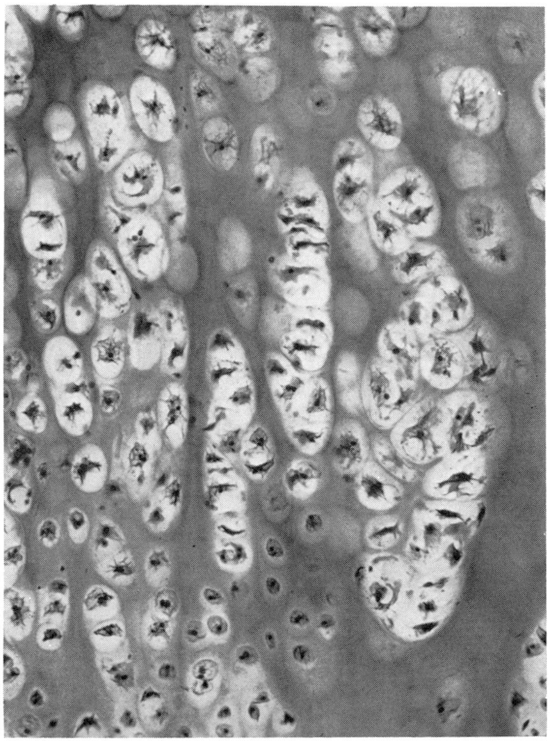

FIG. 2-10. Linear clusters of chondrocytes mimicking the appearance of a normal epiphysis. Individual nuclei are small and multinucleated chondrocytes are rare in the average benign osteochondroma (×110).

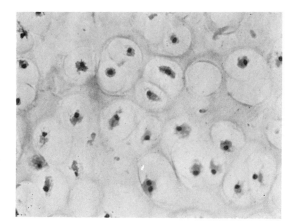

FIG. 2-11. Multinucleated cells occur not infrequently in some of the benign exostoses of childhood (×210).

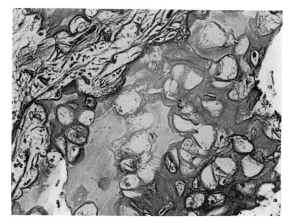

FIG. 2-12. Calcifying foci of degenerating cartilage in the stalk of an osteochondroma (×170).

Treatment

The presence of an osteocartilaginous exostosis is, in itself, insufficient reason for surgical extirpation since malignant transformation occurs in only about 1% of clinically recognized osteochondromas. Removal is indicated if the tumor is unsightly, is producing pain or disability, has roentgenologic features suggestive of malignancy, or shows abnormal increase in size.

Removal of the tumor flush with the bone of origin is the treatment when surgical intervention is indicated. The entire cartilaginous cap should be removed. In some locations, such as a rib, block excision of the affected bone is best, especially if the diagnosis is uncertain.

Although chondrosarcoma will develop in approximately 10% of patients with multiple osteocartilaginous exostoses the tumors are too numerous to allow prophylactic removal. The same general principles should govern removal of a tumor in this condition as in the solitary form of the disease.

Prognosis

Osteochondromas, if benign, are practically always cured by complete excision. Nine tumors (2% of the series) were recurrent when the patients came here or recurred after excision here. These recurrent lesions made a second operation necessary at intervals varying from 1 year to 26 years, although all were benign. Second operations in these cases proved curative. Failure to remove the entire cartilaginous cap or even its overlying periosteum probably explains most recurrences. Sometimes a nearby similar cartilaginous focus is unwittingly left behind and produces a second tumor.

Recurrence suggests the possibility that the original tumor was a chondrosarcoma. Such was the case in some of the earlier "osteochondromas" in our series that have since been reclassified as chondrosarcomas.

Subungual Exostoses

Thirty-seven exostoses removed from the distal portions of the distal phalanges were not included in the data on tumors. Patients with these lesions frequently give such a convincing history of trauma and repeated or continuous infection at the site of the lump that these seem likely to play a part in its genesis. The proliferating fibrocartilaginous tissue capping a growing subungual exostosis resembles callus in its morphologic gradations to mature bony trabeculae, further supporting the likelihood of the tumor's being a response to injury. Sometimes the advancing margin of these lesions is so actively growing as to mimic sarcoma much the way a march fracture may. Attention to the lack of true anaplasia and to the orderly progression to mature bone provides the clues of benignity.

These frequently painful projections from the distal phalanges are usually under the nail and rarely measure more than 1 cm in diameter. Pain and swelling are the result. Ulceration and infection may be present and make subungual melanoma a consideration clinically. Of the 37 tumors, 29 affected the first toe; 3, other toes; 4, the thumb; and 1, the index finger.

Surgical removal effects cure of these exostoses, and they apparently have no premalignant potential.

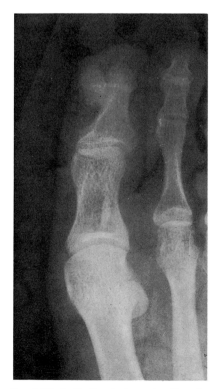 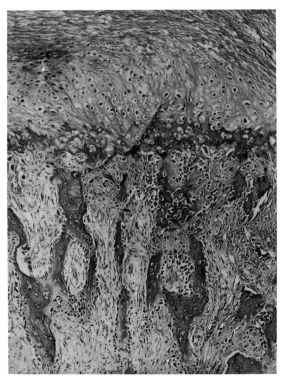

FIG. 2-13. *Left.* Exostosis protruding dorsomedially from the distal phalanx of the first toe. *Right.* Relatively early stage in development of subungual exostosis with proliferating cartilage maturing into bone. Here the orderly progression to bone is evident, although the process is earlier than that depicted in the accompanying roentgenogram (×50).

Sarcomas in Solitary Osteochondroma

Thirteen exostoses, not included in the foregoing data on osteochrondromas, gave rise to chondrosarcomas. The features of these tumors will be further elaborated in the chapter on chondrosarcoma. Roentgenologic, gross, and microscopic evidence indicated the relationship of these malignant tumors to the benign precursor. These 13 tumors comprised 3.1% of all solitary exostoses treated surgically but this figure does not represent accurately the incidence of malignant change since so many benign ones are not treated surgically. Furthermore, it is likely that patients with sarcomatous change gravitate to medical centers.

Two osteogenic sarcomas arose in a parosteal or juxtacortical location but within lesions that bore stigmata of preexisting osteochondroma. One lesion was on the medial aspect and one on the posteromedial aspect of the distal portion of the shaft of the femur but neither was characteristic of ordinary parosteal (juxtacortical) osteogenic sarcoma.

Sarcomas in Multiple Exostoses

None of the 50 patients with multiple exostoses included in Figure 2-1 had sarcomas, but an additional 17 with multiple exostoses have been treated for secondary chondrosarcomas at the Mayo Clinic. Although this represents a 25% incidence of malignant change in the total of 67 patients, the selection factors again make firm conclusions unwise.

Bibliography

1920   Keith, Arthur: Studies on the Anatomical Changes Which Accompany Certain Growth-disorders of the Human Body. I. The Nature of the Structural Alterations in the Disorder Known as Multiple Exostoses. *J. Anat., 54*:101-115.

1943   Jaffe, H. L.: Hereditary Multiple Exostosis. *Arch. Path., 36*:335-357.

1954   Harsha, W. N.: The Natural History of Osteocartilaginous Exostoses (Osteochondroma) *Am. Surgeon, 20*:65-72.

1963   Bethge, J. F. J.: Hereditäre, multiple Exostosen und ihre pathogenetische Deutung. *Arch. orthop. Unfall-Chir., 54*:667-696.

1963   Anastasi, G. W., Wertheimer, H. M., and Brown, J. R.: Popliteal Aneurysm with Osteochondroma of the Femur. *Arch. Surg., 87*:636-639.

1964   Solomon, L.: Hereditary Multiple Exostosis. *Amer. J. Human Genet., 16*:351-363.

1964   Morton, K. S.: On the Question of Recurrence of Osteochondroma. *J. Bone & Joint Surg., 46B*:723-725.

Chapter 3

Chondroma

T HIS BENIGN TUMOR is composed of mature hyaline cartilage. Most commonly, chondromas are centrally located in bone, and such tumors are called "enchondromas." Less often they are distinctly eccentric and bulge the overlying periosteum; this type has been called "periosteal chondroma." In thin or flat bones such as the ribs, scapula, or innominate bone, the exact origin of chondromas, that is, whether central or subperiosteal, often cannot be determined because of destruction of landmarks by the tumor.

Multiple Chondroma

This dysplasia of bone is characterized by failure of normal enchondral ossification with the production of tumefactive cartilaginous masses in the epiphyseal and adjacent regions of the shaft. A few or many bones may be affected. With widespread involvement and a tendency to unilaterality, this condition is often called "Ollier's disease." In addition to tumefaction, there are concomitant bowing and shortening of bones as a result of this disease. In fact, multiple chondroma and fibrous dysplasia both result from disordered ossification, and this relationship is emphasized by lesions containing histopathologic features of both. Patients with multiple chondroma should be sharply distinguished from those with skeletal osteochondromatosis (multiple osteochondromas). Skeletal chondromatosis when associated with angiomas of the soft tissues is called Maffucci's syndrome. Completely reliable figures are not available, but approximately one third of the cases of multiple chondroma are complicated by chondrosarcoma.

Extraosseous Cartilaginous Tumors

Not included in this series are cartilaginous tumors arising in unusual sites such as the larynx and the synovial membranes. These have unusual characteristics, the most significant of which is that their clinical behavior is less aggressive than that suggested by their histology. The same applies to the not uncommon extraosseous cartilaginous tumors of the hands and feet, most of which are small and many of which probably derive from synovium. Frankly malignant extraosseous chondromatus neoplasms are rare.

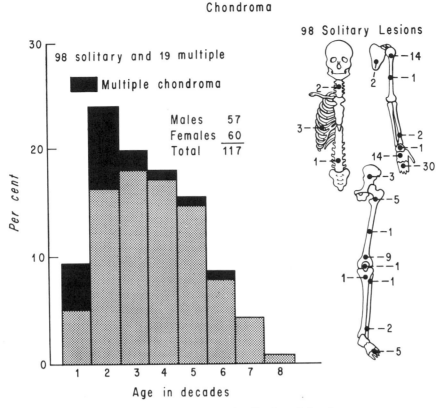

FIG. 3-1. Skeletal, age, and sex distribution of chondromas.

Incidence

Chondromas comprised only 10.4% of the benign tumors of the present series and 3% of the entire series.

Sex

Experience in the present series of cases bears out recorded data which indicate no significant sex predilection. Twelve of the 19 with multiple chondromas were males.

Age

Cases were fairly evenly distributed throughout life. Patients with multiple lesions required operation at an average younger age.

Localization

More than 50% of the tumors were in the hands and feet, chiefly in the phalanges, and 90% of these were in the hands. Chondroma is by far the commonest tumor of the small bones of the hand. One of the three lesions of the innominate bone involved the pubis and two the ilium. The bones most commonly affected by chondrosarcoma are relatively immune to chondroma. None of the rare chondromatous tumors at the base of the skull were encountered in this series. Two intracranial chondromas of meningeal origin were excluded.

CHONDROMA

Symptoms

Many chondromas are asymptomatic, and this can be attributed to their extremely slow rate of growth. Some are discovered accidentally on roentgenographic examination. Pathologic fracture often ushers in the symptoms of the commonly seen chondroma of the distal portions of the extremities. Notable swelling is rarely produced. Pain unassociated with pathologic fracture should arouse the suspicion of malignancy because it suggests that the tumor is invasive.

Physical Findings

Physical examination contributes little to the diagnosis of chondroma of bone. Rarely is there tumefaction. The occurrence of pain or pathologic fracture merely directs one's attention to the appropriate region for roentgenographic study.

Roentgenologic Features

The average chondroma produces a well-circumscribed central region of rarefaction. Any portion of the small tubular bones of the hands and feet may be affected, but the tumor is ordinarily diaphyseal in location. From slight to very prominent stippled or mottled calcification of the tumor is frequently seen, especially in those chondromas occurring in the large tubular bones. Ossification within the lesion may contribute radiopacity. The cortex overlying a chondroma of small bones is often expanded, and the expansion may be eccentric. The presence of calcification within a well-circumscribed rarefying tumor affords strong evidence that the lesion contains hyaline cartilage that is undergoing degenerative change. Some chondromas lie eccentrically, beneath the periosteum, in a well-demarcated cortical defect. Twenty-four of the solitary chondromas in this series were so located.

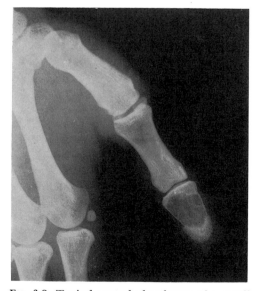

Fig. 3-2. Typical central chondroma of a small bone, in this case affecting the distal phalanx of the thumb.

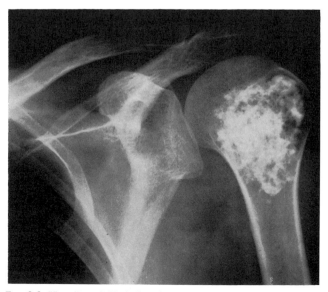

Fig. 3-3. Heavily calcified chondroma. Such density is ordinarily the result of calcification secondary to necrosis.

30

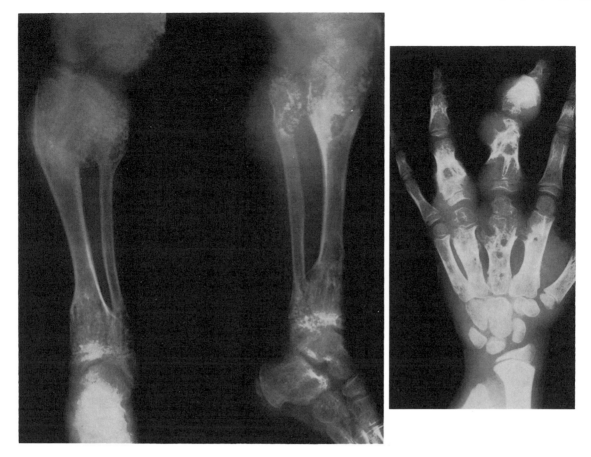

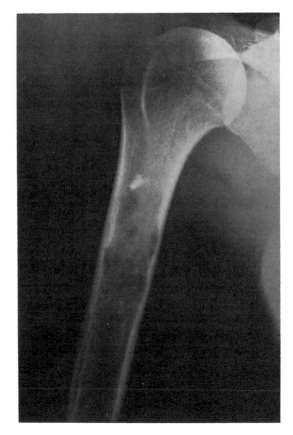

Fig. 3-4. *Above.* Enchondromatosis (Ollier's dyschondroplasia) with multiple, deforming, cartilaginous tumors with punctate calcification in the lesional tissue. (Reproduced with permission from: Pugh, D. G.: *Roentgenologic Diagnosis of Diseases of Bones.* Baltimore, Williams and Wilkins, 1954, pp. 438-442).

Fig. 3-5. *Above, right.* Multiple deforming enchondromas.

Fig. 3-6. *Right.* Chondroma of humerus in 32-year-old woman. Note cortical erosion and focal calcification. The patient was well 4 years after removal of the tumor by curettage.

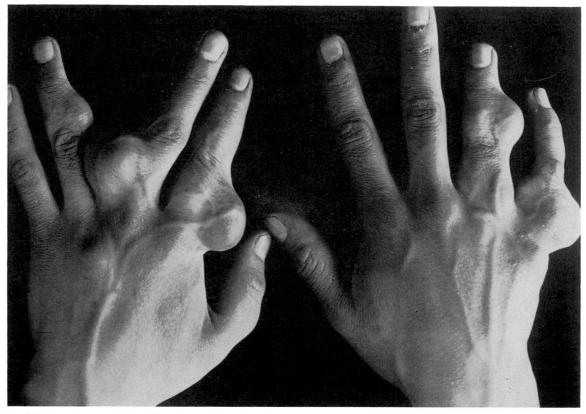

Fig. 3-7. Rare but markedly deforming multiple chondromas, in this case affecting only the hands. This may be a mild manifestation of Ollier's dyschondroplasia. Enchondromas of the hands usually produce no visible swelling. (Reproduced with permission from: Shellito, J. G., and Dockerty, M. B.: *Surg., Gynec & Obst., 86:*465-472, 1948.)

Gross Pathology

The characteristic chondroma is composed of confluent masses of bluish, semitranslucent, hyaline cartilage with a distinctly lobular arrangement. The lobules vary from a few millimeters to a centimeter or more in diameter. The periphery of the lesion may be somewhat indistinct, because ramifications of the cartilaginous tumor sometimes penetrate into adjacent marrow spaces. Some of the tumors are very soft and mucinous. Those characterized by x-ray evidence of punctate areas of calcification have more or less densely calcified masses scattered throughout the tumor, and occasional lesions are heavily calcified and ossified. The gross characteristics of the solitary tumor and of the individual tumors of the multiple variety are similar.

As previously indicated, most chondromas are central in location, but some of them are under the periosteum and produce erosion of the underlying cortex and a bulge in the contour of the bone. These subperiosteal chondromas lie in an excavation in the bone, and their internal limits are marked by a thin sclerotic zone.

Chondromas are characteristically small tumors, and when one encounters a tumor of hyaline cartilage that measures several centimeters in diameter one should check carefully for evidence of malignancy. Lysis of cortex over a central chondroma, especially if associated with extraosseous extension, is an ominous sign and is often indicated in the roentgenogram.

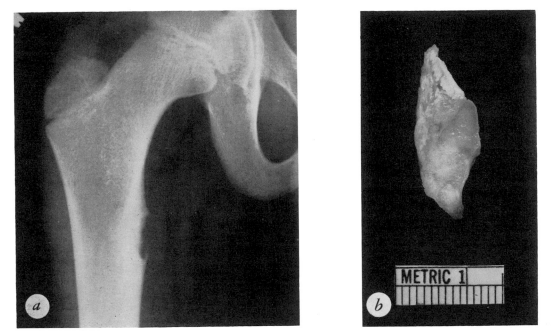

FIG. 3-8. *a.* Typical subperiosteal chondroma lying in a slightly sclerotized concavity in the cortex. *b.* Gross specimen from the same case. The semitranslucent nature of the hyaline cartilage is apparent.

Histopathology

The chondrocytes that make up the cellular component of a chondroma are small cells which lie in lacunar spaces and have a round, regular nucleus similar to that of the chondrocyte seen in nonneoplastic hyaline cartilage. The degree of cellularity varies remarkably in chondromas, some of the enchondromas of the small bones being highly cellular. Hence, cellularity affords little help in differentiating chondroma from chondrosarcoma. Large, oblong lacunar spaces similar to those seen in a growing epiphyseal line and containing a cluster of chondrocytes are sometimes present, and such a finding affords strong presumptive evidence that the lesion is benign. Multinucleated chondrocytes and cells with large nuclei are uncommon and should arouse the suspicion of malignancy. A lobular arrangement is usually apparent microscopically. Finely granular calcific débris or prominent sheets of calcific substance, when present, are apparently at sites of degeneration. The hyaline cartilage may contain foci of enchondral ossification in some of these neoplasms. In others the ground substance has a myxoid or mucinous appearance.

It is necessary to examine numerous fields in these tumors to be certain that there are not areas with sufficient evidence for a diagnosis of malignancy. This is especially true if they are large or if they are located in a long bone near the body, in the pelvic or shoulder girdle, or in a rib. Evidence for chondrosarcoma is sometimes found in only isolated areas within a tumor. The histologic criteria of chondrosarcoma will be detailed in the chapter dealing with that subject. Differentiation of benign from malignant chondromatous tumors of bone requires careful correlation of clinical, roentgenologic, and histopathologic features.

Periosteal chondromas often have an alarming degree of cellular atypia.

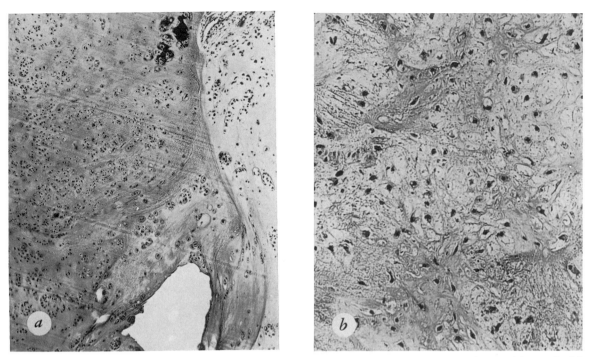

FIG. 3-9. *a*. Chondroma under low magnification showing lobular pattern, clustering of cells, and a small focus of calcification (×65). *b*. Higher magnification to show that each cell has a single small nucleus (×185).

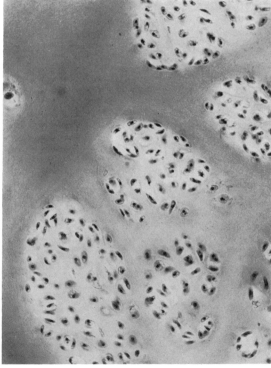

FIG. 3-10. Small, usually single, nuclei are typical of benign chondroma. The cells often occur in clusters (×140).

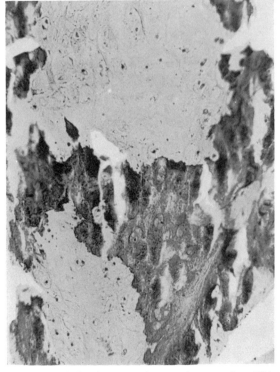

FIG. 3-11. Calcification secondary to degeneration. This is the lesion illustrated in Figure 3-3 (×160).

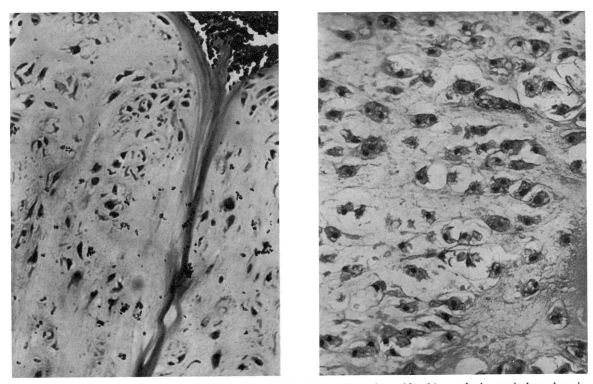

FIG. 3-12. *Left*. Periosteal chondroma. Fair numbers of binucleate cells and considerable cytologic atypia have less significance in chondromas lying in a cortical defect, as in Figure 3-8a. ($\times$175). *Right*. Binucleate cells and cellularity are likewise less ominous in roentgenologically benign-appearing chondromas of the hand such as this one ($\times$350).

Treatment

Curettage, filling the defect with bone chips if necessary, is the usual treatment. After curettage, some recommend chemical cauterization of the cavity and collapse of the cortical bone over the defect. If the tumor is in a small bone such as a rib that can be sacrificed or is in the subperiosteal region of a large bone and it can be excised en bloc with a surrounding portion of normal bone, that is the proper treatment. Such total excision is especially desirable when the possibility of malignancy cannot be excluded preoperatively. Curettage is likely to leave fragments of a lobulated tumor behind so that the tumor can recur even if it is benign.

Prognosis

With the treatment outlined the prognosis in chondroma is good and recurrence is unusual even after curettage. Occasionally, however, a tumor which seemed completely benign recurs, and the recurrent tumor is characterized, in rare instances, by increased anaplasia with obvious evidence of malignancy. Frequently this apparent increase in cellular activity is actually the result of failure of correct interpretation of the original specimen; sometimes the apparent discrepancy is accounted for by the fact that insufficient microscopic sections were made for complete evaluation of the original specimen. Actually in the case of chondroma of the hand, the lesion is so innocuous in the average case that cure can be expected even if the tumor is obviously not completely excised.

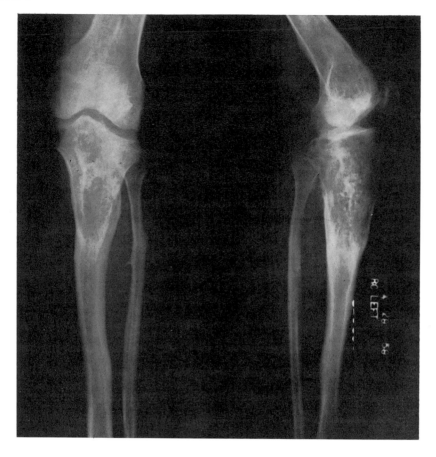

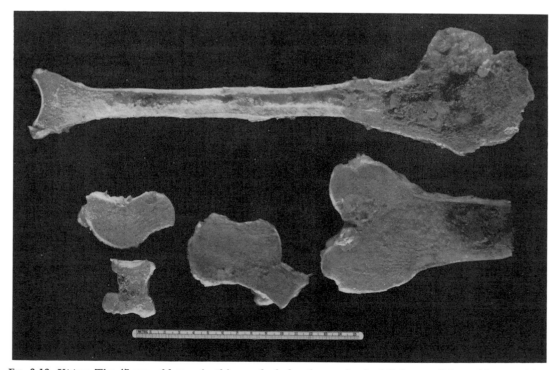

FIG. 3-13. *Upper.* The 47-year-old man in this case had chondromas in the left femur, tibia, and bones of foot. Chondrosarcoma had developed in the tibia. *Lower.* The sarcoma had perforated through the tibial cortex posteriorly. Chondromas were found at the amputation level, in the distal end of the femur, and in several bones of the foot. He died with metastases 58 months later.

36

Multiple Chondroma

Not included in the localization data in Figure 3-1 were 19 patients with benign but multiple chondromas. These patients required operation for a variety of reasons. In five, tissue was removed from a lesion for diagnosis. Deforming tumors were locally excised from the hand in seven patients and from the foot in one. A toe was amputated in one patient, and one or more fingers in three others. One of these latter three patients required disarticulation at the shoulder later for a huge tumor of the humerus, tissue from which is not available for study. One patient required amputation through the femur because of severe and disabling tibial deformity. The final patient required amputation of an affected arm for an associated angiosarcoma of the soft tissues which complicated chronic lymphedema and caused death within a year.

The severity of skeletal chondromatosis varied markedly in this group. The bones of only one hand were involved in five patients and the bones of but one foot in two others. One of the latter had only two tumors. In the hands and feet, nearly all the chondromas were in phalanges, metacarpals, and metatarsals. One patient had chondromas distributed throughout three extremities, and three others had two limbs similarly affected. The remaining eight had diffuse involvement of one extremity, often with involvement of the bones of the ipsilateral shoulder or pelvic girdle. Ribs were involved in one case.

Sarcomas in Multiple Chondroma

In addition to the above 19 patients with skeletal chondromatosis, there were 5 with the same disease complicated by chondrosarcoma. They are included in the data on malignant tumors. One of these patients had three extremities involved with chondromas and the remainder had monomelic disease. Three of the chondrosarcomas occurred in the upper part of the tibia, one in the upper part of the humerus, and one in the distal part of the femur. The patients' ages at the time of diagnosis of sarcoma varied from 38 to 55 years.

Bibliography

1952 Lichtenstein, Louis, and Hall, J. E.:Periosteal Chondroma: A Distinctive Benign Cartilage Tumor. *J. Bone & Joint Surg., 34A*:691-697.

1954 Pugh, D. G.: *Roentgenologic Diagnosis of Diseases of Bones*. Baltimore, Williams and Wilkins, pp. 438-442.

1958 Bean, W. B.: Dyschondroplasia and Hemangiomata (Maffucci's Syndrome). II. *A.M.A. Arch. Int. Med., 102*:544-550.

1962 Murphy, F. P., Dahlin, D. C., & Sullivan, C. R.: Articular Synovial Chondromatosis. *J. Bone & Joint Surg., 44A*:77-86.

1963 Gilmer, W. S., Kilgore, W., & Smith, H.: Central Cartilage Tumors of Bone. *Clinical Orthopedics. No. 26.* J. B. Lippincott Co.

1963 Goethals, P. L., Dahlin, D. C., & Devine, K. S.: Cartilaginous Tumors of the Larynx. *Surg., Gynec. & Obst., 117*:77-82.

Chapter 4

Benign Chondroblastoma

Benign chondroblastoma is one of the neoplasms of bone that has been rescued from the "waste-basket" of giant cell tumors and is now recognized as a distinct entity. The basic proliferating cells of this neoplasm are remarkably similar to those of a true giant cell tumor, but these cells have the ability to produce foci of chondroid matrix, making it reasonable to include chondroblastoma among the tumors of cartilaginous origin. Valls and co-workers have suggested a reticulohistiocytic origin for these tumors, but most people relate them to epiphyseal cartilage.

Although some of the features of this neoplasm were recognized previously, it was not until 1942 that the term "benign chondroblastoma" was introduced and its distinctive clinicopathologic features were delineated. The cellular zones of these tumors ordinarily contain at least a few mitotic figures. These, coupled with the chondroid zones, have frequently led to the erroneous diagnosis of malignant giant cell tumor. Actually, one of the main reasons for recognizing this entity is that clinically it is relatively nonaggressive and readily curable as compared to giant cell tumor.

The present studies and those of others have indicated that there is a close relationship between benign chondroblastoma and chondromyxoid fibroma. In common with most observers, my colleagues and I have recognized no malignant counterpart of benign chondroblastoma.

Benign Chondroblastoma

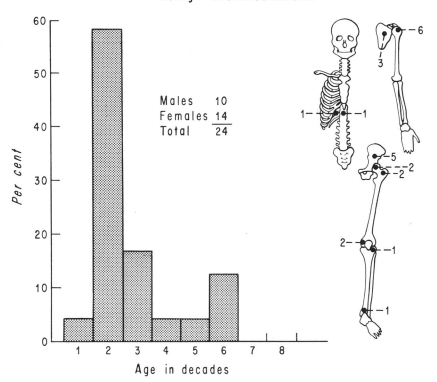

Males 10
Females 14
Total 24

FIG. 4-1. Skeletal, age, and sex distribution of benign chondroblastomas.

Incidence

Less than 1% of this series of bone tumors were chondroblastomas, and they were one sixth as common as were true giant cells tumors.

Sex

Though the Mayo Clinic series contained more females than males, the literature and the more than 40 non-Clinic cases we have seen in consultation indicate that two thirds of the patients are males.

Age

The literature and our non-Clinic referral cases suggest that more than three fourths of chondroblastomas are seen in the second decade of life. Three of our patients were more than 50 and the youngest was 9 years old.

Localization

Chondroblastomas are typically centered in an epiphysis. They are seen most often in the end of a major tubular bone but can appear in any secondary center of ossification such as the greater trochanter. They have been described in a wide variety of bones including those of the hands and feet. The knee region has contributed the most examples.

39

BENIGN CHONDROBLASTOMA

Symptoms

Local pain is the most important and practically a constant symptom of benign chondroblastoma. It is often mild or moderate in degree as evidenced by the fact that patients of the present series had symptoms for 3 months to 16 years before they sought medical attention, and the average duration was slightly more than 2 years. The complaints are ordinarily referred to the adjacent joint region. Tumefaction is usually absent because of the small size of the tumor and the presence of overlying soft tissue.

Physical Findings

Aside from local tenderness which may be present the physical examination is of little diagnostic value. There may be wasting of the muscles in the region of the tumor owing to disuse, and limping may be observed. Some patients have increased fluid in the neighboring joint.

Roentgenologic Features

Characteristically this neoplasm presents with a central region of bone destruction which is usually sharply delimited from the surrounding normal bone by a thin margin of increased bone density. There may or may not be mottled areas of density within the radiolucent zone, depending on the presence and degree of calcification within the tumor. Both trabeculation and active periosteal reaction are rarely seen. The tumor, when it involves the long bones, almost always affects the epiphysis and frequently the adjacent metaphysis. Large chondroblastomas cause bulging and thinning of the cortex of the bone. The most important lesions that should be considered in the differential diagnosis roentgenologically are enchondroma, chondromyxoid fibroma, chondrosarcoma, and benign giant cell tumor.

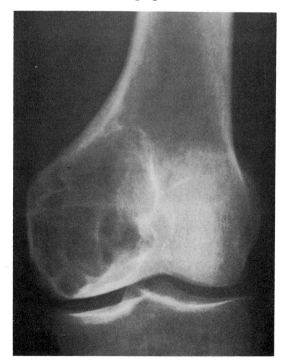

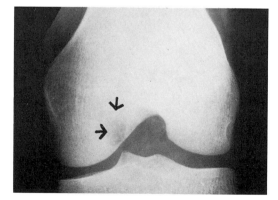

Fig. 4-2. *Above.* Small lytic chondroblastoma of the medial condyle of the femur.

Fig. 4-3. *Left.* Chondroblastoma in the medial condyle of the femur, an asymptomatic lesion in a 54-year-old man found incidentally during angiography. It is well circumscribed and has a slightly sclerotic boundary.

40

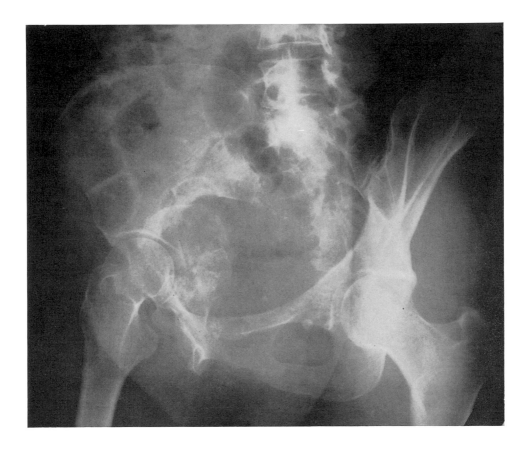

FIG. 4-4. *Above.* Benign chondroblastoma of the right innominate bone in the region of the acetabulum. It has produced obvious expansion into the pelvis. This tumor occurred in a 54-year-old woman and had produced pain for 1 year.

FIG. 4-5. *Right.* Another pertinent lesion, in this case involving the greater trochanter and adjacent neck of the femur of an 18-year-old woman who had had local pain for 4 months.

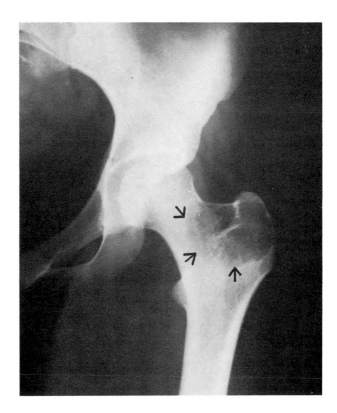

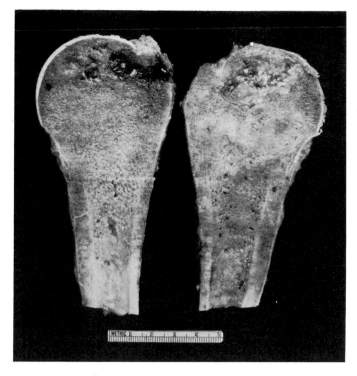

Fig. 4-6. Chondroblastoma of the upper part of the humerus. The lesion is confined to the upper 3 cm of the bone. Excision of the specimen shown was performed because of an erroneous diagnosis of chondrosarcoma. (Reproduced with permission from: Kunkel, M. G., Dahlin, D. C., and Young, H. H.: *J. Bone & Joint Surg., 38A*:817-826, 1956.)

Gross Pathology

Chondroblastomas are ordinarily small. The tumors in this series varied from 1 to 7 cm in greatest diameter. There may be a thin zone of slightly sclerotic bone surrounding the tumor. The lesional tissue itself does not have pathognomonic features. It is grayish pink and may contain zones of hemorrhage or necrosis. In rare instances the chondroïd matrix is so prominent that the tumor has features similar to those of chondroma or chondrosarcoma. Although these tumors often abut on the articular cartilage of a joint, they rarely produce much destruction of this cartilage. An occasional chondroblastoma destroys the bony cortex and produces an extraosseous mass. Minute foci of calcified material may be recognized within the tumor substance. Cystic change, sometimes prominent, is seen on rare occasions.

Although benign chondroblastomas are usually predominantly epiphyseal in location, rare examples have been centered in the metaphyseal region with only a minimal epiphyseal component. This contrasts with the location of the closely related tumor, chondromyxoid fibroma, which almost always is at or near the end of the shaft when a long bone is affected. Both tumors are found, however, in locations that are consistent with the theory that they arise from cells of the epiphyseal cartilaginous plate or from "rests" of these cells.

Histopathology

As indicated by the name of this tumor, its basic proliferating cells are considered to be chondroblasts, that is, cells related to cartilage-forming connective tissue. The round or oval nucleus of this cell is often indented, and the cell borders are ordinarily clearly defined. There is little stroma between the cells except for the zones with chondroid substance. Although mitotic figures are never numerous, they can be found in practically all chondroblastomas. Among the proliferating neoplastic cells are variable numbers of benign multinucleated cells which contain from 5 to 40 or more nuclei. These giant cells of a chondroblastoma are, in general, smaller and less abundant than those of a genuine giant cell tumor of bone. Nuclei of the giant cells resemble closely those of the chondroblasts of the cellular portions of the tumors.

Zones of a chondroid material are the distinctive feature of chondroblastomas, although these zones may be abundant or rare. In two cases of the present series, the chondroid zones overshadowed the cellular zones. Some have likened this ground substance to the chondroid material found in mixed tumors of the salivary glands, but sometimes it closely resembles mature hyaline cartilage. In most chondroblastomas, some islands of this interstitial substance undergo degeneration and subsequent calcification. These calcified portions are characteristically lacelike with residual lacunae where the degenerated chondroblasts had been. Recent evidence has been accumulated which indicates a strong histologic relationship between benign chondroblastoma and chondromyxoid fibroma of bone. Some tumors exhibit zones that are characteristic of each of these neoplasms.

Rare tumors contain typical zones of chondroblastoma and other regions with blood-filled spaces reminiscent of aneurysmal bone cyst; such lesions suggest that the latter process may represent secondary change in a preexisting disease.

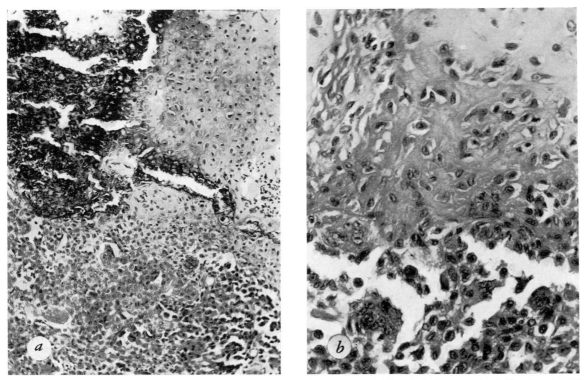

Fig. 4-7. *a.* Typical chondroblastoma with chondroid material in upper half and dark zone of calcification ($\times$130). *b.* Higher magnification to show cell detail and giant cells ($\times$285). (Reproduced with permission from: Kunkel, M. G., Dahlin, D. C., and Young, H. H.: *J. Bone & Joint Surg., 38A*:817-826, 1956.)

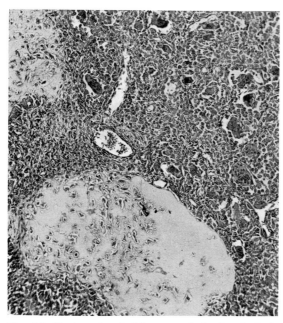

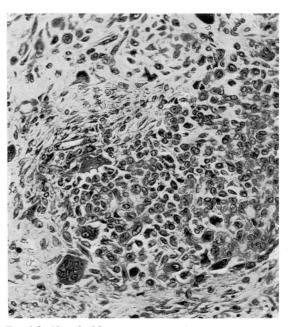

FIG. 4-8. Benign chondroblastoma of the head of the humerus, showing again the relationship of the chondroid islands to the portions that mimic the appearance of genuine giant cell tumor (×100).

FIG. 4-9. Chondroblastomatous zone in recurrence of an originally pure chondromyxoid fibroma removed by curettage 20 months previously (×200). (Reproduced with permission from: Dahlin, D. C.: *Cancer, 9*:195-203, 1956.)

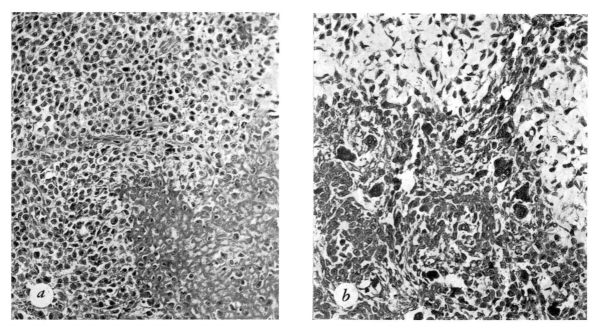

FIG. 4-10. *a.* Benign chondroblastoma in the region of the acetabulum (×145). The roentgenogram in this case is illustrated in Figure 4-4. *b.* Chondromyxoid fibroma of distal metaphysis of femur originally classified as chondroblastoma because of prominent zones such as those dominating this field (×165). (Reproduced with permission from: Kunkel, M. G., Dahlin, D. C., and Young, H. H.: *J. Bone & Joint Surg., 38A*:817-826, 1956.)

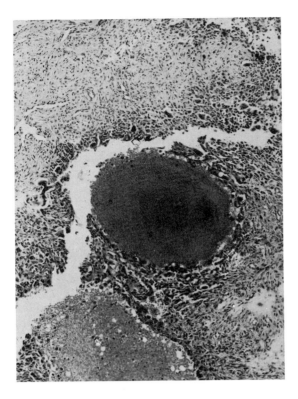

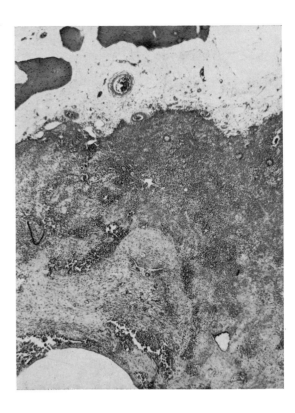

Fig. 4-11. *Above.* Chondroblastoma containing blood-filled spaces in central and lowest portions of picture, producing a resemblance to aneurysmal bone cyst (×60).

Fig. 4-12. *Above, right.* Periphery of chondroblastoma well demarcated from adjacent bone. A cyst is present in the lower left corner (×20).

Fig. 4-13. *Right.* As depicted here, some chondroblastomas contain zones markedly similar to giant cell tumor (×125).

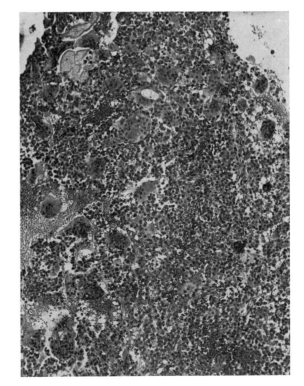

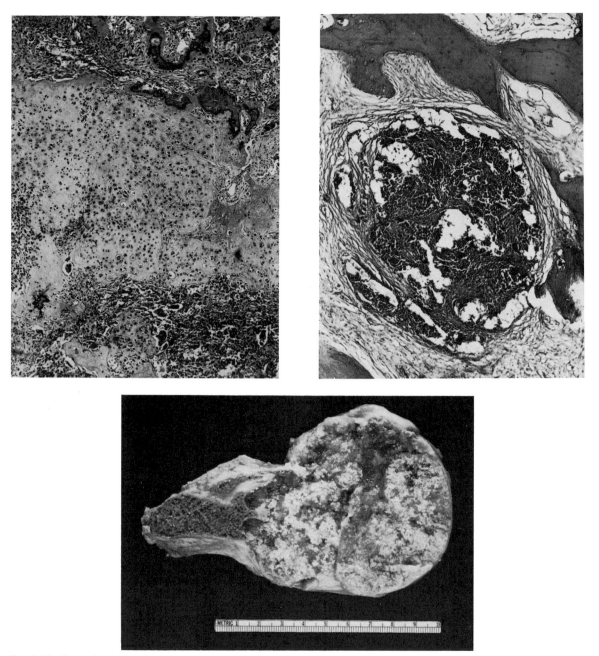

FIG. 4-14. *Above, left.* Benign chondroblastoma of phalanx. Some of its abundant cartilage is differentiating into bone, as is seen especially in the peripheral portions of some of these tumors (×50).

FIG. 4-15. *Above, right.* One of several foci in a recurrent chondroblastoma of the tibia. Such recurrences are unusual and probably result from lobules of tumor that escape the curette (×65).

FIG. 4-16. *Below.* This huge recurrent tumor was excised 10 years after incomplete removal of the benign chondroblastoma seen in Figure 4-4. The patient was well 8 years after excision of this recurrent mass which was, like the original tumor, histologically benign.

Treatment

Because chondroblastomas are so benign and nonaggressive, the main danger is that too radical treatment may be instituted, sometimes because of an erroneous diagnosis. The pathologist who is not conversant with the features of this tumor is likely to mistake it especially for chondrosarcoma or for malignant giant cell tumor. The average tumor of this type is best treated by curettage. Bone grafting of the resultant defect may be necessary. As in the management of other cartilaginous tumors, those chondroblastomas so located that they can be excised completely with a surrounding shell of bone should be so treated. Radiation therapy is unnecessary and probably dangerous.

Prognosis

Practically all chondroblastomas may be eradicated by the treatment outlined above. Even the rare tumor that recurs should be curable by wider local excision. It seems from the available evidence that irradiation is contraindicated. In the two well-documented instances of malignant transformation with which I am familiar, irradiation was part of the primary therapeutic regimen. Ackerman and Spjut mentioned one benign chondroblastoma with metastasis.

Bibliography

1931 Codman, E. A.: Epiphyseal Chondromatous Giant Cell Tumors of the Upper End of the Humerus. *Surg., Gynec. & Obst., 52*:543-548.

1942 Jaffe, H. L., and Lichtenstein, Louis: Benign Chondroblastoma of Bone: A Reinterpretation of the So-called Calcifying or Chrondromatous Giant Cell Tumor. *Am. J. Path., 18*:969-992.

1949 Copeland, M. M., and Geschickter, C. F.: Chondroblastic Tumors of Bone: Benign and Malignant. *Ann. Surg., 129*:724-733.

1951 Hatcher, C. H., and Campbell, J. C.: Benign Chondroblastoma of Bone: Its Histologic Variations and a Report of Late Sarcoma in the Site of One. *Bull. Hosp. Joint Dis., 12*:411-430.

1951 Valls, José, Ottolenghi, C. E., and Schajowicz, Fritz: Epiphyseal Chondroblastoma of Bone. *J. Bone & Joint Surg., 33A*:997-1009.

1956 Kunkel, M. G., Dahlin, D. C., and Young, H. H.: Benign Chondroblastoma. *J. Bone & Joint Surg., 38A*:817-826.

1958 Plum, G. E., and Pugh, D. G.: Roentgenologic Aspects of Benign Chondroblastoma of Bone. *Amer. J. Roentgenol., 79*:584-591.

1962 Ackerman, L. V., and Spjut, H. J.: *Tumors of Bone and Cartilage.* Atlas of Tumor Pathology, Section II, Fascicle 4, Armed Forces Institute of Pathology, Washington, D.C., National Research Council, pp. 15-17.

1964 Welsh, R. A., and Meyer, A. T.: A Histogenetic Study of Chondroblastoma. *Cancer, 17*:578-589.

1965 Steiner, G. S.: Postradiation Sarcoma of Bone. *Cancer, 18*:603-612.

Chapter 5

Chondromyxoid Fibroma

CHONDROMYXOID FIBROMA is a rare and peculiar benign tumor, apparently derived from cartilage-forming connective tissue. Its name, which is cumbersome, has the merit of being highly descriptive and is gaining acceptance for this distinctive tumor. It was described by Jaffe and Lichtenstein in 1948 when they presented eight cases and emphasized the danger of mistaking this benign neoplasm for a malignant lesion, especially chondrosarcoma. The relative rarity of the neoplasm should not lull one into a complacent disregard for it, because anyone dealing with bone tumors must be prepared to interpret and manage any lesion he encounters. The fact is that one cannot ignore even the more complicated ramifications of a useful classification, because he cannot expect to diagnose and treat correctly a tumor with which he is unfamiliar.

Although chondromyxoid fibroma characteristically contains variable amounts of chondroid, fibromatoid, and myxoid components, the fact that certain portions within the tumor resemble hyaline cartilage makes it logical to include this neoplasm among those of cartilaginous derivation.

The rationale of this classification is enhanced by the fact indicated previously that chondromyxoid fibroma and benign chondroblastoma sometimes have a striking histologic similarity.

Many of the tumors referred to in the literature as myxomas and fibromyxomas of bone are, no doubt, examples of chondromyxoid fibroma. The distinctive myxoma (fibromyxoma) of jawbones lacks the lobulation and varied histologic spectrum of chondromyxoid fibroma, has no exact counterpart in the remainder of the skeleton, and is apparently of odontogenic derivation.

The earlier admonition to avoid "overdiagnosing" chondromyxoid fibroma as chondrosarcoma has been taken too seriously by some pathologists. I have seen a number of instances in which errors have been made in the reverse direction with consequent inadequate treatment of chondrosarcoma.

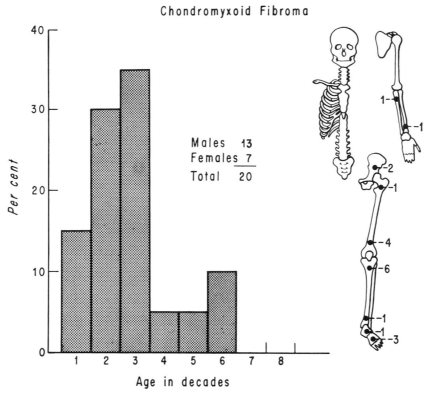

FIG. 5-1. Skeletal, age, and sex distribution of chrondromyxoid fibromas.

Incidence

Chondromyxoid fibroma accounted for but a fraction of 1% of the bone tumors of this series. Reports in the literature indicate that it is less common than chondroblastoma.

Sex

No sex predilection is yet apparent for this tumor.

Age

There is a marked predilection for patients in the second and third decades of life. The youngest in this series was 6 years old.

Localization

The typical chondromyxoid fibroma is located in the metaphyseal region of a bone and may abut on or be a variable distance from the epiphyseal line. Occasionally, a tumor involves both the metaphysis and the epiphysis. This localization suggests that, like benign chondroblastoma, chondromyxoid fibroma possibly arises from the epiphyseal cartilaginous plate. The great majority of the recorded examples of this tumor have been in the long tubular bones, with the tibia contributing about half of all cases. It occurs in other long tubular bones, in small bones of the hands and feet, and in the pelvic girdle, with sporadic examples in such bones as vertebrae, ribs, scapulae, and the mastoid.

CHONDROMYXOID FIBROMA

Symptoms

Pain is by far the most common presenting symptom of patients with chondromyxoid fibroma. Local swelling is occasionally a complaint of patients whose tumors are not camouflaged by a thick layer of overlying tissues. Such tumefaction had been noted by only 3 of the 20 patients in this series. Occasionally these tumors are asymptomatic incidental findings on roentgenograms.

Physical Findings

Physical examination is of little diagnostic aid. Tenderness in the region of the tumor, or a tender or nontender mass, may be found and aid in exact localization.

Roentgenologic Features

The defect is characteristically an eccentric, sharply circumscribed zone of rarefaction that occasionally causes expansion of the bone. The cortical outline was partially absent over three of the tumors of the present series. A chondromyxoid fibroma, especially in a small bone, can produce fusiform expansion of its entire contour.

Trabeculae appear to traverse the defect in most cases, but these are merely the roentgenographic reflection of corrugations on the inner surface of the cavity that contains the tumor. Sometimes the bone adjacent to the tumor is characterized by a thin delimiting line of sclerosis. Although a minority of these neoplasms contain microscopic foci of calcification, these are very rarely reflected in the roentgenographic shadow.

The roentgenologic features of the tumors in this series and of those in additional cases are detailed by Turcotte and co-workers who found that the defect uniformly looks benign.

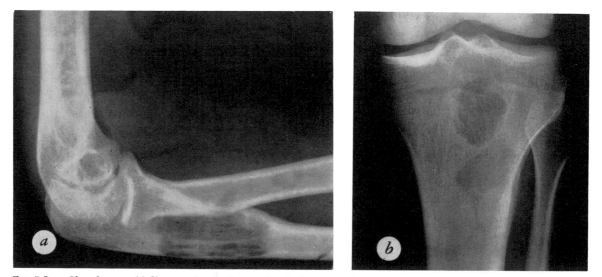

Fig. 5-2. *a.* Chondromyxoid fibroma that had caused pain for 8 months. There was tender swelling of the upper part of the ulna. *b.* This tumor occurred in a 28-year-old man and had produced local pain for 2 years. (Reproduced with permission from: Dahlin, D. C.: *Cancer, 9:*195-203, 1956.)

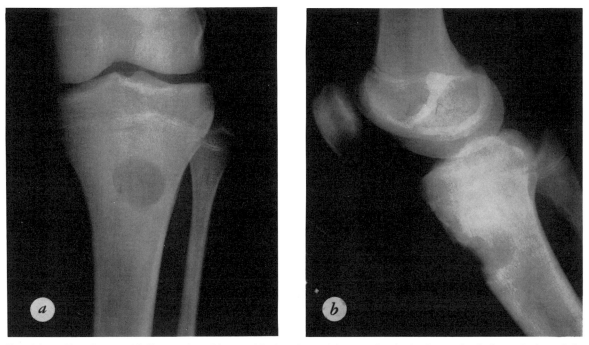

FIG. 5-3. *a.* Chondromyxoid fibroma in a 14-year-old girl who had had local pain for 3 months. *b.* Lateral view of the same lesion. It recurred 20 months after curettage and was then treated by block excision. She is well 11 years after this wider excision. (Reproduced with permission from: Dahlin, D. C.: *Cancer, 9:*195-203, 1956.)

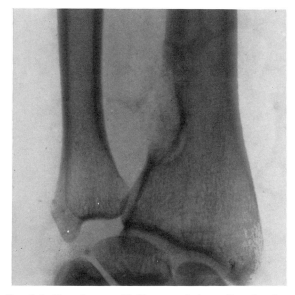

FIG. 5-4. Chondromyxoid fibroma of the radius showing punctate calcification. (Case contributed by Drs. C. R. Dochat, Fowler Robert, and Charles Miller, of Akron, Ohio.)

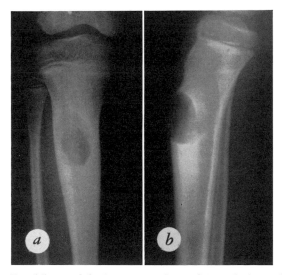

FIG. 5-5. *a* and *b*. Anteroposterior and lateral views of a chondromyxoid fibroma in a 10-year-old boy. Foci of chondroblastoma were present in the tumor. (Reproduced with permission from: Dahlin, D. C.: *Cancer, 9:* 195-203, 1956.)

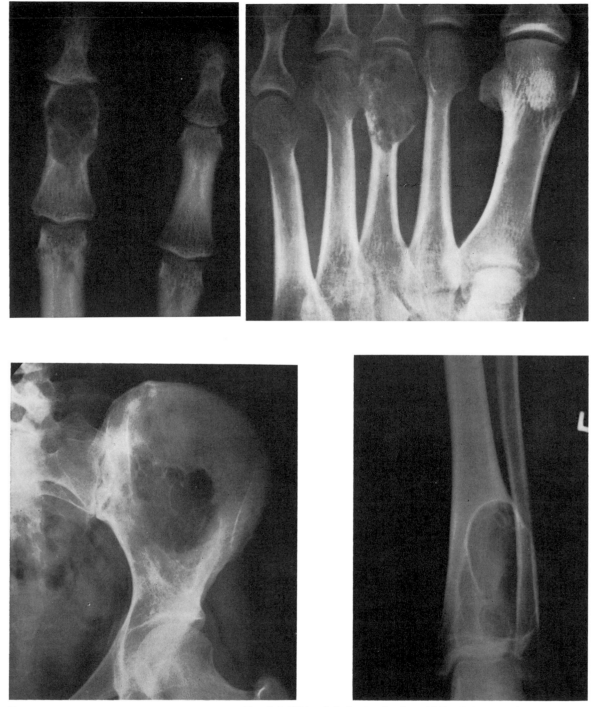

FOUR CHARACTERISTIC CHONDROMYXOID FIBROMAS. FIG. 5-6. *Upper left.* Lesion in the middle phalanx of the third finger with central location. (Courtesy of Dr. R. R. Williams, Middletown, Ohio.) *Upper right.* Tumor in the third metatarsal. *Lower left.* Large defect in the ilium with a trabeculated appearance. (Courtesy of Drs. E. H. Boyer, and J. A. Finer, Youngstown, Ohio.) *Lower right.* Large but typical tumor in the tibia. (Courtesy of Dr. Lorel Stapley, Phoenix, Arizona.) (These four illustrations reproduced with permission from: Turcotte and co-workers: *Am. J. Roentgen., 87*:1085-1095, 1962.)

Gross Pathology

The average tumor of this type is small, those of this series varying in size up to 5 cm in greatest diameter, although larger tumors have been reported. Grossly it may closely resemble hyaline cartilage or appear as a somewhat translucent fibrous mass. In general, the consistency is denser than one would suspect from the histologic appearance. A striking feature is the sharp delimitation from the surrounding bone, a feature which contrasts with what one observes in chondrosarcoma. The surface of the tumor is often distinctly lobulated and the cavity from which it is enucleated frequently is characterized by corrugations that correspond with the tumor lobules. There may be a thin sclerotized zone in the bone immediately adjacent to the neoplasm.

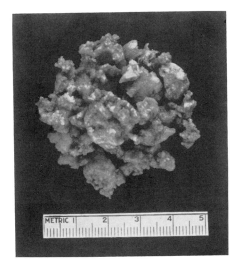

Fig. 5-7. Firm, fibrocartilaginous tissue removed by curettage from a lesion the roentgenogram of which is shown in Figure 5-2b.

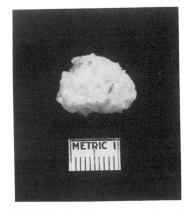

Fig. 5-8. Finely lobulated tumor enucleated from the defect represented in the roentgenograms shown in Figure. 5-3a and b. (Reproduced with permission from: Dahlin, D. C.: *Cancer, 9*:195-203, 1956.)

Histopathology

The name of this tumor indicates the variation observed microscopically in different fields of a given tumor and from tumor to tumor. The gamut includes myxomatous zones, fibrous zones, and fields with a distinctly chondroid appearance. The nuclei of the cells are round, oval, crescentic, or spindle-shaped. Cytoplasmic extensions are often multipolar. The chondroid element may occupy only small foci but it occasionally dominates the histologic picture and introduces the hazard of mistaking the tumor for a chondrosarcoma. Chondromyxoid fibroma characteristically possesses a lobular pattern of growth but this feature is sometimes obscured in microscopic sections prepared from curetted fragments, and the lobules are often only partially separated from each other. A highly characteristic feature is the increased concentration of nuclei observed at the periphery of the lobules and partial lobules. At the edge of the tumor this cellular peripheral zone is sharply demarcated from the surrounding uninvolved tissues. Variable degrees of collagenization of the lobules are observed. Small amorphous foci of calcification are occasionally present and these sometimes have the lacelike quality of the calcification seen in benign chondroblastoma.

CHONDROMYXOID FIBROMA

These may be related to zones of degeneration sometimes present in the lobules. Benign giant cells and phagocytic mononuclear cells may be seen in the tissue between the lobules. As indicated in the preceding chapter, some chondromyxoid fibromas contain cellular foci indistinguishable from microscopic fields in benign chondroblastoma. Rarely one sees a tumor that is difficult to classify strictly into one category or the other.

The most important histologic feature of chondromyxoid fibroma is that the cells in some portions of many of these tumors are large and have nuclei of irregular size and shape, and even contain multiple nuclei at times. These features, if present in a hyaline-cartilage tumor of the chondroma-chondrosarcoma group, would be indicative of malignancy. When one recognizes, however, that these cells are only part of the overall pattern of chondromyxoid fibroma, the benign nature of the lesion is firmly established.

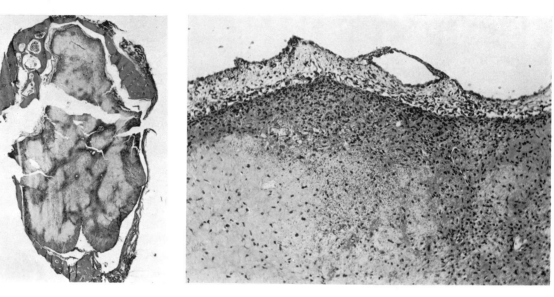

FIG. 5-9. *Above, left.* Cross section of entire tumor which had caused some expansion of a rib (×6). (Reproduced with permission from: Dahlin, D. C.: *Cancer, 9*:195-203, 1956.)

FIG. 5-10. *Above, right.* Periphery of tumor lobule showing characteristic condensation of nuclei beneath rim of compressed adjacent tissue, here located above neoplastic tissue (×130). (Reproduced with permission from: Dahlin, D. C., Wells, A. H., and Henderson, E. D.: *J. Bone & Joint Surg., 35A*:831-834, 1953.)

FIG. 5-11. *Right.* Chondroid zone of the type commonly seen in chondromyxoid fibroma (×200). (Reproduced with permission from: Dahlin, D C., Wells, A. H., and Henderson, E. D.: *J. Bone & Joint Surg., 35A*:831-834, 1953.)

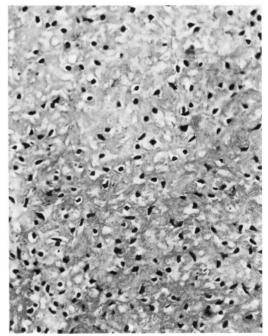

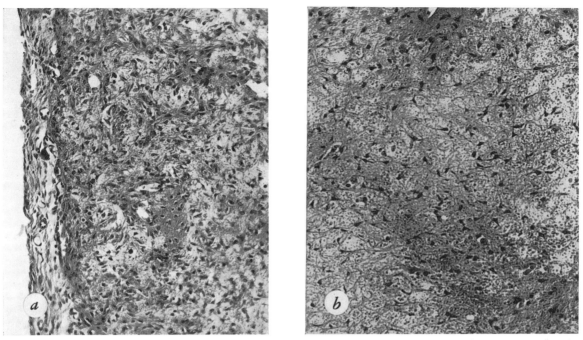

FIG. 5-12. *a.* Well-demarcated periphery showing fibromatoid and chondroid features (×180). *b.* Myxoid zone of the type seen in many chondromyxoid fibromas (×200). (Reproduced with permission from: Dahlin, D. C., Wells, A. H., and Henderson, E. D.: *J. Bone & Joint Surg., 35A*:831-834, 1953.)

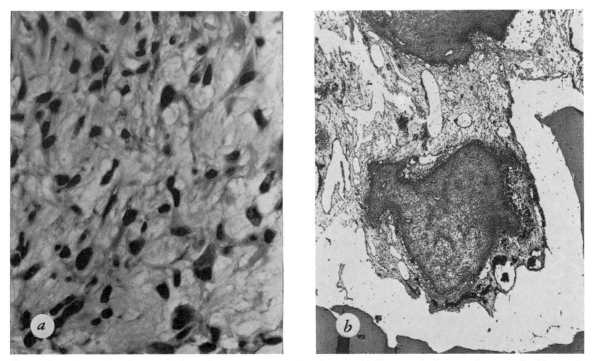

FIG. 5-13. *a.* Focus showing marked nuclear atypism in a chondromyxoid fibroma. Such zones have no significance in a lesion that has the other features of this benign tumor (×520). *b.* Tumor lobule separated, in this plane, from main neoplasm. Such ramifications could be left behind during curettage and thus account for recurrence (×40). (Reproduced with permission from: Dahlin, D. C.: *Cancer, 9*:195-203, 1956.)

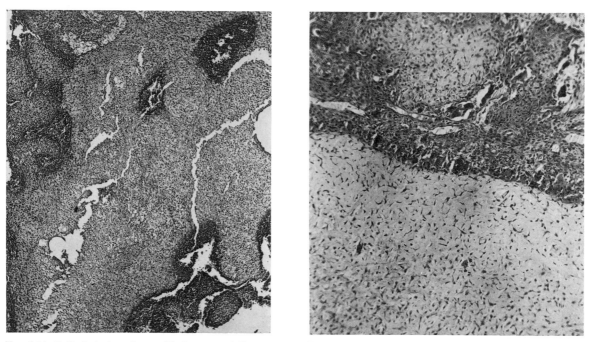

FIG. 5-14. *Left.* Lobules of myxoid tissue partially separated from one another by cellular zones. One of the patterns seen in chondromyxoid fibroma (×25). *Right.* Another variation with very small multipolar cells in the lobules (×100).

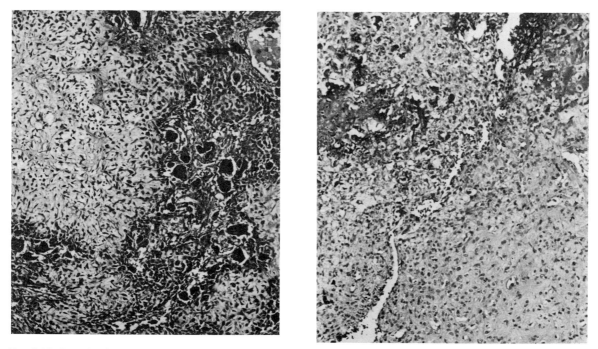

FIG. 5-15. *Left.* Smaller myxoid lobules in a cellular background very reminiscent of benign chondroblastoma (×80). *Right.* Darkly staining calcific foci such as these are seen in a minority of chondromyxoid fibromas (×80).

Treatment

Block excision of the affected area, when feasible, is the best treatment. Curettage, although ordinarily successful, imposes perhaps a 25% risk of recurrence. Radiation therapy is **not** indicated.

Three patients in this series were treated by amputation: one because of the large size of the tumor, one because of a diagnosis of sarcoma, and one because a recurrent lesion treated elsewhere was similarly misinterpreted.

Prognosis

Recurrent tumor developed in six patients in this series. As indicated, one patient was subjected to amputation; the remainder were successfully managed by wider excision. The lobulations on the periphery of these tumors may lead one to leave ramifications behind when treating them by curettage.

Although reference is made by Iwata and Coley and by Gilmer to malignant transformation of chondromyxoid fibroma, their two cases are not convincingly documented. I have not seen such transformation.

Bibliography

1948 Jaffe, H. L., and Lichtenstein, Louis: Chondromyxoid Fibroma of Bone: A Distinctive Benign Tumor Likely to Be Mistaken Especially for Chondrosarcoma. *Arch. Path., 45:* 541-551.

1953 Dahlin, D. C., Wells, A. H., and Henderson, E. D.: Chondromyxoid Fibroma of Bone: Report of Two Cases. *J. Bone & Joint Surg., 35A:*831-834.

1954 Wrenn, R. N., and Smith, A. G.: Chondromyxoid Fibroma. *South. M. J., 47:*848-853.

1956 Dahlin, D. C.: Chondromyxoid Fibroma of Bone, With Emphasis on Its Morphological Relationship to Benign Chondroblastoma. *Cancer, 9:*195-203.

1958 Iwata, S., and Coley, B. L.: Report of Six Cases of Chondromyxoid Fibroma of Bone. *Surg., Gynec. & Obst., 107:*571-576.

1961 Scaglietti, O., and Stringa, G.: Myxoma of Bone in Childhood. *J. Bone & Joint Surg., 43A:* 67-80.

1962 Ralph, L. L.: Chondromyxoid Fibroma of Bone. *J. Bone & Joint Surg., 44B:*7-24.

1962 Benedetti, G. B., Canepa, G., and Garcia, M.: Il fibroma condromixoide dell' osso. Revisione critica delle letterature ed indagini istologiche ed istochimiche su 8 casi. *Arch. "Putti" chir. org. movimento, 17:*44-72.

1962 Turcotte, B., Pugh, D. G., and Dahlin, D. C.: The Roentgenologic Aspects of Chondromyxoid Fibroma of Bone. *Am. J. Roentgenol., 87:*1085-1095.

1962 Gilmer, W. S., Higley, G. B., Jr., and Kilgore, W. E.: *Atlas of Bone Tumors.* Saint Louis, C. V. Mosby Company, pp. 36-39.

Chapter 6

Osteoma

THE ACTUAL OCCURRENCE of true osteoma is so debatable that this tumor was not included in the overall statistical data. Reactive changes from trauma, infection, or invading tumor such as meningioma can cause osseous overgrowth. Since these tumefactions produce the clinical manifestations of a neoplasm they are often erroneously called "osteomas."

Occasional tumors of the skull, especially those involving the paranasal sinuses, are the most nearly bona fide osteomas, and yet there is room for conjecture regarding these. The gamut of fibro-osseous dysplastic lesions that affect these bones runs from soft, purely fibrous lesions to those that are heavily ossified. A few of the dense "ivory" osteomas contain softer zones of fibro-osseous dysplasia. Hence, there is no clear line of distinction between obviously dysplastic lesions and completely osseous tumors that one might wish to call "true osteomas."

Rarely, one encounters a sessile ossified neoplasm on the surface of a bone, a tumor with roentgenologic and pathologic features that relate it closely to the malignant tumor called "parosteal osteogenic sarcoma." These benign counterparts are best regarded as parosteal osteomas.

Skeletal "osteomas" of various bones, but often prominently involving the skull and jaws, are associated with intestinal polyps, fibromatous and other connective tissue lesions, and epidermal cysts in Gardner's syndrome.

The dense bony overgrowths of torus palatinus and torus mandibularis are of unknown etiology but can hardly be considered neoplastic since they have very restricted growth potential. Similar reasoning applies to hyperostosis cranii.

Because of the hodgepodge of tumors included among the "osteomas" no attempt will be made to discuss their features as a group. Some of the characteristics of three pertinent types will be illustrated.

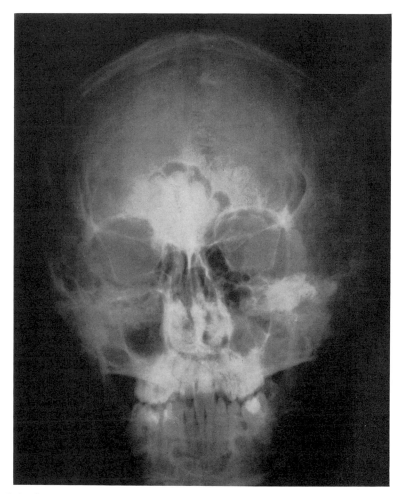

FIG. 6-1. Osteoma of the frontal sinus in a 19-year-old boy. It had produced local tumefaction. Such lesions can produce symptoms by blocking drainage from the sinus or by penetrating into neighboring structures, including the cranial cavity.

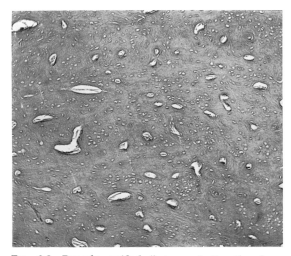

FIG. 6-2. Densely ossified "osteoma." Reactive bony sclerosis can give a similar appearance ($\times$60).

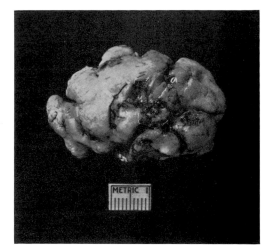

FIG. 6-3. Cross specimen removed from the patient whose roentgenogram is illustrated in Figure 6-1.

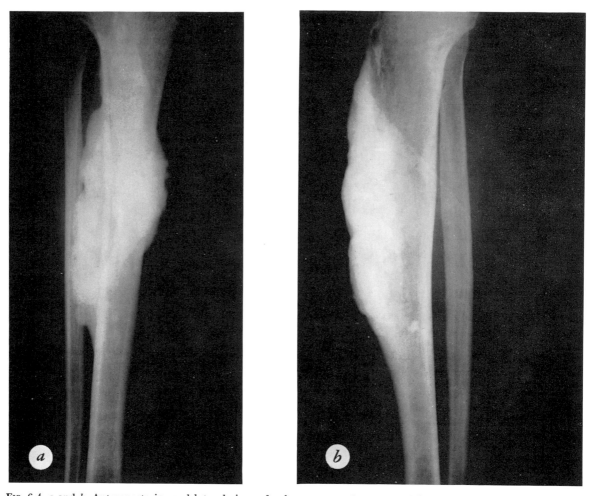

Fig. 6-4. *a* and *b*. Anteroposterior and lateral views of a dense parosteal osteoma of the tibia of a 43-year-old man who had noted gradually increasing swelling for 31 years. This tumor bears a roentgenographic resemblance to parosteal osteogenic sarcoma.

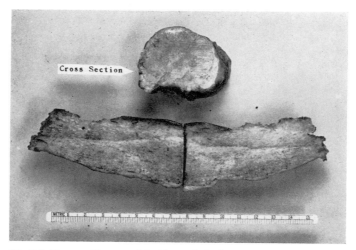

Fig. 6-5. Tumor illustrated in Figure 6-4, above. It was excised along with the subjacent cortex of the bone.

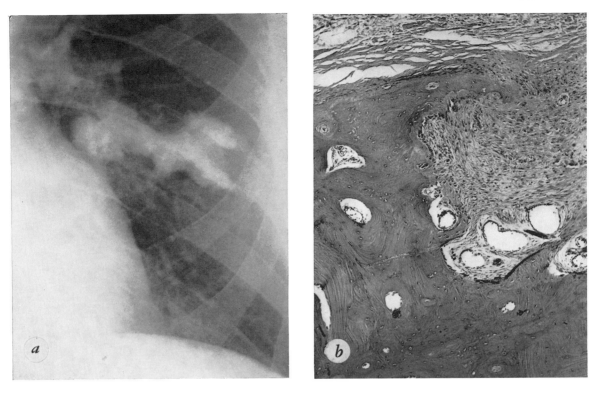

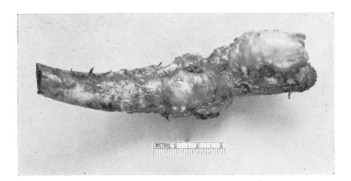

FIG. 6-6. *a.* Irregular sessile osteoma of the eighth rib. This was an incidental finding, having produced no signs or symptoms. *b.* Periphery of the same lesion showing that the osseous tissue appears to be derived from proliferating fibroblasts, apparently by a process of metaplasia. This appearance is reminiscent of what one commonly observes in parosteal osteogenic sarcoma (×70). *c Below.* Excised specimen.

Bibliography

1950   Hallberg, O. E., and Begley, J. W., Jr.: Origin and Treatment of Osteomas of the Paranasal Sinuses. *Arch. Otolaryng., 51:*750-760.

1958   Caughey, J. E.: The Etiology of Hyperostosis Cranii (Metabolic Craniopathy): A Clinical Study. *J. Bone & Joint Surg.,40B:*701-721.

1962   Gardner, E. J.: Follow-up Study of Family Group Exhibiting Dominant Inhertance for a Syndrome Including Intestinal Polyps, Osteomas, Fibromas and Epidermal Cysts. *Am. J. Human Genet.,14:*376-390.

1965   Bullough, P. G.: Ivory Exostosis of the Skull. *Postgrad. M. J.,41:*277-281.

Chapter 7

Osteoid Osteoma

THE MAJORITY OPINION now favors the view that osteoid osteoma is a neoplasm and not the result of some obscure infection or other known specific etiologic agent. This distinctive benign osteoblastic lesion consists of a small oval or round mass, commonly called a nidus. This nidus is often associated with a surrounding zone of sclerotic bone, especially when the lesion develops in a cortical portion of bone. The nidus is the essential part of the tumor, the surrounding sclerosis being a reversible change which disappears after removal of the nidus. As will be illustrated, the major component of this tumor is a meshwork of osteoid trabeculae showing varying degrees of mineralization in a background of more or less vascular fibrous connective tissue.

Certain instances of focal subacute or chronic osteomyelitis in bone produce a clinical and roentgenographic picture that has been confused with that of osteoid osteoma, especially when these inflammatory lesions are associated with a small, discrete, central rarefied focus. Histologically, of course, the lesion produced by inflammation and that by genuine osteoid osteoma are readily distinguished when appropriate sections are made. Osteoid osteomas located immediately beneath articular cartilage have been mistaken for osteochondritis dissecans roentgenologically. Focal islands of idiopathic medullary sclerosis may be the size of a nidus of sclerotic osteoid osteoma but they produce no clinical symptoms.

For a neoplasm, osteoid osteoma has a strangely limited growth potential and tumors more than 1 cm in largest diameter are unusual.

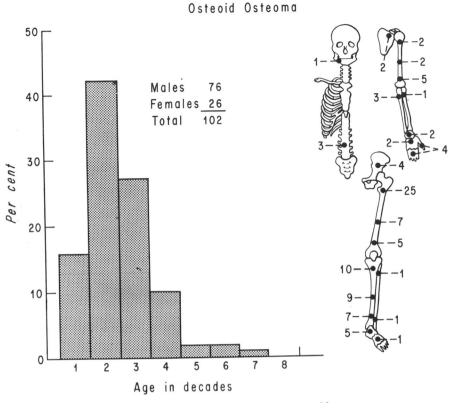

Osteoid Osteoma

Males 76
Females 26
Total 102

Per cent

Age in decades

FIG. 7-1. Skeletal, age, and sex distribution of osteoid osteomas.

Incidence

The 102 osteoid osteomas in the present series comprised 10% of the benign tumors. This is undoubtedly lower than the actual incidence, because this type of tumor was not commonly recognized until recent years.

Sex

The 3 to 1 predominance in males is somewhat higher than in most series.

Age

Paralleling the literature closely, 87% of the patients in this series were aged 5 through 24 years. Four were less than 5, and the youngest was 2 years old.

Localization

At least half the osteoid osteomas occur in the femur or tibia. In long bones they are usually near the end of the shaft. Other fibro-osseous processes in the mandible may simulate osteoid osteoma. In vertebrae the arch is most commonly involved. Some of the vertebral examples, as well as others, in the literature are undoubtedly benign osteoblastomas. The calvarium is apparently spared.

OSTEOID OSTEOMA

Symptoms

By far the most important complaint is pain of gradually progressing severity. Its duration prior to the patient's seeking medical care may vary from weeks to several years. Many have noted that salicylates relieve the pain which otherwise commonly interferes with sleep. The pain is often referred to the adjacent joint region and occasionally it is referred to a site so distant from the lesion that roentgenographic studies are misdirected. In some instances, especially when the bone involved is near the skin, painful local swelling may become evident.

Physical Findings

Dysfunction, often resulting in a limp, is commonly produced by an osteoid osteoma. Atrophy of some muscles of the affected extremity is common. When added to the character of the pain and the decreased muscle stretch reflexes, the atrophy may suggest a neurologic disorder. Two patients with a femoral and one with a tibial osteoid osteoma in this series had been operated on mistakenly for "intervertebral disc."

Scoliosis may result from osteoid osteomas in vertebrae.

Roentgenologic Features

A variable, sometimes extensive, sclerotic zone ordinarily surrounds the nidus and may mask it, necessitating special roentgenographic techniques for its demonstration. Typically the nidus appears as a small, relatively radiolucent zone. Sclerosis of the nidus adds to problems in its recognition. Those without secondary sclerosis may be less or more dense than adjacent bone or may be practically invisible. Sometimes the reactive periosteal laminations of new bone can mimic those of Ewing's tumor.

In some cases the typical clinical symptoms precede the onset of recognizable roentgenographic changes. It should also be emphasized that some osteoid osteomas, especially those in cancellous bone, show little or no perifocal sclerosis. This absence of sclerois in some cases makes the roentgenographic picture of ordinary osteoid osteoma merge with that of benign osteoblastoma, to be discussed in the next chapter.

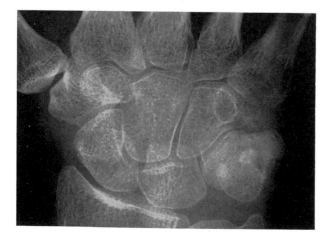

Fig. 7-2. Osteoid osteoma of the triangular bone of the wrist. The center of the nidus is denser than the periphery and there is only slight sclerosis of the bone around the lesion. The other carpal bone involved by osteoid osteoma in this series was the capitate.

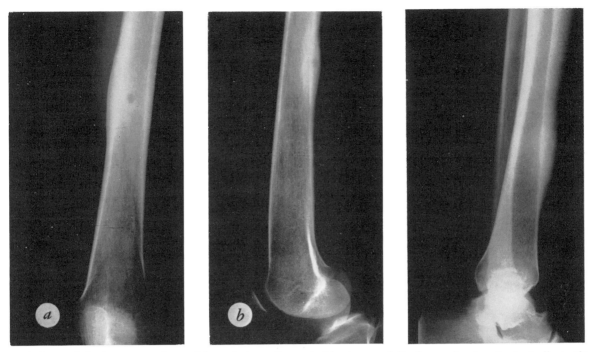

FIG. 7-3. *a* and *b*. Anteroposterior and lateral views of an osteoid osteoma of the femur showing the typically small nidus with considerable sclerosis of the adjacent bone. *Right*. Another typical osteoid osteoma in the cortical region.

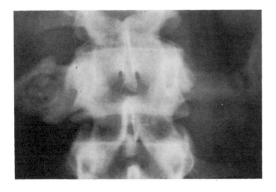

FIG. 7-4. *Above*. Osteoid osteoma of the third lumbar transverse process. This lesion contained some of the more loosely arranged trabeculae as seen in benign osteoblastoma. (Courtesy of Dr. J. E. Holmblad, Schenectady, N.Y.)

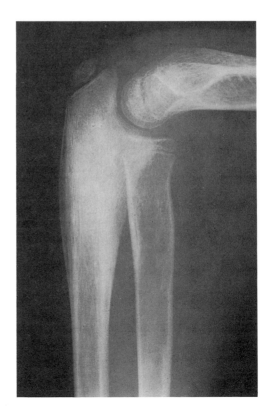

FIG. 7-5. *Right*. Partly because the nidus was not visualized, this osteoid osteoma of the ulna, with its diffuse subperiosteal new bone in layers, was mistaken for Ewing's sarcoma before operation.

Gross Pathology

Whether the osteoid osteoma is found in relatively nonsclerotic cancellous bone or buried in a large region of cortical sclerosis, the actual nidus, upon exposure, usually stands out as a discrete round or oval mass of tissue. It is ordinarily redder than the surrounding bone and can be lifted from its bed. The nidus itself varies in consistency from soft and granular to densely sclerotic, but sclerosis does not correlate with duration of symptoms. Sclerosis, when present, is usually most marked in the central portion of the nidus. Osteoid osteoma has, as previously noted, a peculiarly limited growth potential, which is an unusual feature of true neoplasms. Even when symptoms have been present several years, the nidus rarely exceeds 1 cm in greatest dimension. If the tumor proper measures 2 cm or more in diameter, the general characteristics of the case tend to overlap those of benign osteoblastoma.

When the sclerotic zone including the nidus is chiseled indiscriminately from an affected bone it is difficult or impossible for the pathologist to find the all important central mass of tumor tissue, without which the diagnosis cannot be established. It is important, therefore, that the surgeon remove the nidus intact for satisfactory pathologic appraisal. If the tumor is identified as such and is demonstrated to be completely removed, both the diagnosis and prognosis are established.

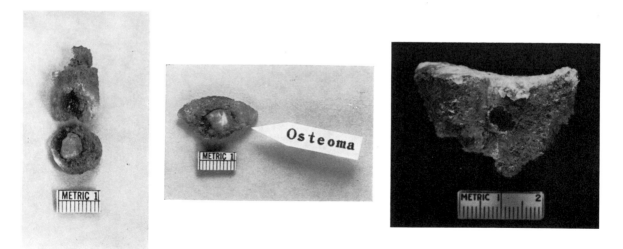

FIG. 7-6. *Left.* Osteoid osteoma removed en bloc from the neck of the femur of a 21-year-old man who had had pain in the hip for 1 year. Photomicrographs of this lesion are shown in Figures 7-9 and 7-12. FIG. 7-7. *Center.* Typical osteoid osteoma from an unusual site, the mandible. This occurred in a 26-year-old woman whose chief complaint was pain in the jaw. FIG. 7-8. *Right.* Red and granular osteoid osteoma, with very thin sclerotic rim, excised from the os calcis of a 7-year-old girl.

Histopathology

Microscopic examination reveals a distinct demarcation between the nidus and the surrounding bone. The surrounding bone may be densely sclerotic but otherwise shows no typical features.

The nidus itself consists of an interlacing network of osteoid trabeculae in which there is a variable amount of mineralization. The trabeculae are usually thin and arranged in a meaningless tangle showing numerous anastomoses. The central part of the nidus ordinarily is the site of the most mineralization and may be converted into atypical bone. Within the trabecular framework, instead of bone-marrow elements, there is a more or less vascular, fibrous connective tissue which contains variable numbers of benign giant cells. The osteoblasts which mantle the osteoid trabeculae in the zones of proliferation are too well differentiated to make one consider osteogenic sarcoma even in a specimen studied out of context.

Attempts to find an anatomic explanation for the pain experienced with this lesion have been unsuccessful.

Benign osteoblastoma typically contains broader and longer osteoid trabeculae. Further, it is, on the average, more vascular than is the ordinary osteoid osteoma. Unfortunately there is no clear line of distinction between these two tumors, and occasional borderline lesions might well be classed in either group. Careful review of the pertinent literature discloses that this is true, and the tumor illustrated in Figure 7-13 is a case in point.

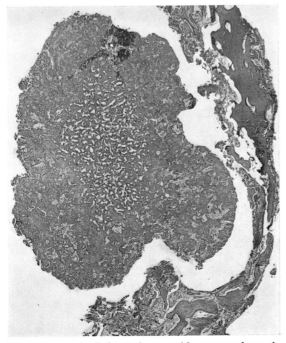

Fig. 7-9. Section of the entire osteoid osteoma shown in Figure 7-6. This tumor was covered by only a thin rim of attenuated cortex (×12).

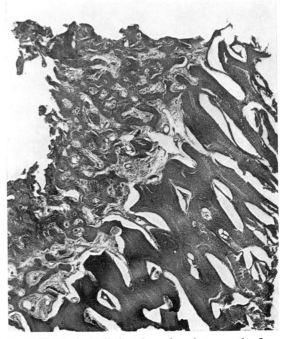

Fig. 7-10. Typical, distinct boundary between the finer trabeculae of the nidus and the sclerotic surrounding bone (×19).

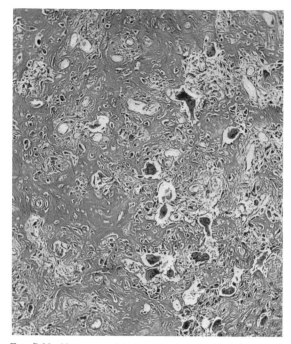

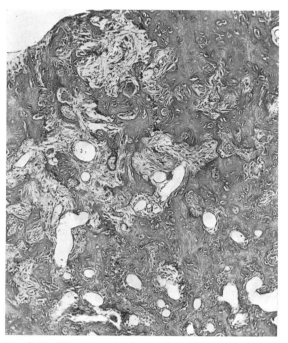

FIG. 7-11. Numerous benign giant cells in the typical ramifying trabeculae of a slightly calcified osteoid osteoma ($\times 110$).

FIG. 7-12. More completely ossified nidus with vascularity still prominent ($\times 90$). This is from the gross lesion seen in Figure 7-6.

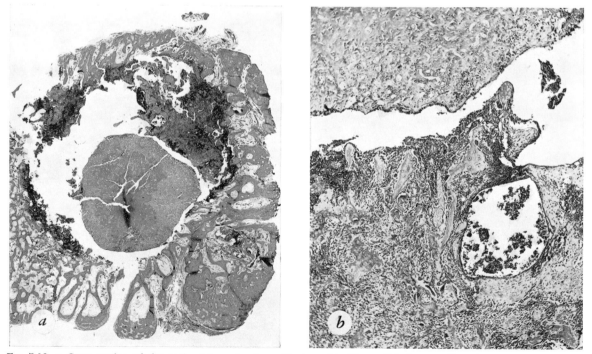

FIG. 7-13. *a*. Cross section of the entire triangular bone illustrated in Figure 7-2. Surrounding the somewhat eccentric dense nidus, there is lesional tissue that is more vascular ($\times 7$). *b*. Higher magnification of the same lesion to show the dense, ordinary nidus of osteoid osteoma above and the looser tissue like that of osteoblastoma below. Also Present were large blood channels reminiscent of aneurysmal bone cyst ($\times 50$).

Treatment

The treatment is complete surgical removal of the nidus. This is best accomplished by en bloc excision of it and some surrounding bone.

Roentgenographic guidance may be necessary at the time of operation. It is not necessary to remove all of the thickened bone around the osteoid osteoma proper, since this zone will resolve spontaneously if the entire nidus is gone.

Prognosis

Complete removal of the focus of tumor tissue results in cure. Incomplete removal of this focus may lead to recurrence of symptoms and the necessity for reoperation. Whether a true osteoid osteoma will resolve without surgical intervention is unknown. The cases in which such a course seems to have occurred have not had pathologic verification of the original diagnosis.

Sometimes the pathologist can identify no nidus of osteoid osteoma after thorough study of an excised specimen or of "shavings" from a region that clinically and by roentgenographic study was characteristic of osteoid osteoma. Interestingly, such patients are usually cured by the surgical procedure, which means that the nidus was somehow lost or that osteoid osteoma has a successful but unnamed mimic.

Bibliography

1935   Jaffe, H. L.: "Osteoid Osteoma": A Benign Osteoblastic Tumor Composed of Osteoid and Atypical Bone. *Arch. Surg., 31*:709-728.

1940   Jaffe, H. L., and Lichtenstein, Louis: Osteoid-osteoma: Further Experience With This Benign Tumor of Bone: With Special Reference to Cases Showing the Lesion in Relation to Shaft Cortices and Commonly Misclassified as Instances of Sclerosing Non-suppurative Osteomyelitis or Cortical-bone Abscess. *J. Bone & Joint Surg., n.s., 22*:645-682.

1947   Sherman, Mary S.: Osteoid Osteoma: Review of the Literature and Report of Thirty Cases. *J. Bone & Joint Surg., n.s., 29*:918-930.

1951   Dockerty, M. B., Ghormley, R. K., and Jackson, A. E.: Osteoid Osteoma: A Clinicopathologic Study of 20 Cases. *Ann. Surg., 133*:77-89.

1955   Rushton, J. G., Mulder, D. W., and Lipscomb, P. R.: Neurologic Symptoms With Osteoid Osteoma. *Neurology, 5*:794-797.

1956   Flaherty, R. A., Pugh, D. G., and Dockerty, M. B.: Osteoid Osteoma. *Am. J. Roentgenol., 76*:1041-1051.

1959   Freiberger, R. H., and Lortman, B. S.: Osteoid Osteoma. A Report of 80 Cases. *Am. J. Roentgenol., 82*:194-205.

1960   Freiberger, R. H.: Osteoid Osteoma of the Spine. A Cause of backache and Scoliosis in Children and Young Adults. *Radiology, 75*:232-236.

1961   Johnston, A. D.: Clinical Problems in Osteoid Osteoma. Evidence of Osteoclastic Aversion to Osteoid. *Bull. Hosp. Joint Dis., 23*:80-94.

1964   Fowles, S. J.: Osteoid Osteoma. *Brit. J. Radiol., 37*:245-252.

Chapter 8

Benign Osteoblastoma (Giant Osteoid Osteoma)

THE LITERATURE concerning this rare, benign tumor is especially confusing. Its osteoblastic nature results in zones often quite like those of an osteoid osteoma, producing a histologic kinship that can scarcely be ignored. Benign osteoblastoma differs, however, in not sharing the markedly limited growth potential of the average osteoid osteoma. Further, it frequently lacks the characteristic pain and the halo of sclerotic bone of the latter tumor. Even so, one occasionally encounters a lesion whose composite features make it fall midway between the two lesions under discussion.

In the literature dealing with neoplasms of the vertebral column, benign osteoblastoma is found under a variety of diagnoses including giant cell tumor, osteoid osteoma, osteogenic (or ossifying) fibroma, and sarcoma. An important reason for recognizing this entity is that it has commonly been mistaken for the much more aggressive, genuine giant cell tumor or even for sarcoma.

One may logically question whether benign osteoblastoma is correctly classed with true neoplasms since some of them regress or become arrested after incomplete surgical removal. Fields within some of these tumors resemble portions of aneurysmal bone cysts. This coupled with a pronounced clinical similarity suggests that both of these processes may be but different manifestations of a reaction to some as yet unknown agent.

The term "giant osteoid osteoma," introduced several years ago, was an attempt to recognize the pathologic similarity of this lesion to osteoid osteoma, at the same time indicating a difference, especially with respect to the size of the average tumor. Benign osteoblastoma has nevertheless become the most widely accepted designation for this tumor.

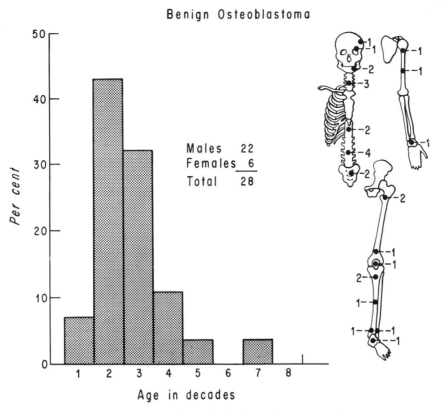

Benign Osteoblastoma

Males   22
Females   6
Total   28

Per cent

Age in decades

Fig. 8-1. Skeletal, age, and sex distribution of benign osteoblastoma.

Incidence

This tumor accounted for less than 1% of the primary tumors of bone in the present series, but it is being diagnosed somewhat more frequently in recent years.

Sex

In this series, in Lichtenstein's (1964), and in that collected by Salzer and Salzer-Kuntschik (1963) the tumor has shown a definite predilection for males.

Age

This tumor appears to be distinctly one of the younger age group, and all but five in this series were in patients in the first 3 decades of life.

Localization

Benign osteoblastoma, in contrast to all other neoplasms of bone except myeloma and chordoma, manifests a distinct predilection for the vertebral column. Eleven in this series affected the spinal column and sacrum. The remainder were in the long bones except for one tumor in the patella, one in the talus, one in the carpal navicular, two in the mandible, one in the roof of the orbit, and one in the temporal bone. Other sites that have been reported involved include rib, scapula, and innominate bone.

BENIGN OSTEOBLASTOMA

Symptoms

Pain, usually at the site of the tumor, is the cardinal symptom. In many instances the pain is due to pressure on adjacent structures, notably the spinal cord or the emerging nerves, and it appears to lack the intrinsic severity of that caused by ordinary osteoid osteoma. Involvement of the spinal cord or nerves may result in weakness or even paraplegia. The pain may be referred to a site distant from the tumor. The lesion develops slowly; the average duration of pain in our original series was 25.8 months before the patient sought medical advice. If the affected bone is not covered by a thick layer of soft tissue, local swelling may be evident. Those patients with a lesion in the lower extremity may experience a limp.

Physical Findings

Physical examination is of little value in the definitive diagnosis of this lesion, but it may reveal a tender mass at the site of the tumor. Atrophy of the adjacent muscles is sometimes seen. Variable neurologic deficits may be noted, depending upon the degree of involvement of the spinal cord or emerging nerves.

Roentgenologic Features

The roentgenologic picture is not as characteristic in this tumor as it is in ordinary osteoid osteoma. In some cases all one observes is bone destruction that is more or less well circumscribed and does not always suggest that the process is benign. In some instances, especially in the long bones, the lesional site is surrounded by a dense sclerotic zone similar to that seen in ordinary osteoid osteoma. The main difference from ordinary osteoid osteoma is that the region of the central nidus is almost always many times larger in these cases. Many benign osteoblastomas arise in bones that are predominantly cancellous and this may help account for the common absence of perifocal sclerosis. Occasionally the tumor is surrounded by a thin layer of bone beneath an expanded periosteum, giving an appearance similar to that of aneurysmal bone cyst; some of

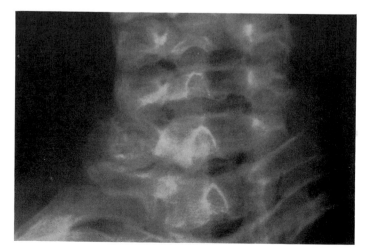

FIG. 8-2. Example of this tumor type. It has produced some expansion of the right transverse process of the seventh cervical vertebra. The excised specimen measured 2 cm in diameter.

Lichtenstein's benign osteoblastomas showed this feature. In older or previously treated lesions, more or less ossification of tumor tissue results in enough radiopacity to cause the roentgenologist to consider that the tumor is an osteoma.

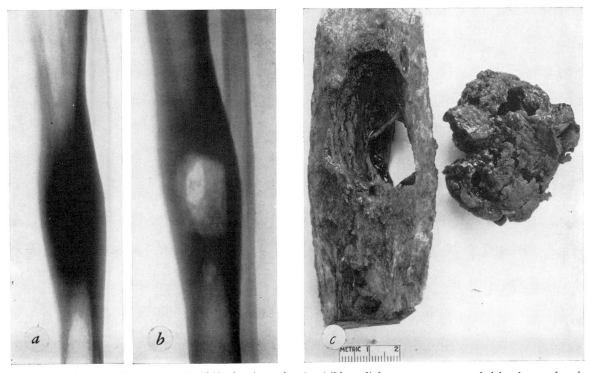

FIG. 8-3. *a.* The left tibia on Sept. 1, 1943, showing a barely visible radiolucent area surrounded by dense sclerotic bone. *b.* Same lesion on Jan. 17, 1946, after three drilling operations elsewhere, each of which brought temporary relief. *c.* Excised tumor and anterior half of tibia. The tumor showed classic features of benign osteoblastoma. (Reproduced with permission from: Dockerty, M. B., Ghormley, R. K., and Jackson, A. E.: *Ann. Surg., 133:*77-89, 1951.)

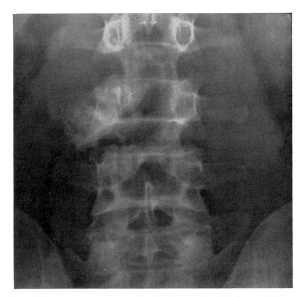

FIG. 8-4. A completely lytic benign osteoblastoma 2.5 cm in diameter was removed 8 years previously from the site of this now sclerotic and asymptomatic tumor.

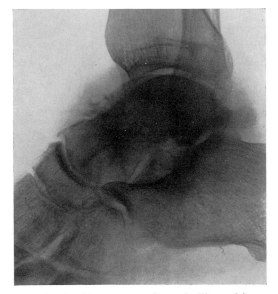

FIG. 8-5. The 32-gm tumor shown in Figure 8-7 was removed from this talus. (Reproduced with permission from: Dahlin, D. C., and Johnson, E. W., Jr.: *J. Bone & Joint Surg., 36A:*559-572, 1954.)

Gross Pathology

The gross pathologic features of this tumor are relatively characteristic. Entire gross specimens are rarely observed because the average lesion is removed by curettement. These tumors are, however, reasonably well circumscribed. The tumor tissue is hemorrhagic, granular and friable, owing to its vascularity and its osteoid component which shows variable degrees of calcification. In some of the older lesions the consistency resembles that of cancellous bone, and decalcification is necessary before microscopic sections can be made. If the tumor bulges from and distorts the contour of the affected bone, its margins are sharply defined. Follow-up studies of some individual cases strongly suggests that young lesions are distinctly lytic, but that they may undergo progressive ossification.

As previously indicated, the bone adjacent to benign osteoblastoma often is not sclerosed. Around the tumor in some cases there is a thin sclerotic rim, and around the tumor proper in others, especially those in the long bones of the extremities, there may be a zone of increased density that is as prominent as that associated with ordinary osteoid osteoma.

Reported tumors have varied up to 10 cm in greatest diameter. Sometimes the vascularity of osteoblastoma is such that hemostasis may be a problem for the surgeon.

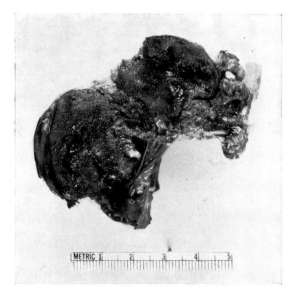

FIG. 8-6. Cut surface of benign osteoblastoma removed from the sacrum of a 22-year-old man who had had local pain for 3 years. It measured 4 by 3.5 by 3 cm. This predominantly lytic lesion involved the left lower part of the sacrum.

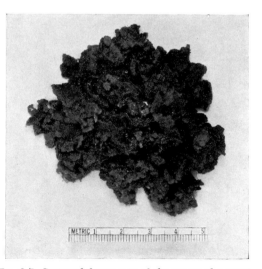

FIG. 8-7. Curetted fragments of the tumor the roentgenogram of which is illustrated in Figure 8-5. (Reproduced with permission from: Dahlin, D. C., and Johnson, E. W., Jr.: *J. Bone & Joint Surg., 36A:* 559-572, 1954.)

Histopathology

The microscopic features of benign osteoblastoma are extremely variable and account for the confusion in the literature regarding this tumor. In what are apparently early lesions one observes actively proliferating connective tissue which may show only slight osteoid formation and numerous giant cells. In the older ones, considerable ossification may be present. This variety accounts for the inclusion of cases of this type among the giant cell tumors, osteogenic fibromas, osteoid osteomas, and osteomas. In the less mature lesions, mitotic figures are found in the actively proliferating cells, some of which may be obviously osteoblastic; hence the occasional confusion of this benign process with osteogenic sarcoma. Most of the benign osteoblastomas contain numerous blood vessels, mainly of dilated capillary type, a feature which poses the question of vascular origin for this tumor.

Some of the lesions under discussion exhibit features of aneurysmal bone cyst. I have observed tumors in which some of the histologic sections were identical with those from an aneurysmal bone cyst, whereas other sections were typical of benign osteoblastoma. This reinforces the interesting speculation as to whether both of these two rather poorly understood processes are related, a possibility that is enhanced by the similar age and skeletal distribution of these two tumors and their similar response to therapy.

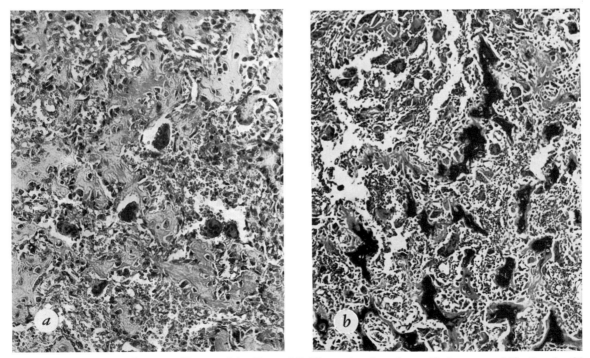

FIG. 8-8. *a.* Benign osteoblastoma illustrated in Figure 8-7. The trabeculae of osteoid show no calcification in this area. Vascularity and benign giant cells are prominent ($\times$170). *b.* Black areas indicate calcification of trabeculae. Giant cells are present ($\times$100). (Reproduced with permission from: Dahlin, D. C., and Johnson, E. W., Jr.: *J. Bone & Joint Surg., 36A:559-572, 1954.*)

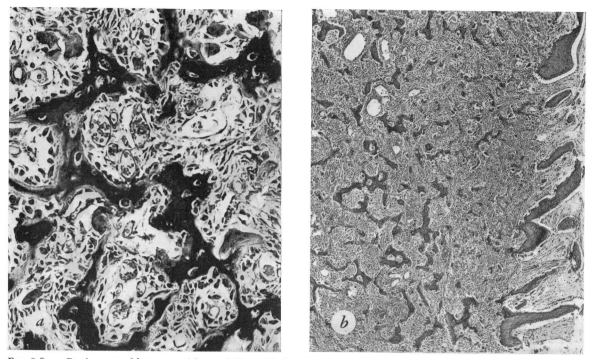

FIG. 8-9. *a.* Benign osteoblastoma with partially ossified trabeculae and prominent vascularity (×200). *b.* Vertebral tumor in this group, showing distinct demarcation from the expanded and attenuated cortex on the right (×35). (Reproduced with permission from: Dahlin, D. C., and Johnson, E. W., Jr.: *J. Bone & Joint Surg., 36A:*559-572, 1954.)

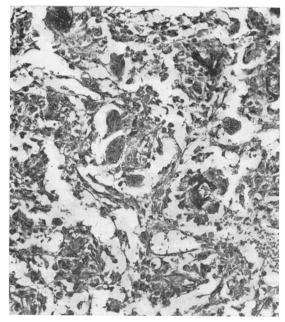

FIG. 8-10. Extremely cellular benign osteoblastoma, presumably an early lesion. This type is likely to be mistaken for sarcoma. There is little osteoid production (×175).

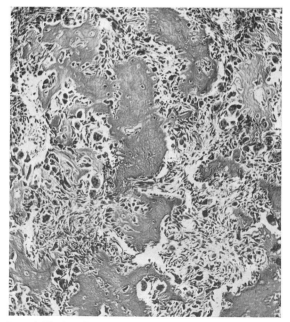

FIG. 8-11. Pertinent lesion involving a vertebra and showing, in this area, rather dense sclerosis. Giant cells are still abundant (×110).

Treatment

The benign nature of benign osteoblastoma dictates that conservative surgical treatment be used. This will usually entail removal of the entire lesion, or as much of it as possible, by curettement, with bone grafting of the defect if indicated. It is doubtful whether radiation therapy is helpful. In some of the cases in the present series, incomplete surgical removal of the lesional part has resulted in cure. The clinical course in the present cases suggests that until surgical intervention has been undertaken the tumefaction usually increases; however, in a 14-year-old girl with an osteoblastoma involving the right half of the sacrum, no treatment was employed following biopsy and she is asymptomatic 7 years later. The tumor was not surgically accessible and it was considered unwise to irradiate her pelvic region. Aegerter and Kirkpatrick describe a very similar case.

Prognosis

Perhaps the main reason for recognizing this rare pathologic entity is that it is not malignant and, as indicated, the response to treatment is nearly always good. Occasional tumors of this type that are incompletely removed will require more than one surgical procedure. The major problem likely to be encountered is that of involvement of the spinal column by a lesion; when this occurs one must direct therapy to preservation of the integrity of the spinal cord and the emerging nerve roots.

The potential hazard of radiation therapy in indicated by one case in this series. A fatal fibrosarcoma developed in the same region 10 years after roentgen therapy for osteoblastoma of the fifth cervical vertebra.

Bibliography

1924 Lewis, Dean: Primary Giant Cell Tumors of the Vertebrae: Analysis of a Group of Cases, With Report of Case in Which Patient Is Well Two Years and Nine Months After Operation. *J.A.M.A., 83:*1224-1229.

1954 Dahlin, D. C., and Johnson, E. W., Jr.: Giant Osteoid Osteoma. *J. Bone & Joint Surg., 36A:*559-572.

1954 Golding, J. S. R., and Sissons, H. A.: Osteogenic Fibroma of Bone: A Report of Two Cases. *J. Bone & Joint Surg., 36B:*428-435.

1956 Jaffe, H. L.: Benign Osteoblastoma. *Bull. Hosp. Joint Dis., 17:*141-151.

1958 Goidanich, I. F., and Battaglia, L.: Osteoblastoma (Fibroma osteogenetico). Neoplasia benigna di Tessuto osteoblastico. Studio clinico, radiografico ed anatomo-patologico di 14 casi. *Chir. org. Movimento, 46:*353-388.

1963 Salzer, M., and Salzer-Kuntschik, M.: Das benigne Osteoblastom. *Langenbecks Arch. klin. Chir., 302:*755-778.

1963 Aegerter, E., and Kirkpatrick, J. A., Jr.: *Orthopedic Diseases.* 2nd Ed. Philadelphia, W. B. Saunders Co., pp. 511-516.

1964 Lichtenstein, L., and Sawyer, W. R.: Benign Osteoblastoma. Further Observations and Report of Twenty Additional Cases. *J. Bone & Joint Surg., 46A:*755-765.

Chapter 9

Giant Cell Tumor (Osteoclastoma)

Giant cell tumor of bone is a distinctive neoplasm of poorly differentiated cells. The multinucleated giant cells apparently result from fusion of the proliferating mononuclear cells, and although they are a constant and prominent part of these tumors, they are likely of less significance than are the mononuclear cells. In fact, these osteoclastlike giant cells, with or without minor modifications, occur in a host of pathologic conditions of bone. The ubiquitous giant cell accounts for the confusion one finds in the older, and in some of the recent, literature on giant cell tumors. Authors have included conditions such as nonosteogenic fibroma, benign chondroblastoma, chondromyxoid fibroma, unicameral bone cysts with a cellular lining, giant cell reparative granuloma (epulis), aneurysmal bone cyst, hyperparathyroidism, giant-cell-containing osteogenic sarcoma, and other entities in the general category of giant cell tumor. Inclusion of these "variants" with their widely divergent biologic behavior has greatly delayed understanding of the clinical features and response to treatment of true giant cell tumor. The exact cell of origin of this neoplasm is unknown.

In addition to the recognized conditions that have been confused with giant cell tumor, one occasionally encounters a benign, more or less fibrogenic, rarefying process that does not fit well into any of the known categories. These rare lesions which contain giant cells and variable amounts of proliferative new bone are apt to be found in the vertebrae or small bones of the hands and feet. They probably represent a peculiar reaction in bone and, fortunately, have a good prognosis.

Malignant giant cell tumor is the subject of chapter 20. This malignant tumor cannot be diagnosed with assurance unless evidence of ordinary benign giant cell tumor exists within the lesion or has been demonstrated previously at the same site. If the stromal cells of a tumor that is rich in benign giant cells are malignant throughout, with features of either osteogenic or fibrosarcoma, the tumor probably bears no relationship to giant cell tumor. The benign giant cells are but an incidental and confusing component. Clinical correlative studies have fortified this concept (Troup and co-workers, 1960).

To further confuse the issue, giant cell tumor can produce metastasis even though cytologically benign. This occurrence is very rare, and only one such case was found in the present series of 155 giant cell tumors.

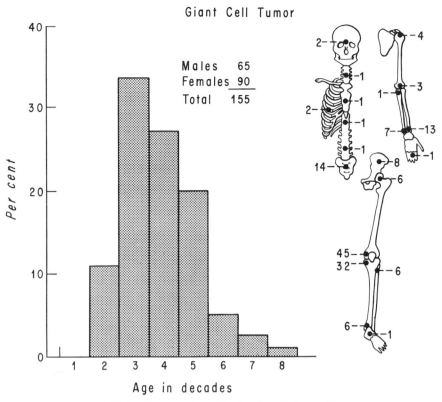

Fig. 9-1. Skeletal, age, and sex distribution of giant cell tumors.

Incidence

The 155 cases in this series represented 3.9% of the total and 15.1% of the benign tumors.

Sex

In many of the recorded series, females have predominated. The ratio in the present series was 90 females to 65 males. This contrasts with the predominance of males in most series of other bone tumors.

Age

When the "variants" of giant cell tumor were excluded, 89% of the neoplasms occurred in patients beyond the age of 19 years, with the peak incidence in the third decade of life. Most of those in the second decade were nearly 20 years of age. Five were in the age group 12 through 14 years.

Localization

Most giant cell tumors are found in the epiphyses of the long bones. More than half of those in the present series occurred about the knee. The sphenoid and ribs accounted for two each and the vertebrae above the sacrum for three. One arose in a tarsal, one in a phalanx, and one in the manubrium. Eight occurred in the ilium and ischium and 14 in the sacrum. It was not possible to segregate any unequivocal giant cell tumors from the numerous giant cell reparative lesions of jawbones. This series reemphasizes that "variants" are commoner than giant cell tumors in vertebrae.

GIANT CELL TUMOR

Symptoms

Pain of variable severity is almost always the predominating symptom. More than three fourths of the patients in the present series had noted swelling in the affected region. Less common symptoms included weakness, limitation of motion of a joint, and symptoms of pathologic fracture.

Physical Findings

A hard, sometimes crepitant and sometimes painful mass is found in more than 80% of patients. There may be atrophy of muscles due to disuse, effusion into the adjacent joint, or local heat and redness.

Roentgenologic Features

According to Gee and Pugh, 1958, these features may be summarized as those of an expanding zone of radiolucency situated eccentrically in the end of a long bone of an adult. Such an appearance is neither specific for giant cell tumor nor produced by all such tumors. The roentgenographic appearance may have been altered by pathologic fracture or by previous therapy. The margin between tumor and normal bone is characterized by gradual alteration of density and there is no reactive sclerosis at this junction in untreated tumors. Gee and Pugh were unable, after studying the available original roentgenograms of 62 of the patients in the present series, to correlate the roentgenographic features with the subsequent behavior of the tumors. A tumor not in the end of a tubular bone lacks specific roentgenographic signs.

Metaphyseal lesions are almost certainly not giant cell tumors, but two of the tumors in this series spared the epiphysis, and a very few similar cases have been reported.

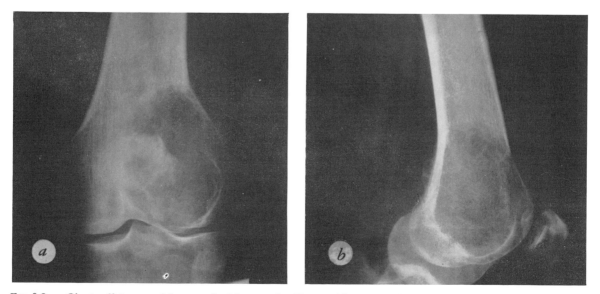

FIG. 9-2. *a*. Giant cell tumor of lower end of femur of a 21-year-old woman who had noted local pain for 9 months. *b*. Lateral view of same tumor.

Giant cell tumor may occur in a lesion of Paget's disease, a rare complication that seems to have a predilection for bones of the skull and face. Only one neoplasm in the present series, an iliac tumor, developed in osteitis deformans.

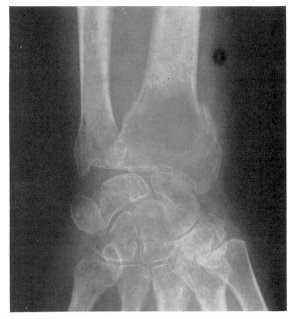

FIG. 9-3. Giant cell tumor affecting a 61-year-old woman who had had local pain for 2.5 months.

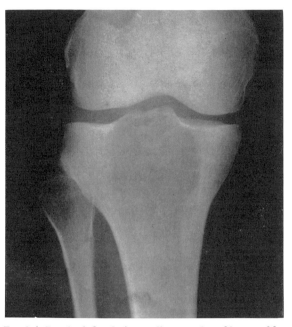

FIG. 9-4. Poorly defined giant cell tumor in a 32-year old woman who had noted local pain for 2 months.

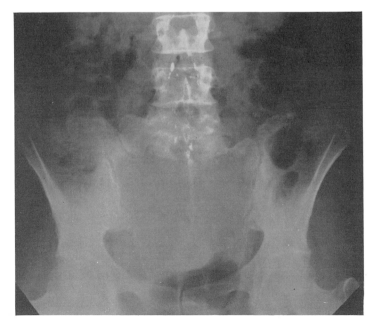

FIG. 9-5. Extensive sacral destruction by a giant cell tumor in a 36-year-old woman who had had low back pain for 9 months.

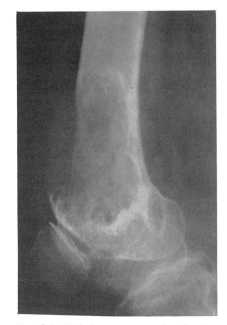

FIG. 9-6. Third recurrence of a benign giant cell tumor.

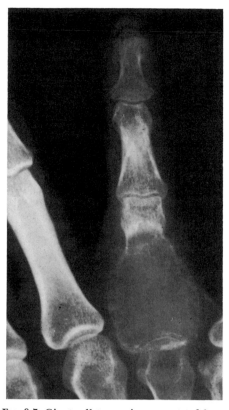

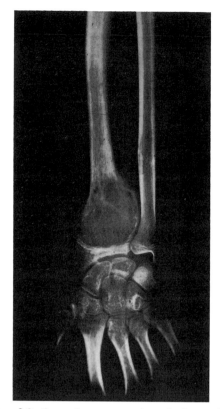

FIG. 9-7. Giant cell tumor in an unusual location, the first phalanx of the fourth finger. (Case contributed by Dr. Richard Lester of Durham, No. Carolina.)

FIG. 9-8. One of two metaphyseal giant cell tumors in the present series. This occurred in an 18-year-old man who had noted swelling for 3 months.

Gross Pathology

The tumor tissue is characteristically soft, friable, and gray to red. Firmer portions may be seen as the result of previous fracture, treatment, or degeneration, all of which may cause fibrosis and osteoid production. Small cystic or necrotic portions, sometimes filled with blood, may be present but these ordinarily constitute an insignificant feature of untreated lesions not modified by previous fracture. This cystification may be sufficiently prominent in recurrent neoplasms to cause them to be confused with aneurysmal bone cysts. The aggressive nature of giant cell tumors accounts for their immense size when they had been neglected. Intact gross specimens show variable degrees of expansion of the bone with corresponding attenuation or destruction of the cortex. The remainder of the osseous structures in the region of the tumor is completely replaced. The tumor practically always extends to the articular cartilage and its boundaries are only moderately well demarcated from adjacent bone and cartilage. Even with very large lesions the periosteum is rarely breached.

Multicentric giant cell tumors are extremely rare; one patient in this series developed a giant cell tumor of the upper tibia 16 months after excision of one from her sphenoid.

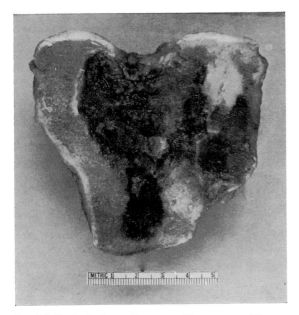

Fig. 9-9. Excised giant cell tumor of lower part of femur. Tumor has been modified by two previous operations that included bone grafting, which accounts for white zones.

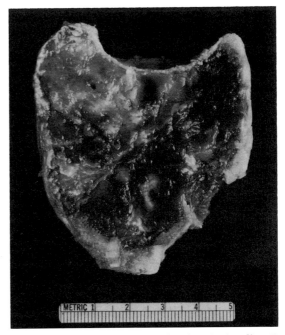

Fig. 9-10. Giant cell tumor of distal end of radius. It had produced pain for 1.5 years and had not been treated. Dark zones were brown owing to hemosiderin pigment.

Histopathology

The basic, proliferating cell has one round to oval or even spindle-shaped nucleus. In the fields that are diagnostic of true giant cell tumor these nuclei are surrounded by an ill-defined cytoplasmic zone, and no discernible intercellular substance is being produced. Mitotic figures can be found in practically every lesion, and in some they are numerous. These nuclei lack the hyperchromatism and variation in size and shape characteristic of sarcoma. However, one does occasionally encounter an osteogenic sarcoma with unusually small malignant cells and an abundance of benign giant cells. Such tumors may pose a difficult problem in differentiation from giant cell tumor histologically, but they are nearly always metaphyseal in location and in a younger age group. Histochemical methods for separating giant cell tumor from its variants have not proved of value (Schajowicz, 1961), so the pathologist must make the separation on the subtle cytologic and histologic features.

Evidence that the giant cells derive from fusion of the mononuclear cells includes the marked similarity of their nuclei. In certain areas, especially following fracture or unsuccessful treatment, some of the proliferating cells show metaplasia to a type capable of producing collagen or even osteoid tissue. Cartilaginous differentiation is unusual, and its presence is indicative of benign chondroblastoma, especially if it is disposed in discrete islands. Zones containing numerous foam cells or phagocytized iron pigment apparently result from old hemorrhage or necrosis. Necrotic foci may be present and sometimes extensive. Tiny fragments of tissue containing a few giant cells are inadequate for verification of true giant cell tumor; thus aspiration biopsy has limited usefulness in the diagnosis of this neoplasm.

Malignant change in giant cell tumor is discussed under prognosis and in chapter 20.

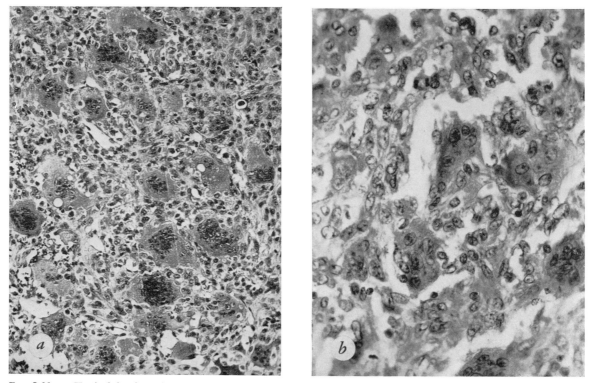

FIG. 9-11. *a.* Typical benign giant cell tumor with no definite intercellular substance and with prominent multinucleated cells (×160). *b.* Note marked similarity of nuclei of mononuclear and multinucleated cells. One can scarcely define the boundaries of the giant cells (×420). (Reproduced with permission from: Williams, R. R., Dahlin, D. C., and Ghormley, R. K.: *Cancer,* 7:764-773, 1954.)

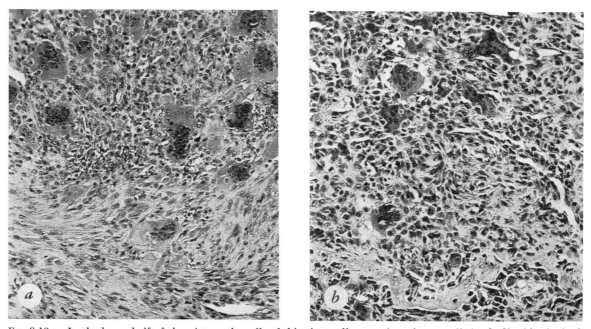

FIG. 9-12. *a.* In the lower half of the picture the cells of this giant cell tumor have become distinctly fibroblastic. Such fibrogenic zones that contain scattered multinucleated cells are seen in many conditions of bone (×160). *b.* Osteoid trabecula in a giant cell tumor. Such foci may be present even before therapy or fracture alters the tumor (×185). (Reproduced with permission from: Williams, R. R., Dahlin, D. C., and Ghormley, R. K.: *Cancer,* 7:764-773, 1954.)

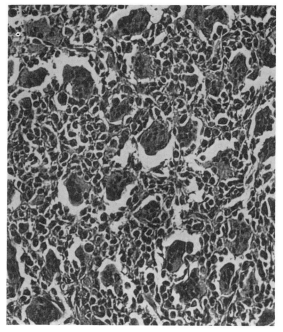

FIG. 9-13. Sacral giant cell tumor (×200). Tissue from the case illustrated in Figure 9-5.

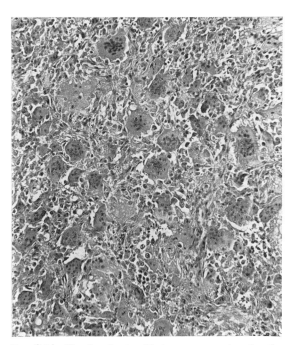

FIG. 9-14. Classic giant cell tumor occurring in the sphenoid of a 25-year-old woman (×100).

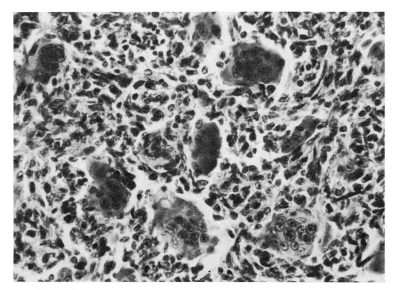

FIG. 9-15. Giant cell tumor of dorsal vertebral body. Thorough sampling revealed no histologic evidence of a variant such as aneurysmal bone cyst or osteoblastoma, both of which are considerably more common than true giant cell tumor in vertebrae above the sacrum (×365).

GIANT CELL TUMOR

Treatment

Removal of the tumor by curettage is the most widely accepted type of therapy. Many advocate chemical or thermal cautery of the walls of the cavity, and the defect is ordinarily filled with bone chips. Total excision of the tumor and its surrounding shell of bone and periosteum is sometimes the treatment of choice, especially when a small bone such as the fibula or radius is involved. Some believe that total excision is indicated even at the knee, although it ordinarily results in loss of function of the joint. Bone grafting is usually required after such excisions. In some of the massive lesions with marked destruction of juxta-articular bone, primary amputation is necessary. Some believe that, after multiple recurrences, amputation or radical excision should be considered because of the hazard of malignant transformation.

Irradiation as primary or adjunctive therapy has its advocates but is falling into disfavor because of its potential danger of inducing malignant transformation and the recognition that true giant cell tumors are radioresistant. Irradiation should be reserved for those giant cell tumors not amenable to surgical excision.

When malignant change has occurred, the treatment is that indicated for radioresistant sarcoma.

Prognosis

Long-term follow-up is essential in assessing the results of therapy for giant cell tumor, since malignant change has developed nearly 30 years after primary treatment. Several studies have shown the recurrence rate to be 50% or more, and sarcoma complicates the course in approximately 10%.

Curettage was followed by recurrence in more than 50% of the cases in the present series. Size of tumor, bone involved, preoperative duration of symptoms, cauterization of tumor cavity, bone grafting, cellular appearance, and adjunctive irradiation therapy have had no recognizable influence on the recurrence rate.

Amputation or total excision has been uniformly curative, but amputation is indicated as primary treatment only for huge, neglected giant cell tumors.

Secondary malignant change is usually in the form of pure fibrosarcoma or osteogenic sarcoma. It was found in 14 of the 155 cases in the present series. Ten of the 14 malignant tumors in this series occurred an average of 6 years after verification of benign giant cell tumor and therapy which included irradiation in all but 1 instance. Eight of these 10 patients died as a result of metastasis, and 2 were cured by amputation. In 1 of the 10 patients a rapidly lethal fibrosarcoma appeared 1½ years after curettage and bone grafting without irradiation. Three patients had sarcomas present in portions of typical benign giant cell tumors at the time of their first operation. The fourteenth patient had foci of anaplastic osteogenic sarcoma in an otherwise typical giant cell tumor; curettage and radiation had been performed elsewhere 8 months previously and that tissue was not available for study.

Original sections from those benign giant cell tumors that recurred or from which secondary

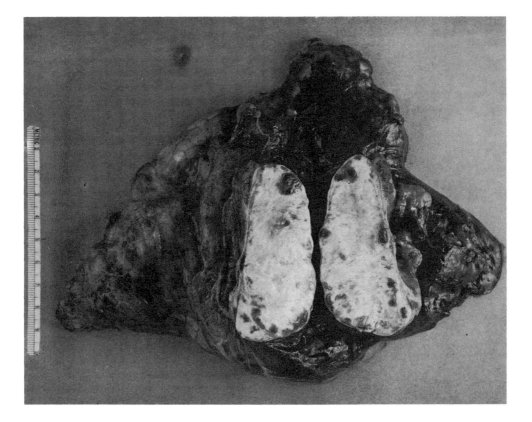

FIG. 9-16. *Above*. Solitary metastatic benign giant cell tumor nodule excised with right lower pulmonary lobe and portion of attached diaphragm. This lesion appeared nearly 6 years after curettage, grafting, and irradiation of a giant cell tumor of the distal end of the radius. No residual tumor was present in the radius. The patient has remained well for nearly 8 years since pulmonary resection. *Right*. Pulmonary nodule which appeared identical to the original benign giant cell tumor of the radius (×200). (Reproduced with permission from: Pan, P., Dahlin, D. C., Lipscomb, P. R., and Bernatz, P. E.: *Proc. Staff Meet., Mayo Clin., 39*:344-349, 1964.)

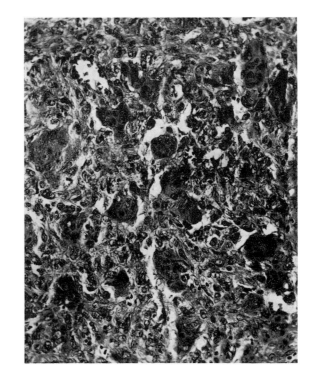

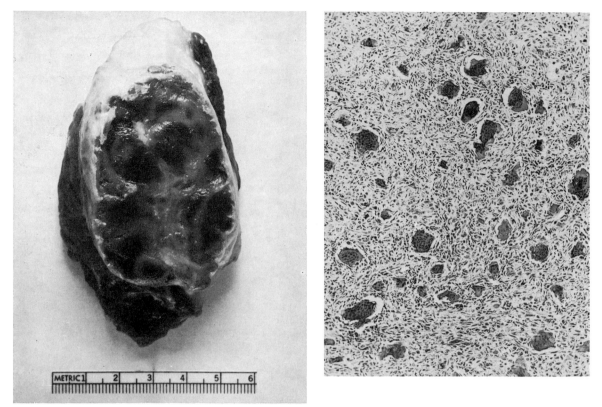

Fig. 9-17. *Left.* Circumscribed recurrence of benign giant cell tumor excised from the muscles adjacent to the distal end of the femur of a 22-year-old woman. There was no definite evidence of recurrence of the primary lesion of the distal portion of the femur, which had been treated by curettage and grating more than 4 years before, by irradiation during the ensuing year, and by curettage and grafting again a year prior to excision of this lesion. Such recurrence in soft tissues was very unusual in this series. Interestingly, a thin shell of bone had developed from the tumor cells at the periphery of the mass, a phenomenon that occurs sometimes in the rare metastases of benign giant cell tumor. *Right.* The microscopic appearance of this recurrence in soft tissue appeared identical to that of the original benign giant cell tumor of the femur ($\times$110). (Reproduced with permission from: Johnson, E. W., Jr.: *Am. J. Surg., 109:* 163-166, 1965.)

sarcomas developed were histologically indistinquishable from those cured by one surgical procedure. Grading of these tumors as to degree of malignancy has been of no prognostic value in the author's hands.

Metastasis from benign giant cell tumor, with the metastatic deposit appearing benign, has been documented adequately less than a dozen times, and only one instance was encountered in the present series.

Bibliography

1940   Jaff, H. L., Lichtenstein, Louis, and Portis, R. B.: Giant Cell Tumor of Bone: Its Pathologic Appearance, Grading, Supposed Variants and Treatment. *Arch. Path., 30*:993-1031.

1947   Aegerter, E. E.: Giant Cell Tumor of Bone: A Critical Survey. *Am. J. Path., 23*:283-297.

1949   Willis, R. A.: The Pathology of Osteoclastoma or Giant-Cell Tumour of Bone. *J. Bone & Joint Surg., 31B*:236-240.

1953   Shuffstall, R. M., and Gregory, J. E.: Osteoid Formation in Giant Cell Tumors of Bone. *Am. J. Path., 29*:1123-1131.

1953   Compere, E. L.: The Diagnosis and Treatment of Giant-cell Tumors of Bone. *J. Bone & Joint Surg., 35A*:822-830.

1953 Jaffe, H. L.: Giant-cell Tumor (Osteoclastoma) of Bone: Its Pathologic Delimitation and the Inherent Clinical Implications. *Ann. Roy. Coll. Surgeons England, 13:*343-355.

1954 Williams, R. R., Dahlin, D. C., and Ghormley, R. K.: Giant-cell Tumor of Bone. *Cancer, 7:*764-773.

1956 Dahlin, D. C., Ghormley, R. K., and Pugh, D. G.: Giant Cell Tumor of Bone: Differential Diagnosis. *Proc. Staff Meet., Mayo Clin., 31:*31-42.

1956 Murphy, W. R., and Ackerman, L. V.: Benign and Malignant Giant-Cell Tumors of Bone. A Clinical-Pathological Evaluation of Thirty-one Cases. *Cancer, 9:*317-339.

1957 Bullock, W. K., and Luck, J. V.: Giant Cell Tumor-like Lesions of Bone. *California Med., 87:*32-36.

1958 Coley, B. L., Higinbotham, M. L., and Kogura, T.: Giant Cell Tumor of Bone. *Am. J. Surg., 96:*479-491.

1958 Gee, V. R., and Pugh, D. G.: Giant-Cell Tumor of Bone. *Radiology, 70:*33-45.

1959 Johnson, E. W., Jr., and Dahlin, D. C.: Treatment of Giant-Cell Tumor of Bone. *J. Bone & Joint Surg., 41A:*895-904.

1960 Troup, J. B., Dahlin, D. C., and Coventry, M. B.: The Significance of Giant Cells in Osteogenic Sarcoma: Do They Indicate a Relationship between Osteogenic Sarcoma and Giant Cell Tumor of Bone? *Proc. Staff Meet., Mayo Clin., 35:*179-186.

1961 Schajowicz, F.: Giant-Cell Tumors of Bone (Osteoclastoma). A Pathological and Histochemical Study. *J. Bone & Joint Surg., 43A:*1-29.

1961 Sherman, M., and Fabricius, R.: Giant-Cell Tumor in the Metaphysis in a Child. Report of an Unusual Case. *J. Bone & Joint Surg., 43A:*1225-1229.

1961 Goldner, J. L., and Forrest, J. S.: Giant Cell Tumor of Bone. *South. M. J., 54:*121-133.

1962 Hutter, R. V. P., Worcester, J. N. Jr., Francis, K. C., Foote, F. W. Jr., and Stewart, F. W.: Benign and Malignant Giant Cell Tumors of Bone. A Clinicopathological Analysis of the Natural History of the Disease. *Cancer, 15:*653-690.

1962 d'Aubigne, R. M., and Mazabraud, A.: A propos de 22 observations de "vraies" tumeurs à cellules géantes. *Lyon chir., 58:*389-403.

1963 Edeiken, Jack, and Hodes, P. J.: Giant Cell Tumors vs. Tumors with Giant Cells. *Radiol. Clin. N. Am., 1:*75-100.

1963 Hutter, R. V. P., Foote, F. W. Jr., Frazell, E. L., and Francis, K. C.: Giant Cell Tumors Complicating Paget's Disease of Bone. *Cancer, 16:*1044-1056.

1964 Pan, P., Dahlin, D. C., Lipscomb, P. R., and Bernatz, P. E.: "Benign" Giant Cell Tumor of the Radius with Pulmonary Metastasis. *Proc. Staff Meet., Mayo Clin., 39:*344-349.

1964 Jewell, J. H., and Bush, L. F.: "Benign" Giant-Cell Tumor of Bone with A Solitary Pulmonary Metastasis. A Case Report. *J. Bone & Joint Surg., 46A:*848-852.

1964 Tate, R. G.: Giant Cell Tumour of Bone. *Canad. J. Surg., 7:*25-42.

1964 Bradshaw, J. D.: The Value of X-ray Therapy in the Management of Osteoclastoma. *Clin. Radiol., 15:*70-74.

1964 Mnaymneh, W. A., Dudley, H. R., and Mnaymneh, L. G.: Excision of Giant-Cell Bone Tumor. *J. Bone & Joint Surg., 46A:*63-75.

1965 Lichtenstein, L.: *Bone Tumors.* St. Louis, C. V. Mosby Co., pp. 139-159.

Chapter 10

Fibroma (Nonosteogenic Fibroma of Bone, Metaphyseal Fibrous Defect, Fibrous Cortical Defect) and "Xanthoma"

THE ABOVE TERMS all apply to the same basic histopathologic process in bone. The spontaneous resolution of most of these lesions and their relationship to the growing portions of bones support the concept that they represent faulty ossification rather than neoplasm. Roentgenographic evidence of cortical defects may be found in approximately a third of growing children, most commonly in the femur. A small fraction of these pose a sufficient diagnostic problem or produce severe enough symptoms to require operation. Strangely, a few of these fibroblastic masses, histologically indistinguishable from the innocuous ones, continue to grow and may produce pathologic fracture of even a major tubular bone. Patients may have multiple fibrous defects in one or more extremities.

Despite the innocuous clinical behavior of this lesion, its component of benign multinucleated cells still frequently results in its being erroneously considered to be a genuine giant cell tumor of bone.

The so-called periosteal desmoid appears to be a hypocellular variant of this group of fibrous defects; perhaps it results from trauma.

Desmoplastic fibroma is a locally aggressive benign neoplasm which will be discussed in the chapter dealing with fibrosarcoma of bone.

Congenital generalized fibromatosis, a rare condition, may produce rarefactions in bone, but these desmoplastic proliferations are quite different from the fibromas under discussion.

It is pertinent to point out that one occasionally sees fibrous defects of bone that lack the cellularity and roentgenologic features of typical fibroma. The exact nature of some of these is obscure. Some may result from old trauma, hemorrhage, or infection and some may represent the end stage or scar of an ordinary fibroma or of fibrous dysplasia. Several such lesions were encountered in the files of the Mayo Clinic, but they have been excluded from the data in Figure 10-1 and from the discussion which follows.

Xanthoma or xanthofibroma is a term that has been employed for some of the fibromas that have a prominent lipoid component. Aside from such fibromas, one occasionally encounters a small or large osseous lesion that is predominantly xanthic. Some aspects of this problem are elaborated in this chapter.

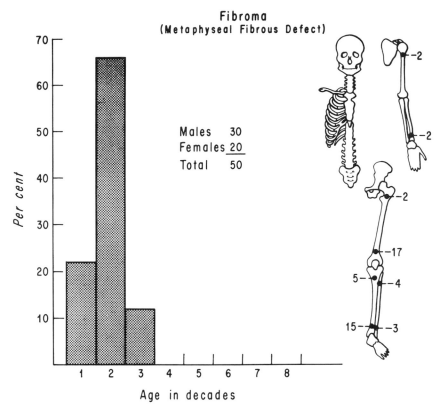

Fig. 10-1. Skeletal, age, and sex distribution of fibromas.

Incidence

Although fibromas constituted less than 5% of the benign bone tumors in this series, their true incidence is much greater because the vast majority of them never come to operation. The data in Figure 10-1. like the other data in this book, derive from surgical cases only.

Sex

Males predominated in the present series, which is in keeping with the findings of others. In my earlier series, which included some of the nondescript fibrous scars in bone, there was a female predominance.

Age

Fibroma in its classic form is almost exclusively a disease of childhood and adolescence. The oldest patient in this series was 25 years of age.

Localization

Every fibroma in this series was in the metaphyseal portion of a long bone of a limb. Only four were in an upper extremity. This distribution is in keeping with the findings of others.

FIBROMA

Symptoms

This lesion is commonly silent clinically and is discovered accidentally when a region is subjected to roentgenographic study for unrelated reasons. Local pain, usually of short duration, is sometimes produced. Occasionally, especially in slender tubular bones such as the fibula, pathologic fracture ushers in the clinical symptoms.

Physical Findings

Physical examination is of little diagnostic value in fibroma of bone. In rare instances slight swelling may be observed if the affected bone is near the surface of the body.

Roentgenologic Features

Most fibromas present a characteristic roentgenographic appearance which is virtually pathognomonic. When a large tubular bone is affected, the lesion is practically always eccentrically located and often produces some bulging of the cortical outline which is usually very thin over the defect.

The tumor begins in the metaphysis, near or at the epiphyseal line, and appears to migrate toward the center of the bone as the epiphyseal region grows away from it. The inner boundary of the lesion often is demarcated by a thin or prominent scalloped line of sclerosis. Trabeculae frequently appear to traverse the defect and give it a multilocular appearance; these trabeculae are, however, nearly always incomplete and the appearance is actually produced by the shadows of corrugations on the inner surface of the cavity housing the tumor. Sometimes a fibroma has a poorly delimited periphery with no surrounding sclerosis. In thin bones the entire width of the bone may be involved. Central lesions may simulate fibrous dysplasia or simple bone cysts.

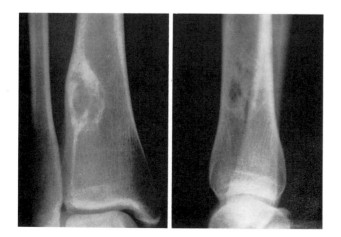

FIG. 10-2. *Left.* Fibroma of distal part of tibia with classic features except for somewhat more than usual sclerosis. *Right.* Lateral view of same lesion.

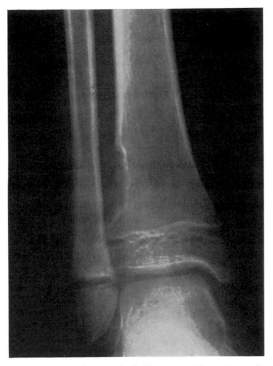

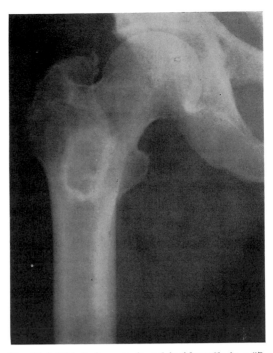

FIG. 10-3. Another typical fibroma, although small. This one was found incidentally on roentgenographic study of the ankle of an 8-year-old girl.

FIG. 10-4. This lesion was found incidentally in a 57-year-old man. It consisted of dense fibrous tissue with a sclerosed border. The genesis of this process is obscure and it was not included with the fibromas.

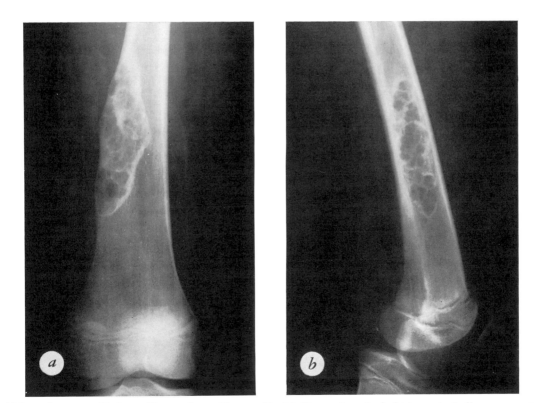

FIG. 10-5. *a.* An unusually large fibroma in an 11-year-old girl. Its roentgenologic features, including an appearance of trabeculation, bulging of the cortical outline, and a distinct inner boundary, are typical. *b.* Lateral view of the same lesion makes it appear to be a basically central one. (Roentgenograms of this case were provided through the courtesy of Drs. P. K. Odland, G. L. Thomas, and M. B. Llewellyn, of Janesville, Wisconsin.)

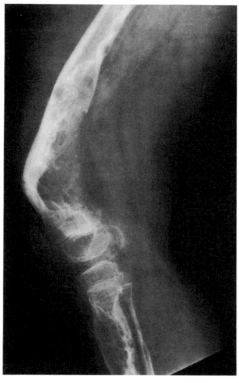

Fig. 10-6. Multiple nonosteogenic fibromas which had produced multiple fractures of the femur. The resultant deformity later necessitated amputation. Note that there is involvement of the tibia and fibula also.

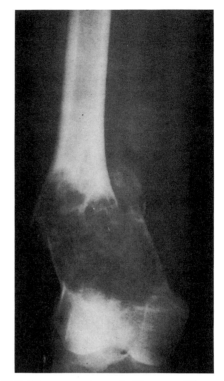

Fig. 10-7. Huge nonosteogenic fibroma with associated pathologic fracture of distal metaphyseal region of femur of 14-year-old girl. Curettage and grafting resulted in healing with some shortening of femur. (Case contributed by Dr. A. R. Haugen, San Bernardino, Calif.)

Gross Pathology

As indicated by the roentgenogram, the cortex is ordinarily attenuated but intact over a fibroma unless fracture has occurred. The lesions vary in greatest diameter, some reaching 5 cm or more. The long axis tends to parallel that of the affected bone. The tumor itself is usually distinctly demarcated from the surrounding bone, and sometimes consists of multiple discrete lobules of soft tissue surrounded by walls of bone and showing more or less confluence. The pathologist ordinarily receives curetted fragments of more or less fibrous, fleshy tissue. It is often completely or partially yellow, depending on its lipid content. It may contain enough hemosiderin to make it distinctly brown.

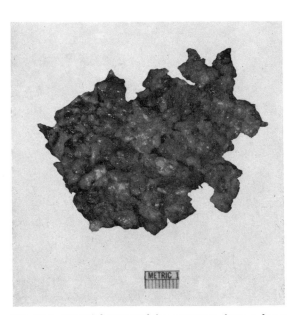

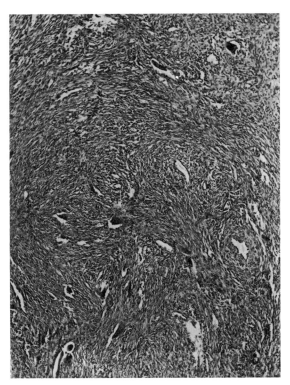

FIG. 10-8. Material removed by curettage from a large fibroma of the lower part of the tibia. Lighter zones represent foci with many foam cells. The gross appearance is, on the whole, not diagnostic.

FIG. 10-9. Classic appearance of nonosteogenic fibroma. Note cell-rich fibroblastic tissue disposed in somewhat whorled bundles. Giant cells are sparser than in the average giant cell tumor (×50).

Histopathology

Microscopic examination reveals a dominant, cellular, fibroblastic connective-tissue background with the cells arranged in whorled bundles. The fibrogenic characteristic aids in differentiation from genuine giant cell tumors which, in sections from diagnostic portions, are not fibrogenic. Benign multinucleated cells, containing fewer nuclei on the average than do those of giant cell tumor, are irregularly distributed throughout the lesion. Nests of lipophages, which appear to be converted fibroblasts, are sometimes seen. They rarely dominate or even form a prominent part of the picture, but one encounters an occasional lesion in bone that has the roentgenographic appearance of fibroma but shows extreme lipidization. Giant cells are uncommon in the foci of foam cells. Hemosiderin pigmentation of variable degree may be seen in the cytoplasm of the fibroblasts.

Occasional fibromas are active enough that mitotic figures may be found with comparative ease. The benign quality of the nuclei should allay the fear that one is dealing with a malignant tumor in such cases.

A fibroma associated with pathologic fracture may have undergone so much necrosis and hemorrhage that identification is difficult.

Small foci of osseous metaplasia may be found in some fibromas, even in some of those not complicated by fracture. This is contrary to much of what is said in the literature, but this finding has led to the suggestion that fibroma and fibrous dysplasia are related processes.

95

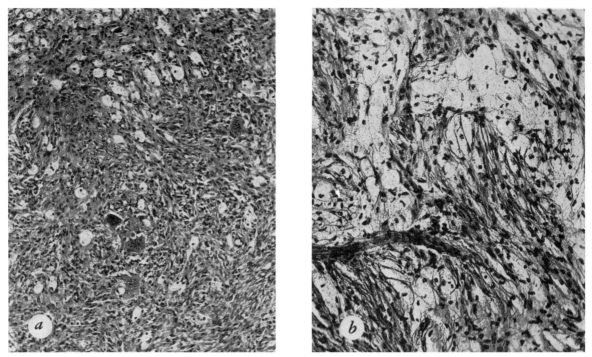

FIG. 10-10. *a.* Essential features of a fibroma, including fibroblastic connective tissue and benign giant cells. In addition, there are foam cells scattered throughout (×110). *b.* Prominent nests of foam cells in a fibroblastic stroma (×200).

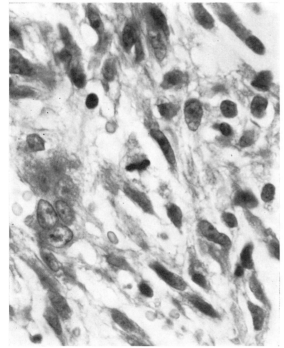

FIG. 10-11. Some fibromas, such as this one, exhibit worrisome cellular activity as evidenced by occasional mitotic figures (×800).

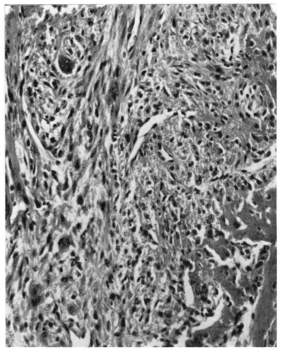

FIG. 10-12. Rarely, fibromas produce foci of osteoid, as at lower right, even without previous fracture (×210).

"Xanthoma" of Bone

In the total series of bone tumors were 27 that were composed predominantly of xanthic material in the form of masses of cholesterol and clusters of lipophages. These lesions often contained considerable hemosiderin. Fairly definite clinical and roentgenologic evidence indicated that a few of these were fibromas (fibrous defects) of bone, and portions of the histologic picture supported this concept. Four others were in the correct location and age group for giant cell tumor and were so categorized; zones within them supported this diagnosis microscopically. These four lesions suggest that giant cell tumor may sometimes become degenerative and quiescent. A few of these "xanthomas" were undoubtedly markedly degenerative and probably ancient lesions of fibrous dysplasia. Some were likely simple bone cysts altered by time and organization of hematomas within them. This group of "xanthomas" provided evidence to suggest that aneurysmal bone cyst may become senescent, lose its typical features, and contain nondescript, lipid-laden fibrous tissue. Lesions of hyperparathyroidism may show marked fatty degeneration. Several of these tumors had no features by which their fundamental nature could be surmised. Sometimes prior surgical or radiation therapy masked the basic pathology.

With recognition of the likelihood that "xanthoma" of bone is always a secondary phenomenon in some preexisting process, it is necessary to acknowledge that one may encounter such tumors. They are not related to the lipid-storage disorders such as Gaucher's disease nor are they part of the histocytosis X complex which includes eosinophilic granuloma, Schüller-Christian disease and Letterer-Siwe's syndrome.

These "xanthomas" are benign, and conservative surgical treatment has been effective for almost

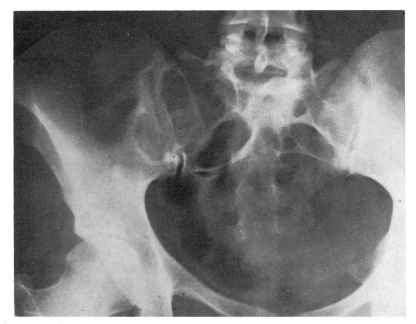

FIG. 10-13. "Xanthoma" producing well-circumscribed rarefaction in the right side of the sacrum and adjacent ilium. This occurred in a 23-year-old woman who had noted sciatica for 1 year. Her condition was markedly improved 5 years after curettage of the lesion. The pathology is illustrated in figures 10-14 and 10-15.

all of them. A very few resemble the so-called fibrous xanthomas or histiocytomas; even the malignant variant of this ill-defined neoplasm is suggested by an occasional tumor.

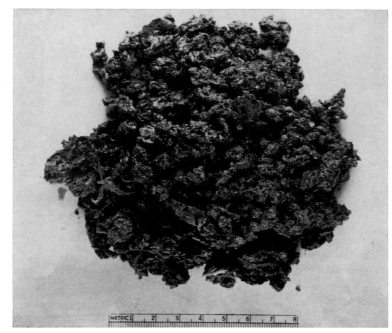

FIG. 10-14. Slightly fibrous hemorrhagic-appearing xanthic material curetted from the defect shown in Figure 10-13. This specimen is dark because it had been fixed prior to photography, but the volume is apparent.

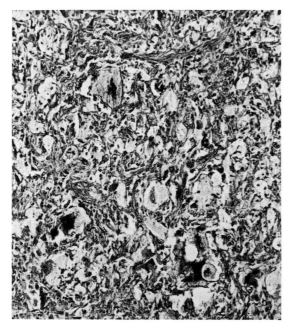

FIG. 10-15. The tissue shown in Figure 10-14 had this appearance throughout. Foam cells were interspersed with degenerating giant cells and some fibroblasts. The basic process in this "xanthoma" was not apparent (×125).

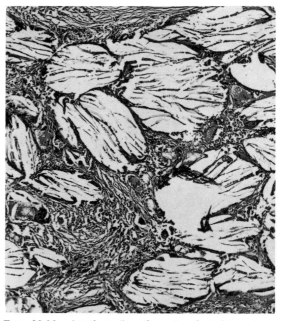

FIG. 10-16. Another "xanthoma" of indeterminate pathogenesis. This was a large lesion which showed cholesterol clefts throughout. Giant cells related to these clefts were prominent (×65).

Treatment

If one is confident of the roentgenologic diagnosis and the structural integrity of the bone is not in question, no treatment need be employed and the progress of the lesion can be followed by repeat roentgenograms. If the diagnosis is uncertain, one can accomplish diagnosis and therapy with one surgical procedure. This tumor is readily eradicated by conservative surgical means, curettage ordinarily being employed. Bone grafting of the defect may be desirable if the lesion is large. Radiation therapy is contraindicated for two reasons, namely the inherent sarcoma-producing potential of this form of therapy and the frequent proximity of the fibroma to a growing epiphyseal line.

Prognosis

As indicated, conservative surgical treatment, when necessary, is curative. Many lesions have been shown to undergo spontaneous regression. It has been observed that fracture through one of these lesions heals but the defect in the bone usually persists.

Bibliography

1942   Jaffe, H. L., and Lichtenstein, Louis: Non-osteogenic Fibroma of Bone. *Am. J. Path., 18:* 205-221.

1945   Hatcher, C. H.: The Pathogenesis of Localized Fibrous Lesions in the Metaphyses of Long Bones. *Ann. Surg., 122:*1016-1030.

1949   Ponseti, I. V., and Friedman, Barry: Evolution of Metaphyseal Fibrous Defects. *J. Bone & Joint Surg., 31A:*582-585.

1951   Kimmelstiel, P., and Rapp, I.: Cortical Defect Due to Periosteal Desmoids. *Bull. Hosp. Joint Dis., 12:*286-297.

1955   Caffey, J.: On Fibrous Defects in Cortical Walls of Growing Tubular Bones. *Advances Pediat., 7:*13-51.

1955   Devlin, J. A., Bowman, H. E., and Mitchell, C. L.: Non-osteogenic Fibroma of Bone: A Review of the Literature With the Addition of Six Cases. *J. Bone & Joint Surg., 37A:*472-486.

1956   Cunningham, J. B., and Ackerman, L. V.: Metaphyseal Fibrous Defects. *J. Bone & Joint Surg., 38A:*797-808.

1956   Maudsley, R. H., and Stansfeld, A. G.: Non-osteogenic Fibroma of Bone. (Fibrous Metaphysial Defect). *J. Bone & Joint Surg., 38B:*714-733.

1961   Kauffman, S. L., and Stout, A. P.: Histiocytic Tumors (Fibrous Xanthoma and Histiocytoma) in Children. *Cancer, 14:*469-482.

1961   Condon, V. R., and Allen, R. P.: Congenital Generalized Fibromatosis. Case Report, with Roentgen Manifestations. *Radiology, 76:*444-448.

1964   Morton, K. S.: Bone Production in Non-osteogenic Fibroma. An Attempt to Clarify Nomenclature in Fibrous Lesions of Bone. *J. Bone & Joint Surg., 46B:*233-243.

1964   Gordon, I. R. S.: Fibrous Lesions of Bone in Childhood. *Brit. J. Radiol., 37:*253-259.

1964   O'Brien, J. E., and Stout, A. P.: Malignant Fibrous Xanthomas. *Cancer, 17:*1445-1455.

Chapter 11

Vascular Tumors

Hᴇᴍᴀɴɢɪᴏᴍᴀꜱ ᴏꜰ ʙᴏɴᴇ play a minor role in a consideration of lesions requiring surgical procedures for diagnosis or therapy. The alterations commonly interpreted as hemangiomas of the vertebrae, by the roentgenologist are practically always asymptomatic and are probably zones of telangiectasis rather than true hemangiomas. Most bona fide hemangiomas in bone are solitary lesions. Hemangiomas may affect two or more bones of a single extremity, sometimes involving the overlying soft tissues as well, and sometimes producing serious malformation and dysfunction. Diffuse skeletal hemangiomatosis (Wallis and co-workers, 1964) is a rare disorder with the lesions most commonly seen in the spine, ribs, pelvis, skull, and shoulders. When such hemangiomatosis affects soft tissues as well as bones, the prognosis is poor; otherwise the osseous process tends to become stabilized with variable degrees of lytic and sclerotic change.

"Disappearing" or "phantom" bone disease, also called massive osteolysis and Gorham's disease, is now linked with the angiomas of bone. This relatively rare condition, which usually occurs in children or young adults, is characterized by the dissolution, in whole or in part, of one or several adjacent bones. The affected bones show a cavernous angiomatous permeation as the prominent pathologic feature. The process is self-limited but the extent of progression is unpredictable.

Hemangioendothelioma or hemangiosarcoma of bone encompasses a somewhat nebulous group of tumors which vary from debatably malignant capillary and cavernous proliferations to highly lethal endothelial sarcomas sometimes of multicentric origin.

Hemangiopericytoma, another rather poorly understood neoplasm with poorly defined histologic delineation, occurs as a very rare primary lesion of bone. Glomus tumor may erode bone or even arise within it.

Lymphatic vascular proliferations are also described as producing solitary or multiple zones of rarefaction of the skeleton.

The foregoing statements suggest the wide range of the clinical and pathologic spectrum of vascular proliferations in bone. A well-defined and lucid classification of these disorders is not available. Accordingly, portions of the brief discussion to follow will be in general terms.

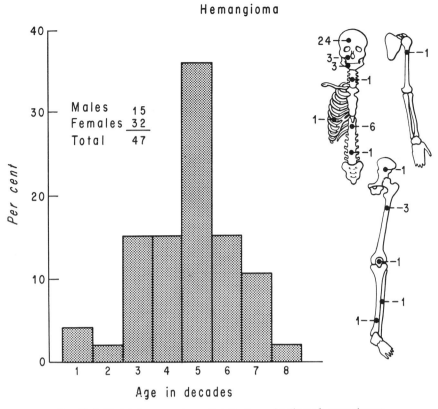

Fig. 11-1. Skeletal, age, and sex distribution of solitary hemangiomas.

Incidence

The 47 solitary hemangiomas in the present series comprised less than 1.2% of the total tumors. The total series also included one patient with multiple hemangiomas of bones of a lower extremity, six examples of massive osteolysis, seven hemangiosarcomas, and four hemangiopericytomas.

Sex

More than twice as many females as males had solitary hemangiomas.

Age

According to most reports, hemangiomas are usually found in adults. In this series, more than one third were found in the fifth decade of life.

Localization

Nearly 70% of these solitary hemangiomas were in the cranium or vertebrae. Six affected the jaws. Three of the hemangiosarcomas involved lumbar vertebrae, one the ischium, one the pubis, and two had multicentric skeletal foci. A vertebra, a rib, the ischium, and the sacrum provided the four hemangiopericytomas. Two of the six patients with massive osteolysis had the pelvic region affected, one a leg and part of the pelvis, one a leg, one the thoracic region, and one the forearm.

101

VASCULAR TUMORS

Symptoms

Many of the hemangiomas of the calvarium in this series were asymptomatic and discovered during roentgenographic study for other reasons. Those hemangiomas that produce expansion of bone and new bone formation may result in notable swelling. Local pain is sometimes a feature. There may be fractures, including compression fractures of vertebrae. Severe hemorrhage may be encountered during surgical procedures. Patients with massive osteolysis have pain and disability commensurate with the degree of osseous involvement. Malignant vascular tumors have the nonspecific pain and swelling common to all malignant processes in bone.

Physical Findings

Physical examination usually contributes no specific information. Occasionally soft-tissue or cutaneous hemangiomas provide evidence suggesting the nature of the osseous disease. It should be remembered, however, that such nonosseous hemangiomas are also part of the Maffucci syndrome which includes skeletal chondromatosis.

Roentgenologic Features

Hemangiomas in vertebrae characteristically cause rarefaction with exaggerated vertical striations or a coarse honeycombed appearance. In the skull, hemangiomas produce a well-circumscribed zone of rarefaction which may have a honeycombed appearance and is often associated with outward expansion of the bony profile. This expanded zone may show striations of bone radiating outward from the center of the lesion. In other bones, hemangiomas produce rarefactions that may have features like those described above. When hemangioma of soft tissues coexists it may contain phleboliths. The defects in diffuse skeletal hemangiomatosis often contain sclerotic foci. Massive osteolysis does not respect boundaries, and adjacent bones often disappear. A diagnostic sign is a tapering down of the bone at the edge of the zone of complete resorption. Hemangiosarcomas produce solitary or multiple destructive lytic areas.

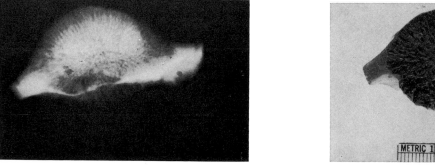

Fig. 11-2. *Left.* Roentgenogram of hemangioma excised from calvarium. Expansion inwardly as well as outwardly has occurred, and striations are prominent. *Right.* Specimen of same hemangioma, showing honeycombing and radiating spicules of bone.

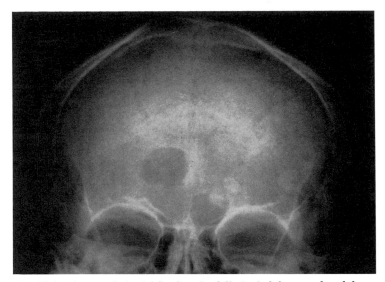

FIG. 11-3. Characteristic, fairly sharply delimited defect produced by a cavernous hemangioma of the skull. Although a sunburst appearance has been attributed to hemangiomas that have expanded bones, such an ominous appearance has been unusual in the experience of the Mayo Clinic.

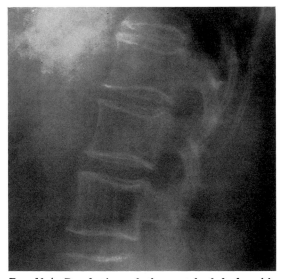

FIG. 11-4. Rarefaction of the vertebral body with exaggerated vertical striation, changes commonly attributed to hemangioma in this location. (Reproduced with permission from: Pugh, D. G.: *Roentgenologic Diagnosis of Diseases of Bones.* Baltimore, Williams & Wilkins, 1954, pp. 559AS-559AV.)

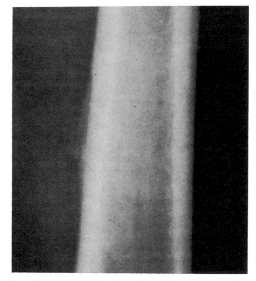

FIG. 11-5. Painful subperiosteal cavernous hemangioma near midshaft of femur. In this unusual location it has eroded the cortex slightly and caused some reactive new bone.

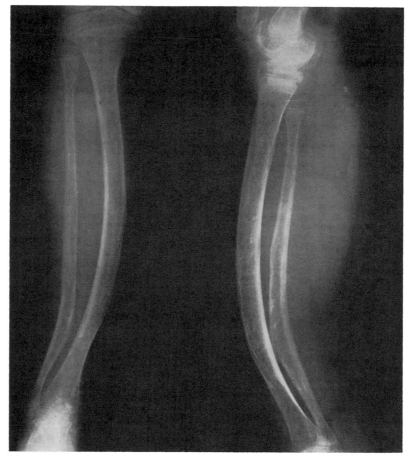

Fig. 11-6. Massive diffuse hemangioma of deep soft tissues of leg associated with multicentric cavernous hemangioma of tibia, fibula, and bones of foot in an 8-year-old girl. Amputation was necessary because of increasing disability and failure to control the tumor by other means.

Gross Pathology

On exposure a hemangioma is apt to be blue, and a honeycombed feature may be obvious. Cellular angiosarcomas and hemangiopericytomas are often gray to white, grossly simulating other sarcomas.

Histopathology

Interpretation of vascular lesions of bone is complicated by the fact that it is difficult to know when a conglomeration of vascular channels is in fact a hemangioma instead of a hamartomatous malformation. Assessing the literature is made all but impossible because of the large number of unconvincing photomicrographs. If the blood has escaped, hemangioma can simulate lymphangioma to further complicate the problem. In fact, hemangioma and lymphangioma may coexist as I have observed in examples of massive osteolysis. Most hemangiomas of bone are basically cavernous in type, although sometimes a capillary component is present and may even be dominant.

Some angiosarcomas of bone with their component of spindle-shaped vasoformative cells are readily recognizable as such, but the borderline between benign and malignant capillary proliferations is not always easily drawn. Highly cellular angiosarcomas may have few or no spaces to suggest their endothelial derivation. On the other hand, sarcomas of other basic types may possess a confusing vascular component.

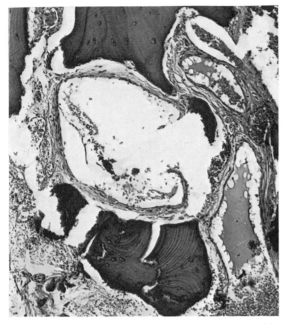

FIG. 11-7. Cavernous hemangioma of the skull. Thin-walled large blood vessels are interspersed among the osseous trabeculae (×95). This is the same case as that represented in Figure 11-3.

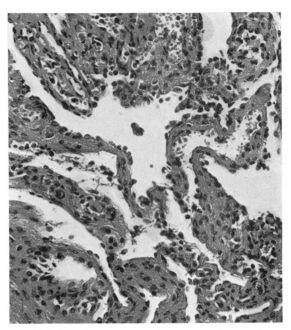

FIG. 11-8. Mixed capillary and cavernous hemangioma that had expanded the ascending ramus of the mandible. This lesion was originally classed erroneously as hemangiopericytoma (×200).

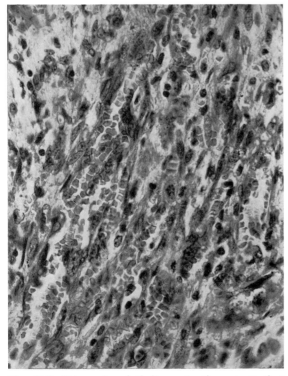

FIG. 11-9. Hemangioendothelioma (angiosarcoma) that had caused destruction of the second lumbar vertebra of a 38-year-old man (×360).

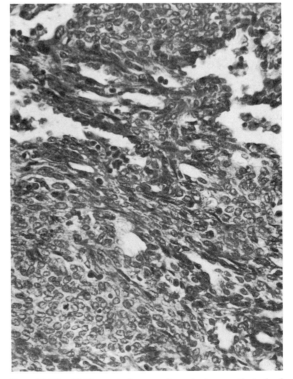

FIG. 11-10. Malignant hemangiopericytoma that had produced a destructive, slightly expansile defect in the ischium (×300).

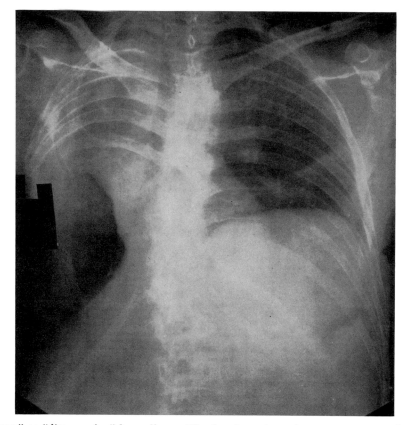

FIG. 11-11. "Phantom" or "disappearing" bone disease. The female patient whose roentgenogram is shown above had difficulties that began with pathologic fracture of a rib 5 years before this picture was taken. Eight years after onset, having lost all or part of most of her right ribs and the ninth, tenth, and eleventh thoracic vertebrae, she succumbed to the effects of this destruction of her thoracic cage.

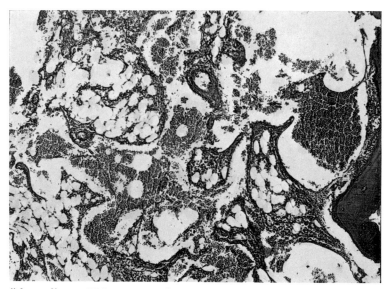

FIG. 11-12. "Phantom" bone disease. This cavernous hemangioma pattern was found in one of the ribs procured for biopsy in the case illustrated above in Figure 11-11. This histologic appearance is characteristic of that found routinely in massive osteolysis or "phantom" bone disease ($\times 65$).

Fig. 11-13. *Right.* Angiosarcoma with malignant destruction of fibula of 8-year-old boy. The other bones about the knee and foot were considered unremarkable.

Fig. 11-14. *Below.* Amputated specimen with destruction of fibula (near scale) but also showing multicentric foci of angiosarcoma in femur, tibia, and bones of foot. Malignant tissue had permeated the bone in all of the dark zones. The patient died of the sarcoma within 6 months.

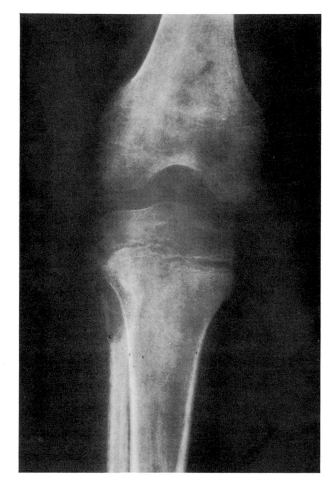

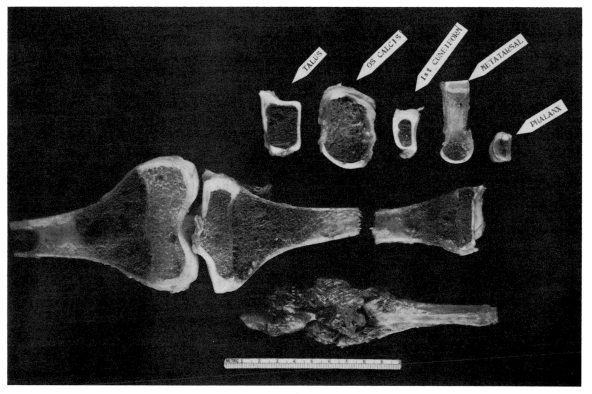

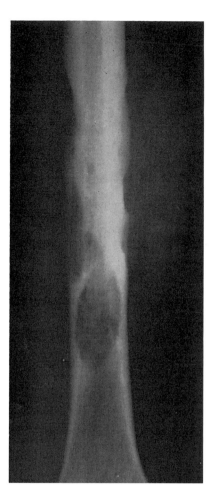

FIG. 11-15. *Left*. Hemangiosarcoma of large portion of femoral shaft, showing multiple zones of central and cortical destruction with tumor extending into adjacent soft tissue.

FIG. 11-16. *Below, left*. Microscopic appearance of part of tumor illustrated in Figure 11-15. Here the angiosarcoma is reasonably well differentiated, with plump, malignant endothelial cells producing spaces, some of which contain blood (×200).

FIG. 11-17. *Below, right*. In other regions the angiosarcoma of Figure 11-15 is highly anaplastic, as shown here. Transitions from the well-differentiated zones were observed. The anaplastic portions taken out of context may have been misinterpreted as some other sarcoma (×300). (Case contributed by Dr. Manuel Sarmina, Findlay, Ohio, who stated that the patient was well 27 months after disarticulation at the hip.)

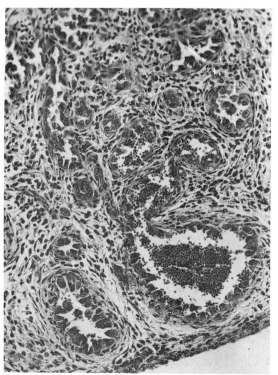

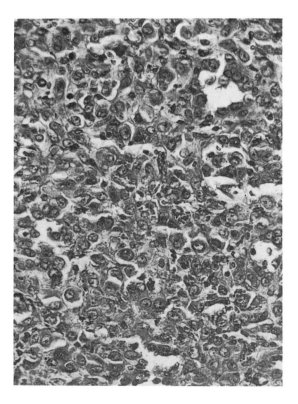

Treatment

Hemangiomas usually respond well to conservative surgical procedures. Radiation may be required for those in inaccessible sites. The unpredictable course of massive osteolysis has made the results of treatment difficult to assess, but reconstructive surgical procedures and radiation have been employed. The consensus favors surgical excision or ablation for malignant vascular tumors in accessible sites and radiation for the remainder. The reader is referred to pertinent references listed below for additional information.

Bibliography

1942   Thomas, Atha: Vascular Tumors of Bone: A Pathological and Clinical Study of Twenty-seven Cases. *Surg., Gynec. & Obst., 74*:777-795.

1954   Pugh, D. G.: *Roentgenologic Diagnosis of Diseases of Bones.* Baltimore, Williams & Wilkins, pp. 559AS-559AV.

1955   Gorham, L. W., and Stout, A. P.: Massive Osteolysis (Acute Spontaneous Absorption of Bone, Phantom Bone, Disappearing Bone): Its Relation to Hemangiomatosis. *J. Bone & Joint Surg., 37A*:985-1004.

1955   Cohen, J., and Craig, J. M.: Multiple Lymphangiectases of Bone. *J. Bone & Joint Surg., 37A*:585-596.

1957   Kleinsasser, O., and Albrecht, H.: Die Hämangiome und Osteohämangiome der Schädelknochen. *Langenbecks Arch. Deutsch Z. Chir., 285*:115-133.

1958   Jaffe, H. L.: *Tumors and Tumorous Conditions of the Bones and Joints.* Philadelphia, Lea & Febiger, pp. 224, 341.

1961   Sherman, R. S., and Wilner, D.: The Roentgen Diagnosis of Hemangioma of Bone. *Am. J. Roentgenol., 86*:1146-1159.

1961   Krueger, E. G., Sobel, G. L., and Weinstein, C.: Vertebral Hemangioma with Compression of Spinal Cord. *J. Neurosurg., 18*:331-338.

1962   Goidanich, I. F., and Campanacci, M.: Vascular Hamartomata and Infantile Angioectatic Osteohyperplasia of the Extremities. *J. Bone & Joint Surg., 44A*:815-842.

1962   Spjut, H. J., and Lindbom, A.: Skeletal Angiomatosis. Report of Two Cases. *Acta path. et microbiol. scandinav., 55*:49-58.

1962   Mackenzie, D. H.: Intraosseous Glomus Tumours. Report of Two Cases. *J. Bone & Joint Surg., 44B*:648-651.

1962   Hartmann, W. H., and Stewart, F. W.: Hemangioendothelioma of Bone. Unusual Tumor Characterized by Indolent Course. *Cancer, 15*:846-854.

1964   Halliday, D. R., Dahlin, D. C., Pugh, D. G., and Young, H. H.: Massive Osteoloysis and Angiomatosis. *Radiology, 82*:637-644.

1964   Lund, B. A., and Dahlin, D. C.: Hemangiomas of the Mandible and Maxilla. *J. Oral Surg., 22*:234-242.

1964   Wallis, L. A., Asch, T., and Maisel, B. W.: Diffuse Skeletal Hemangiomatosis. Report of Two Cases and Review of Literature. *Am. J. Med., 37*:545-563.

1965   Bundens, Jr., W. D., and Brighton, C. T.: Malignant Hemangioendothelioma of Bone. Report of Two Cases and Review of the Literature. *J. Bone & Joint Surg., 47A*:762-772.

Chapter 12

Lipoma and Liposarcoma

Dᴇsᴘɪᴛᴇ ᴛʜᴇ ᴀʙᴜɴᴅᴀɴᴄᴇ of adipose connective tissue in bone marrow, lipomas of bone are extremely rare. Child in 1955 described one involving the os calcis and found only three intraosseous lipomas reported in the literature. A few additional cases have been reported since. Lipomas of soft tissues adjacent to bone, sometimes even apparently arising in or under the periosteum, may cause erosion of bone but such is rare. Discrete, small collections of adipose connective tissue that might possibly be considered neoplastic are sometimes seen in vertebrae.

Liposarcoma of bone can occur, as evidenced by the case described by Dawson in 1955. She found that several of the eight cases she collected from the literature were difficult to accept. Goldman in 1964 described a case and accepted only three of those reported after Dawson's as being adequately documented. No unequivocal liposarcoma of bone was found in the present series. In one case there was extensive malignant destruction of a humerus by liposarcoma but the patient had a large retroperitoneal mass which may have been the primary site. Liposarcomas of soft-tissue origin sometimes produce skeletal metastasis that may mimic primary sarcoma of bone.

Tumors containing the large, sometimes vacuolated, pleomorphic cells that make one think of liposarcoma have been included among the osteogenic sarcomas in the Mayo Clinic series. This was done because foci of similar pleomorphic cells occur in many tumors that are obviously osteogenic sarcomas.

Lipoblastic tumors, apparently of a hamartomatous nature, can diffusely involve soft tissues and bone of an extremity as described by Kauffman and Stout (1959).

Only four lipomas were found in this total series of bone tumors, making the incidence 1 per 1,000 cases. Two produced radiolucent zones each 1.5 cm in maximal diameter in a parietal and a frontal bone respectively. The third lesion may have represented merely a localized focus of osteoporosis. It had produced a poorly defined 4 by 3 cm region of rarefaction visible in the roentgenogram of the upper part of the shaft of a femur. The fourth, illustrated in Figures 12-1 and 12-2, was located beneath the periosteum of the ulna. The patients' ages ranged from 31 to 69 years. Three were men. Three of the lipomas were incidental findings but the ulnar example had produced a mass.

110

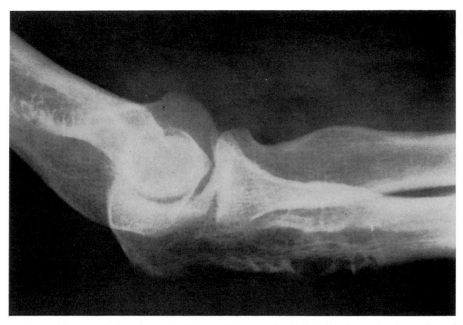

Fig. 12-1. Lipoma of the ulna of a 44-year-old man who had had a lump in the region of involvement for 30 years. He had no complaints referable to the lesion. The roentgenologist interpreted the process as probably neoplastic and suggested the possibility of its being malignant. (Reproduced with permission from: Caruolo, J. E., and Dahlin, D. C.: *Proc. Staff Meet., Mayo Clin., 28*:361-363, 1953.)

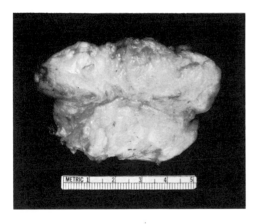

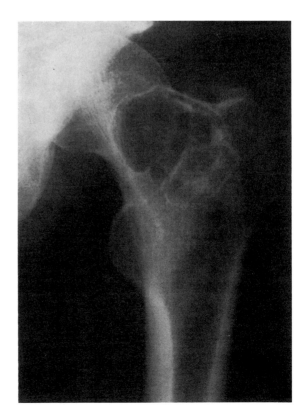

Fig. 12-2. *Above.* Lipoma excised from the region of involvement shown in Figure 12-1. The tumor was found beneath the periosteum and it had produced irregular, partially loculated erosion of the cortex.

Fig. 12-3. *Right.* Lipoma of neck and trochanteric region of femur. Note sclerotic discrete borders. This occurred in a 62-year-old man who had had pain in the hip for 5 months. The patient was well 4 years after curettage and bone grafting. (Contributed by Dr. J. A. Holbert, Coos Bay, Oregon.)

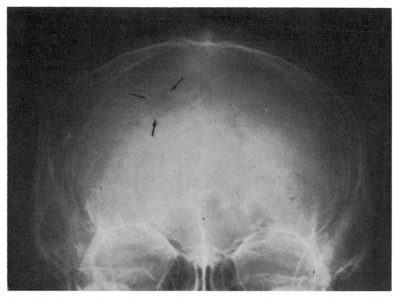

FIG. 12-4. Lipoma involving the left frontal bone of a 31-year-old man. This lesion, which measured 1.5 by 1.5 by 0.4 cm when excised, was apparently an incidental finding on a roentgenogram taken because of the patient's complaint of headache of 2 years' duration.

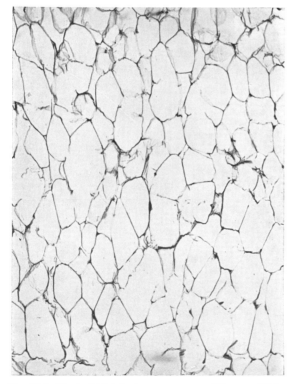

FIG. 12-5. Typical histologic appearance of lipoma. This picture is representative of the tissue seen in the cases depicted in Figures 12-1, 2, 3, and 4 (×120).

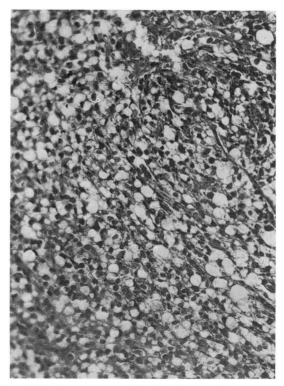

FIG. 12-6. Liposarcoma which had destroyed the upper half of the right humerus of a 38-year-old woman. She also had an abdominal mass which may have been the primary site. The vacuolated cells took a strongly positive stain for fat (×200).

Treatment

Treatment of the rare lipoma one may encounter in bone should be conservative. The necessity for surgical intervention is ordinarily dictated by failure to make a correct preoperative diagnosis.

The available evidence indicates that prompt ablative surgical treatment is the one of choice for liposarcoma. There are too few reported cases to provide statistics on prognosis.

Bibliography

1953   Fairbank, H. A. T.: A Parosteal Lipoma. *J. Bone & Joint Surg., 35B:*589.

1953   Caruolo, J. E., and Dahlin, D. C.: Lipoma Involving Bone and Simulating Malignant Bone Tumor: Report of Case. *Proc. Staff Meet., Mayo Clin., 28:*361-363.

1955   Child, P. L.: Lipoma of the Os Calcis: Report of a Case. *Am. J. Clin. Path., 25:*1050-1052.

1955   Dawson, Edith K.: Liposarcoma of Bone. *J. Path & Bact., 70:*513-520.

1956   Mastragostino, S.: Tumori lipoblastici primitivi dello Scheletro. *Chir. org. movimento, 44:*18-36.

1957   Mastromarino, R., and Assennato, G.: Lipoma intraosseo. *Ortop. e traumatol., 25:*1077-1084.

1957   Newman, C. W.: Fibrolipoma of the Mandible. Report of Case. *J. Oral Surg., 15:*251-252.

1957   Smith, W. E., and Fienberg, R.: Intraosseous Lipoma of Bone. *Cancer, 10:*1151-1152.

1957   Skinner, B. G., and Fraser, R. G.: Medullary Lipoma of Bone. *J. Canad. A. Radiol., 8:*19-21.

1959   Kauffman, S. L., and Stout, A. P.: Lipoblastic Tumors of Children. *Cancer, 12:*912-925.

1961   Retz, L. D.: Primary Liposarcoma of Bone. Report of a Case and Review of the Literature. *J. Bone & Joint Surg., 43A:*123-129.

1962   Fleming, R. J., Alpert, M., and Garcia, A.: Parosteal Lipoma. *Am. J. Roentgenol., 87:*1075-1084.

1962   Ackerman, L. V., and Spjut, H. J.: *Tumors of Bone and Cartilage.* Atlas of Tumor Pathology, Section II, Fascicle 4, Armed Forces Institute of Pathology, Washington, D.C., National Research Council, pp. 163-164.

1963   Catto, M., and Stevens, J.: Liposarcoma of Bone. *J. Path. & Bact., 86:*248-253.

1964   Moon, N., and Marmor, L.: Parosteal Lipoma of the Proximal Part of the Radius. A Clinical Entity with Frequent Radial-Nerve Injury. *J. Bone & Joint Surg., 46A:*608-614.

1964   Goldman, R. L.: Primary Liposarcoma of Bone. Report of a Case. *Am. J. Clin. Path., 42:*503-508.

Chapter 13

Neurilemmoma and Related Tumors

Nᴇᴜʀᴏɢᴇɴɪᴄ ᴛᴜᴍᴏʀs of bone are rare. Fifteen cases of neurilemmoma arising in bone were collected from the literature and their own material by Samter and co-workers in 1960. These neurilemmomas characteristically produce a discretely outlined zone of rarefaction which may have a sclerotic border. Pain or swelling may be present. The tumor is apt to be yellow or brown owing to lipid and hemosiderin in it, and cystic degeneration may be present. The microscopic appearance is like that of its exceedingly more numerous counterpart in soft tissues; palisading of the spindle-shaped nuclei is the most obvious diagnostic clue. Marked nuclear polymorphism may result apparently from degenerative changes in this benign tumor. Secondary bony changes due to erosion by a neurilemmoma of soft-tissue origin, especially along the spinal column or in the cranium, are sometimes seen.

Neurofibromatosis has been found to be associated with a variety of skeletal changes which occurred in approximately half of a large group of cases studied at the Mayo Clinic by Hunt and Pugh in 1961. These changes included erosive defects in bone caused by contiguous neurogenic tumors, disorders of bone growth associated with hypertrophy of overlying soft tissues, dysplasia of vertebral bodies with scoliosis, defects of the posterior orbital wall, congenital bowing, and pseudarthrosis. Intraosseous neurofibromas are distinctly rare. Some of the osseous defects described in patients with Recklinghausen's disease have been coincidental, unrelated processes.

Malignant tumors of neurogenic origin (malignant schwannomas) have rarely been described as arising in bone, and the evidence in reported cases is not altogether convincing. The inherent characteristics of a malignant growth make it difficult to verify the exact tissue of origin in a questionable case. Gross relationship to a nerve is important in establishing the neurogenic origin of a sarcoma. In any event the problem is academic since the treatment for such a sarcoma would be the same as for fibrosarcoma of bone.

Seven benign neurogenic tumors of bone were encountered in the present series of nearly 4,000 tumors. All arose within the osseous substance and produced well-defined cystlike rarefactions roentgenographically. Four were in the mandible, one at the glenoid in the scapula, one in a rib, and one in the distal portion of the shaft of the femur. The seven patients ranged from 19 to 64 years but only three were more than 25 years of age. Four of the patients were women. The femoral tumor, although only 8 mm in diameter, had produced pain for 5 years. Two others had caused notable pain and the mandibular tumors gave local swelling. All responded satisfactorily to conservative surgical therapy. One of the mandibular tumors is perhaps best classed as a neurofibroma; it occurred in a patient with Recklinghausen's disease. The remainder are distinctly neurilemmomas.

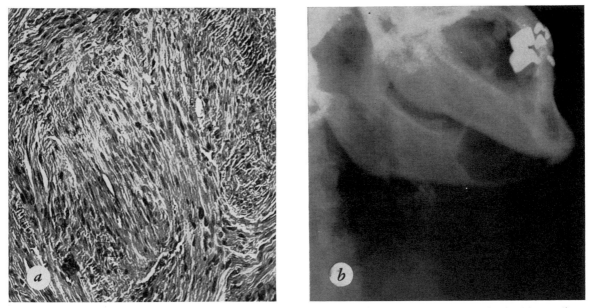

FIG. 13-1. Neurilemmoma of the mandible. *a.* Tissue section ($\times$180). *b.* An expanding lesion is evident. This neurilemmona was found in a 64-year-old woman and the clinical history suggested that it had been present for 20 years.

Bibliography

1934　Peers, J. H.: Primary Intramedullary Neurogenic Sarcoma of the Ulna. Report of a Case. *Am. J. Path., 10:*811-819.

1939　Gross, P., Bailey, F. R., and Jacox, H. W.: Primary Intramedullary Neurofibroma of the Humerus. *Arch. Path., 28:*716-718.

1940　De Santo, D. A., and Burgess, E.: Primary and Secondary Neurilemmoma of Bone. *Surg., Gynec. & Obst., 71:*454-461.

1943　Green, W. T., and Rudo, Nathan: Pseudarthrosis and Neurofibromatosis. *Arch. Surg., 46:*639-651.

1950　McCarroll, H. R.: Clinical Manifestations of Congenital Neurofibromatosis. *J. Bone & Joint Surg., 32A:*601-617.

1952　Güthert, H.: Ein malignes Neurinom des Knochens. *Zentralbl. allg. Path., 88:*185-188.

1953　Jones, H. M.: Neurilemmoma of Bone. *Brit. J. Surg., 41:*63-65.

1953　Adams J. P., and Golden, J. L.: Fibrous Lesions of Bone. *South. M. J., 46:*529-536.

1957　Wilber, M. C., and Woodcock, J. A.: Ganglioneuromata in Bone. *J. Bone & Joint Surg., 39A:*1385-1388.

1958　Jaffe, H. L.: *Tumors and Tumorous Conditions of the Bones & Joints.* Philadelphia, Lea & Febiger, pp. 240-255.

1960　Samter, T. G., Vellios, F., and Shafer, W. G.: Neurilemmoma of Bone. Report of 3 Cases with a Review of the Literature. *Radiology, 75:*215-222.

1961　Hunt, J. C., and Pugh, D. G.: Skeletal Lesions in Neurofibromatosis. *Radiology, 76:*1-20.

1962　Ackerman, L. V., and Spjut, H. J.: *Tumors of Bone and Cartilage.* Atlas of Tumor Pathology, Section II, Fascicle 4, Armed Forces Institute of Pathology, Washington, D.C., National Research Council, pp. 247-249.

1963　Divertie, M. B., and Dahlin, D. C.: Neurilemmoma of Rib. Report of a Case. *Dis. Chest, 44:*635-637.

Chapter 14

Myeloma

T HIS TUMOR of hematopoietic derivation is the most common neoplasm of bone in the present series. Furthermore its relative incidence is increasing; nearly 55% of the 1,323 new patients with malignant bone tumors seen and verified pathologically at the Mayo Clinic in the 9 years from 1956 through 1964 had myeloma. This neoplasm is composed of plasma cells showing variable degrees of differentiation. The neoplastic process is usually multicentric and often involves bone marrow so diffusely that it may be diagnosed in the great majority of cases by marrow aspiration.

Most patients with myeloma have predominant hematologic problems, and their therapy is managed by hematologists or by cancer chemotherapists and radiotherapists. The discussion in this chapter is oriented toward the problems as encountered in surgical material. The complex hematologic and protein disturbances will not be elaborated, but some of the pertinent literature is indicated in the bibliography.

Extraskeletal infiltrates of myeloma cells in a wide variety of tissues may occur in patients with multiple myeloma, but they are rarely a prominent feature. Solitary extramedullary myeloma (plasmacytoma), nearly 80% of which tumors occur in the upper air passages and oral cavity, is curable in the majority of cases by local therapy, which has included electrocoagulation or excision, irradiation, or combinations of these. A minority of patients with these extramedullary plasma cell tumors develop multiple myeloma.

Renal involvement with manifestations of renal insufficiency is an important complication of myeloma that may be the immediate cause of death. Not myelomatous infiltration but blockage of the tubules by proteinaceous casts is the histologic finding. Much less important is the occasional development of renal amyloidosis, "metastatic" calcification of the kidneys in those with severe skeletal demineralization, or pyelonephritis.

"Solitary" Myeloma

Occasionally one sees a single osseous focus of myeloma which is associated with normal sternal marrow and with few or none of the abnormal laboratory findings so characteristic of multiple myeloma. Patients with such lesions usually develop multiple myeloma, but sometimes only after a latent period of 5 to 10 years or even longer. Some become long term "cures." "Solitary" myeloma in bone must be distinguished from a focus of chronic osteomyelitis with abundant plasma cells. The distinction is aided by the proliferation of fibroblasts and capillaries as part of the response to inflammation and the sprinkling of polymorphonuclear leukocytes and histiocytes in the latter condition.

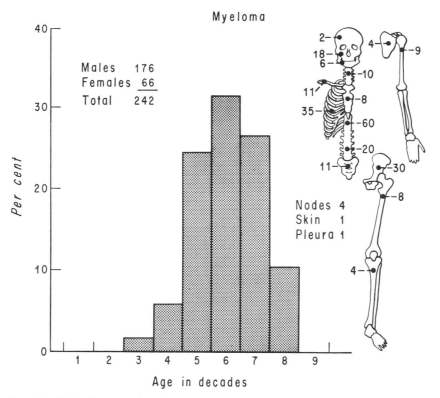

Fig. 14-1. Skeletal, age, and sex distribution of 242 surgical cases (1,044 cases diagnosed by marrow aspiration not included).

Incidence

The total of 1,286 myelomas of bone comprised 43% of the malignant bone tumors in this series. The major reasons for operation in the surgical series included the presence of an indeterminate osseous lesion or compression of the spinal cord.

Sex

Nearly 73% of the 242 surgical patients were men.

Age

The graph above accents the well-known rarity of myeloma before the fifth decade of life.

Localization

The bones that contain hematopoietic marrow in adults harbor most of the recognizable myeloma nodules. Although the data tabulated above are selected, since they are based on surgical cases only, the distribution shown is similar to that observed at necropsy except that the skull is usually involved by the time myeloma has caused the patient's death. The group of "solitary" myelomas had a skeletal distribution much like that depicted above, but the 25 vertebral examples indicate a predilection for this area.

MYELOMA

Symptoms

Pain of an increasing nature is the most common complaint of patients with myeloma, and it is most often centered in the lumbar or thoracic spinal regions. On the average, the pain is of less than 6 months' duration prior to the time the patient is admitted, but sometimes it has been present for several years. Weakness and loss of weight occur during the course of the disease in nearly every case of myeloma. Pathologic fracture, with abrupt onset of symptoms, is common and the majority of such fractures involve the vertebral column. Neurologic symptoms, usually from involvement of the spinal cord or nerve roots secondary to pathologic fracture or extraosseus extension of the neoplastic tissue, are frequently observed. Complaints referable to renal involvement may be encountered. Less common symptoms include palpable tumor, hemorrhagic tendency, anemia and fever.

Physical and Laboratory Findings

Physical findings may reflect secondary changes resulting from generalized malignant disease with replacement of bone marrow. Local pain or tenderness, with or without palpable tumor, and neurologic dysfunction may be elicited.

Smears of peripheral blood often show excessive rouleau formation and have been reported as containing myeloma cells in from 10 to 73% of cases. Rarely, plasma cell leukemia develops. Moderate to severe anemia is the rule. Erythrocyte sedimentation rate is notoriously rapid. Hypercalcemia occurs in from 20 to 50% of patients. With perseverance, Bence Jones proteinuria can be found in over half the cases. Evidences of renal insufficiency or amyloidosis, which may be generalized, sometimes develop. Levels of serum alkaline phosphatase are rarely elevated.

Electrophoretic studies of serum and urinary proteins provide critical diagnostic information because of elevation of various globulin fractions. Kyle and co-workers found the electrophoretic patterns diagnostic of "myeloma proteins" in nearly 75% of 165 patients with myeloma. A majority of those with nondiagnostic serum electrophoretic patterns had diagnostic changes in the urinary proteins. Only 15 of 6,051 serum patterns in nonmyeloma patients showed changes typical of myeloma and the majority of these had either macroglobulinemia or amyloidosis. The complexities of these protein studies have been elaborated by Osserman and Takatsuki (1963).

Roentgenologic Features

These features result from replacement of osseous structures by the myelomatous masses. The first and most extensive changes usually occur in the ribs, vertebrae, skull, and pelvis. Classically there are "punched-out" areas of bone destruction which vary up to 5 cm in diameter and about which there is no surrounding zone of sclerosis. Expansion of the affected bone may produce a "ballooned-out" appearance, especially in the ribs. A variable degree of osteoporosis is common, and pathologic fracture, especially of vertebrae, is often seen. From 12 to 25% of patients with myeloma are reported to have no discernible foci of bone destruction. Some of these, on close scrutiny, will be found to have diffuse demineralization of portions of the skeleton. Metastatic carcinoma, reticulum cell sarcoma, and hyperparathyroidism can produce bone lesions that simulate

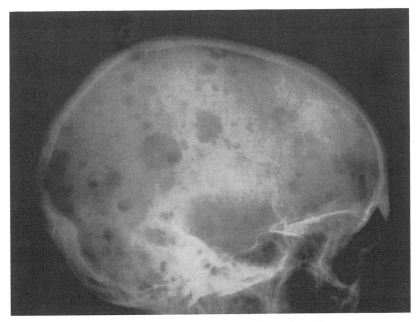

FIG. 14-2. Myeloma in one of the most commonly affected sites. There are numerous discrete foci of osseous destruction.

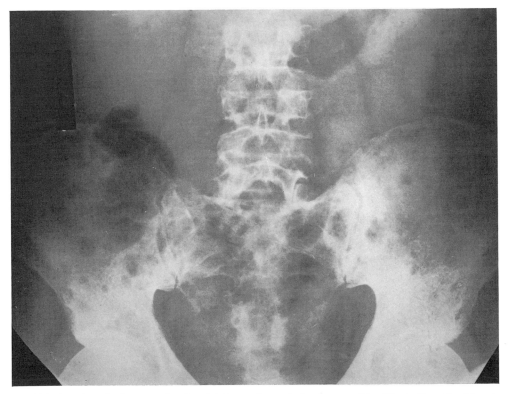

FIG. 14-3. Another classic example of multiple myeloma. As in the preceding illustration, the discrete foci of rarefaction are not associated with sclerosis of bone. (Reproduced with permission from: Pugh, D. G.: *Roentgenologic Diagnosis of Diseases of bones.* Baltimore, Williams & Wilkins, 1954. pp. 487-492.)

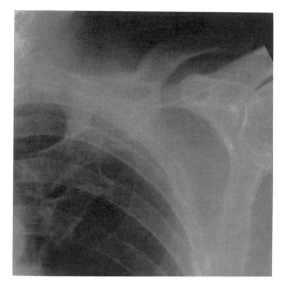

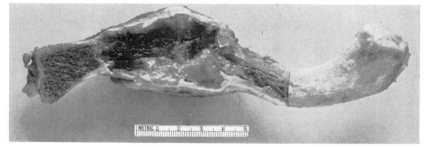

FIG. 14-4. *Left*. Expansile lesion of the clavicle. This proved to be myeloma of the "solitary" type. A fracture, apparently pathologic, occurred through this region in September 1950, and again in January 1953. The clavicle was excised in April 1953. When last heard from 11 years later the patient was alive and well. *Below*. Excised specimen from the case illustrated on the left.

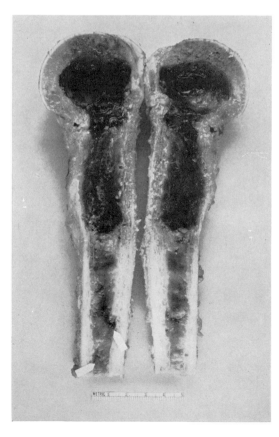

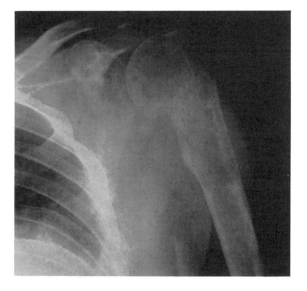

FIG. 14-5. *Above*. Destruction of humerus produced by "solitary" myeloma. Forequarter amputation was performed on Nov. 11, 1953. Sixteen months later, signs of dissemination were present. An erroneous diagnosis of reticulum cell sarcoma was made at the time of amputation. *Left*. Gross specimen in the same case. This lesion dramatically demonstrated the occasional difficult problem of differentiating myeloma from reticulum cell sarcoma. See also Figure 14-8.

those of myeloma. "Solitary" myeloma lesions of bone are classically destructive but they too may produce expansion of the bone's contour. Only one patient in this series had sclerosing lesions.

Gross-Pathology

The myelomatous masses are classically soft, gray, and friable, resembling the tissue of a malignant lymphoma. As with other invasive tumors, more marrow will be seen to be involved than is indicated by the roentgenologic changes. Expansion of the affected bone and, even more commonly, extraosseous extension of the tumor contribute to damage to adjacent structures. Extraosseous lesions are sometimes grossly discernible in other portions of the hematopoietic system, notably in the lymph nodes and spleen. Nodes containing myeloma were removed from eight patients in this surgical series. As indicated, pathologic fracture may be present and often results in damage to the spinal cord. In very rare instances enough amyloid is formed by the tumor to be grossly obvious. An unusual combination of sclerosis and lysis involved almost an entire femur in this series; amputation was performed for plasma cell myeloma which complicated chronic osteomyelitis of 40 years' duration.

Histopathology

Typically, one sees sheets of closely packed cells with little intercellular substance. These cells have abundant cytoplasm which tends to be granular and basophilic. The cell outlines are distinct and the nucleus is characteristically round or oval and eccentric. Two or even three nuclei are sometimes observed. When one studies a series of cases of myeloma, gradations are found to exist, these apparently reflecting the maturity or degree of differentiation of the cells. At one extreme are tumors with cells closely resembling the plasma cells seen in inflammatory conditions; these show prominent clumping of chromatin, sometimes producing the "wheel-spoke" appearance. With decreasing differentiation, nucleoli become large and clumping of chromatin is less marked. Cytoplasmic vacuoles increase in prominence and the cell boundary becomes indistinct. Finally the nuclei may have grooves and lobules, and at the other extreme is a tumor that may be indistinguishable from reticulum cell sarcoma. In fact, some myelomas have foci that are quite like reticulum cell sarcoma and some even contain multinucleated cells of such size that the diagnosis of Hodgkin's sarcoma may be considered. The occasional shading together of these tumors should not be surprising since all three very likely are basically of reticuloendothelial derivation.

Mitotic figures are rare in the average myeloma. The similarity of the cells comprising the solid sheets in this tumor contrasts with the multiplicity of cell types in the occasional chronic inflammatory focus that superficially resembles myeloma. The inflammatory pseudoneoplasm often contains a prominent capillary network that aids in differentiation.

Amyloidosis is related to the altered proteins as evidenced by its occurrence in approximately 10% of patients with myeloma. Its distribution with generalized deposition simulates that of primary systemic amyloidosis, a diagnosis which depends on the exclusion of myeloma as well as the more obvious causes of amyloidosis. Amyloid deposits are sometimes found within the myelomatous proliferations and may be so abundant as to mask the neoplasm.

Bayrd's article in 1948 describes the cytologic details of myeloma cells as seen in marrow smears.

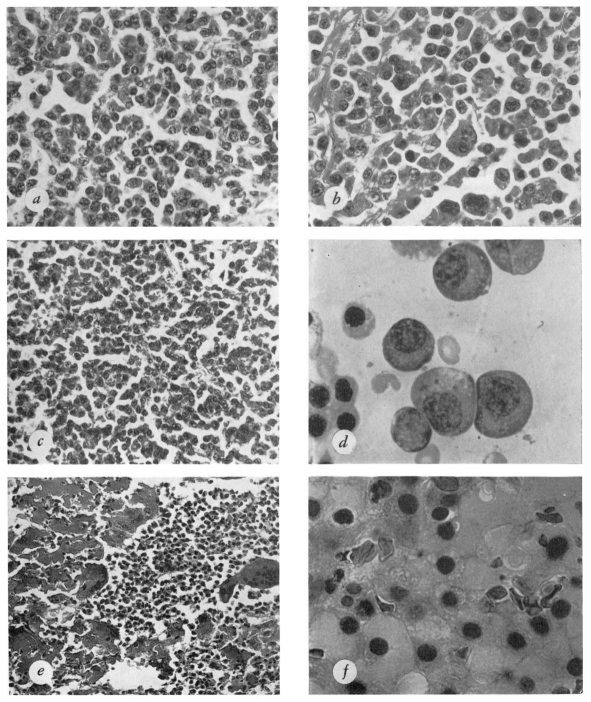

FIG. 14-6. *a*. Relatively well-differentiated myeloma with characteristic eccentric nuclei and abundant cytoplasm (×380). *b*. Highly malignant myeloma at the same magnification as in *a*. Note the large nuclei and the multinucleated giant cells (×380). *c*. Same tumor as that illustrated in *a* (×265). *d*. Wright-stained smear of sternal marrow containing typical myeloma cells (×850). *e*. Amyloid masses in a myeloma nodule. Note benign giant cell reaction commonly seen around amyloid masses (×175). *f*. Myeloma cells that contain amyloid or a precursor. This is an extremely rare finding (×800). (Figure 14-6*e* reproduced with permission from: Dahlin, D. C., and Dockerty, M. B.: *Am. J. Path.*, 26:581-593, 1950.)

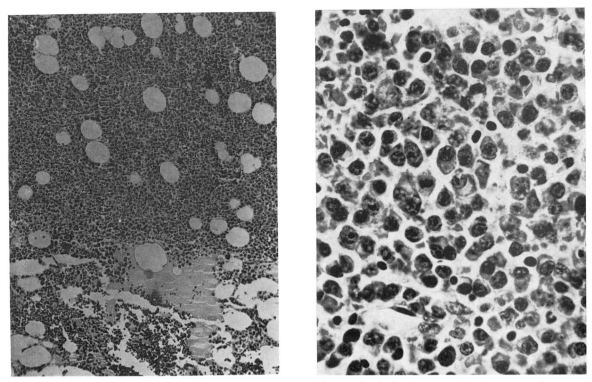

FIG. 14-7. *Left.* Myeloma nodule in section of bone marrow. It has replaced the hematopoietic elements and most of the fat (×100). *Right.* Higher magnification showing characteristic well-defined cytoplasm of myeloma cells and nuclear anaplasia as manifested by large nucleoli (×700).

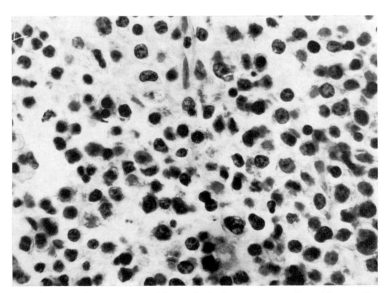

FIG. 14-8. Anaplastic tumor with cytologic features suggesting either malignant lymphoma or myeloma. In rare instances an absolute distinction cannot be made on a single specimen of tissue (×525).

MYELOMA

Treatment

The mode of treatment in myeloma varies, depending upon whether the disease is "solitary" or disseminated.

For localized myeloma irradiation is the treatment of choice. Excision (total if possible) or at least diagnostic biopsy should precede irradiation. Aspiration biopsy has been used successfully in a number of Mayo Clinic patients with vertebral involvement. In the patients with severe neurologic symptoms, decompression of the spinal cord may be necessary prior to irradition. Therapy must be directed at preservation of the spinal cord since many patients with a "solitary" lesion may live several years before dissemination occurs. Amputation may have to be considered for patients with a solitary lesion of myeloma in an extremity.

Chemotherapy has now proved of value in the management of patients with multiple myeloma. Cytoxan (cyclophosphamide) and Alkeran (l-phenylalanine mustard) are the currently most effective agents (Bayrd, 1966). They have been able to effect subjective and objective improvement. It may be desirable to use irradiation in conjunction with chemotherapy if focal myelomatous proliferations produce a significant problem in a patient with multiple myeloma. General supportive measures are necessary.

Prognosis

Inanition, anemia, involvement of the spinal cord, and renal failure are the major factors contributing to the death of patients with disseminated myeloma, and the average patient succumbs within 2 years after diagnosis. The Study Committee of the Midwest Cooperative Chemotherapy Group (1964) found that 10% of patients with multiple myeloma survived 56 months. In the present series of surgical cases in which the disease was not in a solitary focus at the time of diagnosis, somewhat more than 10% have survived at least 5 years. Accurate prediction of survival time in a given case is not possible.

Occasional patients die from the effects of a complicating systemic amyloidosis.

"Solitary" myeloma, as many authors have stressed, is the forerunner of disseminated myelomatosis. The current series reemphasizes that such dissemination may be long delayed and perhaps is not inevitable. Of 34 patients with "solitary" skeletal myelomas treated before 1960, 18 were alive 5 years later. Seven of these died at intervals varying from 5 to 20 years after diagnosis, and 11 were living at intervals that varied from 7 to 24 years. This series attests to the value of local therapy for this disease. Cohen and co-workers (1964) have elaborated some facets of the problem in a study of vertebral myelomas not as strictly localized as the "solitary" lesions in the current study. They found that the degree of cellular anaplasia did not affect the patient's chance of prolonged survival and that elevated serum globulin levels and Bence Jones proteinuria were not necessarily associated with short survival.

Bibliography

1948 Lumb, G., and Prossor, T. M.: Plasma Cell Tumours. *J. Bone & Joint Surg., 30B*:124-152.

1948 Bayrd, E. D.: The Bone Marrow on Sternal Aspiration in Multiple Myeloma. *Blood, 3*:987-1018.

1950 Dahlin, D. C., and Dockerty, M. B.: Amyloid and Myeloma. *Am. J. Path., 26*:581-593.

1950 Churg, Jacob, and Gordon, A. J. Multiple Myeloma: Lesions of the Extra-osseous Hematopoietic System. *Am. J. Clin. Path., 20*:934-945.

1953 Svien, H. J., Price, R. D., and Bayrd, E. D.: Neurosurgical Treatment of Compression of the Spinal Cord Caused by Myeloma. *J.A.M.A., 153*:784-786.

1953 Bruce, K. W., and Royer, R. Q.: Multiple Myeloma Occurring in the Jaws. A Study of 17 Cases. *Oral Surg., 6*:729-744.

1954 Pugh, D. G.: *Roentgenologic Diagnosis of Diseases of Bones*. Baltimore, Williams & Wilkins, pp. 487-492.

1955 Carson, C. P., Ackerman, L. V., and Maltby, J. D.: Plasma Cell Myeloma: A Clinical, Pathologic and Roentgenologic Review of 90 Cases. *Am. J. Clin. Path., 25*:849-888.

1959 Glenchur, Harry, Zinneman, H. H., and Hall, W. H.: A Review of Fifty One Cases of Multiple Myeloma: Emphasis on Pneumonia and other Infections as Complications. *A.M.A. Arch. Int. Med., 103*:173-183.

1960 Engels, E. P., Smith, R. C., and Krantz, Simon: Bone Sclerosis in Multiple Myeloma. *Radiology, 75*:242-247.

1960 Kyle, R. A., Bayrd, E. D., McKenzie, B. R., and Heck, F. J.: Diagnostic Criteria for Electrophoretic Patterns of Serum and Urinary Proteins in Multiple Myeloma. *J.A.M.A., 174*:245-251.

1960 Feinleib, M., and MacMahon, B.: Duration of Survival in Multiple Myeloma. *J. Nat. Cancer Inst., 24*:1259-1269.

1962 Silverman, L. M., and Shklar, Gerald: Multiple Myeloma: Report of a Case. *Oral Surg., 15*:301-309.

1962 Webb, H. E., Harrison, E. G., Masson, J. K., and ReMine, W. H.: Solitary Extramedullary Myeloma (Plasmacytoma) of the Upper Part of the Respiratory Tract and Oropharynx. *Cancer, 15*:1142-1155.

1963 Osserman, E. F., and Takatsuki, K.: Plasma Cell Myeloma: Gamma Globulin Synthesis and Structure. A Review of Biochemical and Clinical Data, With the Description of a Newly-Recognized and Related Syndrome, "H-Gamma-2-Chain (Franklin's) Disease." *Medicine, 42*:357-384.

1964 Study Committee of the Midwest Cooperative Chemotherapy Group: Multiple Myeloma. General Aspects of Diagnosis, Course, and Survival. *J.A.M.A., 188*:741-745.

1964 Cohen, D. M., Svien, H. J., and Dahlin, D. C.: Long-Term Survival of Patients With Myeloma of the Vertebral Column. *J.A.M.A., 187*:914-917.

1965 Herskovic, T., Andersen, H. A., and Bayrd, E. D.: Intrathoracic Plasmacytomas. Presentation of 21 Cases and Review of Literature. *Dis. Chest, 47*:1-7.

1965 Council on Drugs: An Alkylating Agent for Multiple Myeloma. Melphalan (Alkeran). *J.A.M.A., 191*:547-549.

1966 Bayrd, E. D.: Personal Communication to the Author.

Chapter 15

Malignant Lymphoma of Bone
(Reticulum Cell Sarcoma)

Prior to the classic article by Parker and Jackson in 1939, reticulum cell sarcomas of bone were generally "lumped" with Ewing's tumors. The remarkably better prognosis as well as clinical implications makes it important to recognize this special tumor. The discussion in this chapter is oriented to the problems of lymphoma of the skeleton as encountered by the surgical pathologist, the surgeon, and the therapist. Detailed considerations of lymphoma in general and leukemia are purposely avoided.

Although the term "reticulum cell sarcoma" is commonly employed for the tumor under discussion, it is a misnomer since relatively few pertinent tumors are composed solely of this type of cell. A mixture of reticulum cells, lymphoblasts, and lymphocytes is so common in these neoplasms that it is a diagnostic aid. Furthermore, lymphocytic and Hodgkin's lymphomas can produce primary lesions in bone. For these reasons, the term "malignant lymphoma" better categorizes the entire group. These tumors are morphologically identical to their soft-tissue counterparts.

When malignant lymphoma is responsible for an osseous lesion, one of three clinical conditions may be found. First, careful study of the patient may reveal no evidence of disease elsewhere, and the osseous lesion can be presumed to be primary. Of the 195 cases in this series, 101 fell into this category. This "primary" variety affords the best opportunity for successful therapy. Second, similar disease may be found in other osseous or in soft-tissue sites and one must assume that the bony lesion in question may be a region of secondary involvement. Sixty-six cases of the series were in this category. Third, a patient with known lymphomatous disease elsewhere may have tissue removed from a metastatic osseous focus for one reason or another. Although such obviously secondary skeletal involvement is commonly seen at autopsy, especially in reticulum cell sarcoma and Hodgkin's disease, only 28 examples were encountered in this surgical series.

Focal infiltrates in leukemia may mimic the histologic appearance of malignant lymphoma. Osseous manifestations are apt to be prominent in acute leukemias, especially in childhood. In nearly 10% of patients with acute leukemia the clinical course is dominated by symptoms referable to the bones and joints. The lower extremity is most commonly affected. Juxtaepiphyseal rarefactions, focal or extensive osteolytic zones, periosteal elevation with new bone deposition, and generalized rarefaction are among the roentgenographic findings.

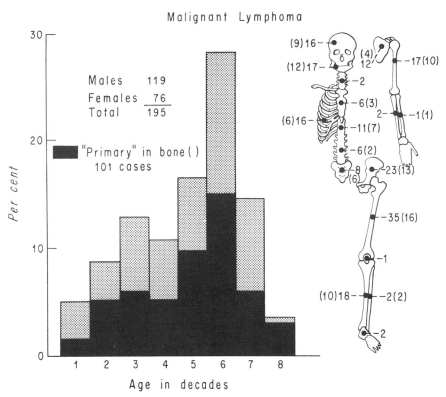

FIG. 15-1. Skeletal, age, and sex distribution of malignant lymphoma of bone. Those "primary" in bone are indicated in parenthesis.

Incidence

Malignant lymphoma comprised 6.6% of the malignant group in this series. The 101 that were "primary" in bone comprised only 3.4%.

Sex

Males predominated in a ratio of approximately 3:2 in the "primary" and in the total group. This is in general agreement with the literature.

Age

This neoplasm can occur at any age but is rare in the very young. The age distribution for those presumably primary in bone parallels that of the overall group.

Localization

When a malignant lymphoma arises in certain specific sites such as the antrum or along the spinal column, it is often impossible to prove an osseous origin. Some 40 patients with involvement of the antrum and one or more of its bony walls are excluded from the above data because an origin from bone could not be verified. Likewise, the majority of surgical patients with lymphoma affecting the spinal cord or its emerging nerves are excluded because proof of osseous disease was not available. The distribution of the "primary" cases was similar to that of the entire group.

MALIGNANT LYMPHOMA

Symptoms

Pain, swelling, and subsequent disability are the cardinal features of any malignant tumor of bone, including lymphoma. Pain of variable intensity is practically a constant feature, and occasionally it has been present for several years, although ordinarily its duration is measured in months. Neurologic symptoms commonly occur when these tumors affect the spinal column. Many have emphasized that patients with even extensive solitary malignant lymphomas have a surprising sense of well-being and absence of general complaints so commonly associated with malignant disease. Pathologic fracture may occur. One patient in this series developed malignant lymphoma in a focus of old chronic osteomyelitis of the tibia.

Physical Findings

A mass in the region of the tumor, which may be tender or warm, is the main finding, and this is often associated with disability of the affected part. Enlarged regional lymph nodes may be found. One should search for signs of disseminated malignant lymphoma, such as involvement of multiple bones, distant lymph nodes, and other soft-tissue structures. Because of the occasional similarity of tumefactions due to malignant lymphomas and those due to leukemia, it is important to study the peripheral blood of these patients.

Roentgenologic Features

Roentgenologically, the lesions frequently appear to be very extensive, often involving 25 to 50% of the affected bone and in some cases involving the entire shaft. Bone destruction is the predominant feature of primary reticulum cell sarcoma. The areas of destruction give the bone a mottled and patchy appearance in many cases, and sometimes its outline is entirely lost. The diseased bone blends imperceptibly with the adjacent normal bone. Approximately half the patients in this series have shown evidence of some reactive proliferation of new bone that is not laid down by the tumor cells themselves. Nearly every malignant lymphoma produces destruction of cortical bone, and approximately 25% are associated with some thickening of the cortex. There is often obvious soft-tissue extension of the tumors and sometimes there is calcification in the soft-tissue mass. In approximately one fourth of the cases there is evidence of pathologic fracture.

Irregular sclerosis of the affected site is sometimes a marked feature and adds to the confusion of reticulum cell sarcoma with chronic osteomyelitis that sometimes occurs. Disseminated malignant lymphomatous involvement of the skeleton may simulate osteoblastic metastatic carcinomatosis.

Wilson and Pugh, who studied the Mayo Clinic series, concluded that the roentgenograms varied so much that their appearance could not be regarded as characteristic. Although the radiologist can frequently suspect the diagnosis of reticulum cell sarcoma, other lesions including osteogenic sarcoma, Ewing's tumor, eosinophilic granuloma, and chronic osteomyelitis cannot always be excluded with certainty.

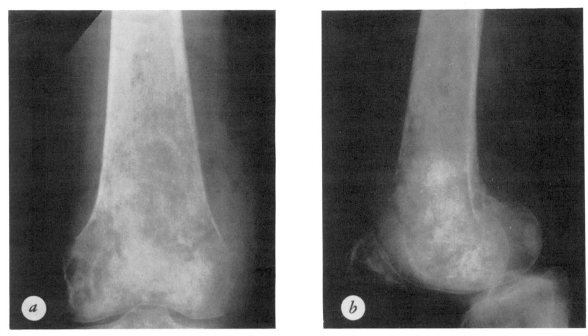

FIG. 15-2. Anteroposterior (a) and lateral (b) views of primary malignant lymphoma destroying lower portion of femur. There is blotchy sclerosis in area of destruction. (Figure 15-2a reproduced with permission from: Ivins, J. C., and Dahlin, D. C.: *J. Bone & Joint Surg.*, *35A*:835-842, 1953.)

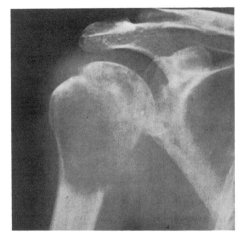

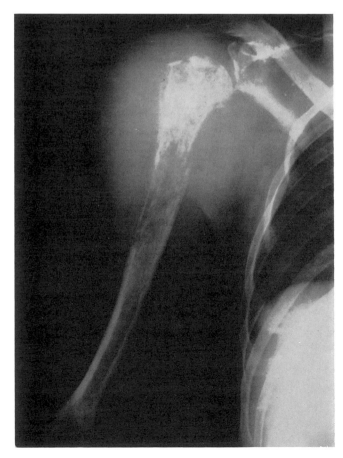

FIG. 15-3. *Above.* Hodgkin's lymphoma primary in upper end of humerus. Note markedly lytic destruction. *Right.* Typical destruction produced by primary lymphoma. This one is of mixed type, is extensive, has disrupted the cortex, has resulted in zones of sclerosis, and has a large soft-tissue component.

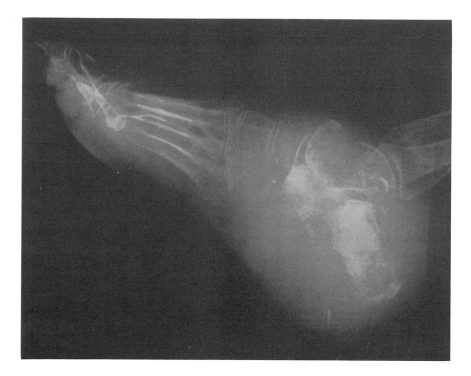

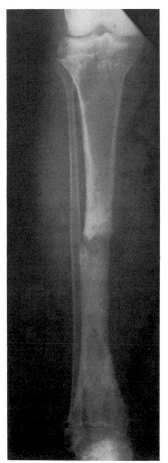

FIG. 15-4. *Above.* Reticulum cell sarcoma producing marked destruction of the tarsal bones of a 65-year-old woman. Inguinal nodes were enlarged and biopsy material from one of these presented the characteristic pattern of malignant lymphoma of the reticulum cell type.

FIG. 15-5. *Left.* This tumor of the right tibia developed at the site of recurrent osteomyelitis of 20 years' duration. Specimens from the tibia, the associated soft-tissue mass, and a right inguinal node all showed the rare complication, reticulum cell sarcoma. The patient died with generalized lymphoma 14 months later.

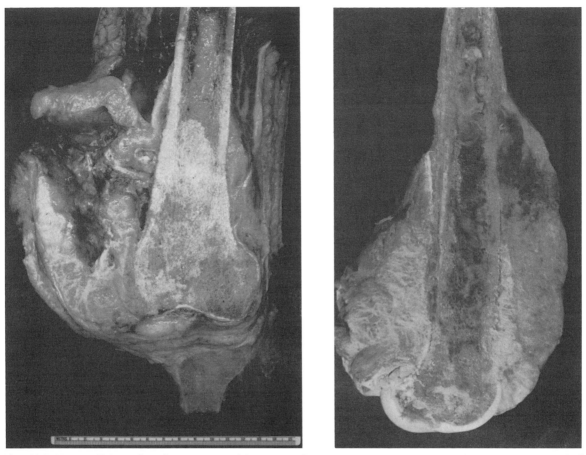

FIG. 15-6. Two maliginant lymphomas removed by amputation. *Left.* This nearly "pure" reticulum cell sarcoma had been considered an "inflammatory" lesion at the time of previous biopsy. At the time of amputation it had grown through the skin. Despite postoperative radiation therapy to the groin and pelvis, the patient died in 2 years. *Right.* This malignant lymphoma of mixed cell type, also involving the lower portion of a femur, was treated the same way and the patient survived 27 years. (Reproduced with permission from: McCormack, L. J., Ivins, J. C., Dahlin, D. C., and Johnson, E. W., J.: *Cancer* 5:1182-1192, 1952.)

Gross Pathology

The gross features of primary malignant lymphoma of bone are not pathognomonic, but some of them warrant mention. Although any portion, and frequently a large part, of a long bone may be involved, the main mass of the tumor and its extraosseous extension, if present, are most often in or near the metaphyseal region. A variable amount of soft-tissue extension is practically always present by the time diagnosis is made. The bone itself at the affected site is destroyed to a variable extent, and not infrequently one sees white areas of necrosis or zones of secondary sclerosis. Residual osseous trabeculae are frequently admixed with tumor, imparting a firm and gritty consistency. When a reticulum cell sarcoma extends into the soft tissues, it produces a soft mass that is friable and simulates the appearance of malignant lymphomas arising in soft tissues. The margins of a malignant lymphoma in the bone as well as in the adjacent soft tissues are ordinarily indistinct. Regional lymph nodes may be involved and, as indicated above, there may be any of the gross pathologic evidences of disseminated malignant lymphoma.

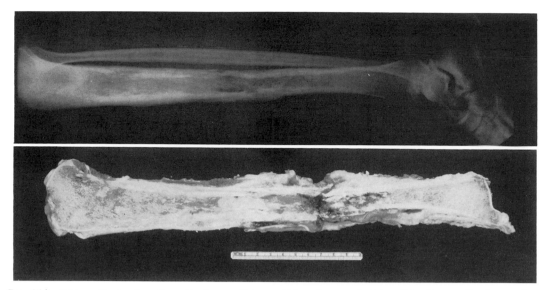

Fig. 15-7. *Upper*. Predominantly reticulum cell type of lymphoma of right tibia. *Lower*. Specimen after amputation. Although practically the entire length of the bone is involved, there is very little extension into the soft tissue. Three years later the left tibia was similarly affected, as shown in Figure 15-15.

Histopathology

The basic proliferating cell in tumors of this type is the reticulum cell. It characteristically has a grooved or folded nucleus, one or more distinct nucleoli, and indistinct, irregular cytoplasmic boundaries. Cytoplasmic processes may extend outward from the cell bodies. Reticulum cells overshadow all others in some of these tumors, but the great majority contain variable numbers of lymphoblasts and lymphocytes, and sometimes these cells dominate the histologic picture. On rare occasions one encounters a pure lymphocytic malignant lymphoma that is apparently primary in bone. Occasional highly malignant reticulum cell sarcomas of bone contain multinucleated cells of the Reed-Sternberg type, and these tumors quite logically fall into the category of Hodgkin's sarcoma. Even the granulomatous form of Hodgkin's disease can present as a primary tumor of bone. In no less than 12 of the 195 cases in this series the tissue contained Reed-Sternberg cells, and in 7 of these the tumor was apparently primary in bone.

Since the cells of the average malignant lymphoma lie in a reticular framework, there is a tendency for an alveolar grouping, a feature which is often prominent even under low magnification. This helps differentiate reticulum cell sarcoma from Ewing's tumor in which large masses of cells are associated with no fibrillar intercellular material. Special stains for reticulum accentuate the network in which the cells lie. In my experience, however, this stain has been of little value for diagnosis because those tumors that appear atypical when stained with ordinary dyes contain an equivocal amount of stainable reticulum. There is no discernible difference between malignant lymphoma that begins in bone and malignant lymphoma that begins elsewhere in the body.

The large numbers of lymphocytic cells present in some of these tumors may lead to the diagnosis of an inflammatory process, an error especially likely to occur if one has only a small amount of material for biopsy or if the tumor is infected as it is apt to be in malignant lymphoma of the jaws.

It must be admitted that certain anaplastic small cell tumors lie in a gray zone between lymphoma and Ewing's sarcoma. A practical plan is to make the diagnosis of Ewing's sarcoma if the cells are so anaplastic that they cannot be categorized in the reticulum cell-lymphocyte series with certainty. The histiocytes of histiocytosis X may be difficult to differentiate from reticulum cell sarcoma, especially if cytologic features are distorted by decalcification, but in the average case the cells of histiocytosis X are obviously benign.

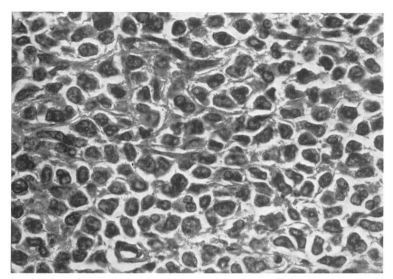

Fig. 15-8. Classic reticulum cell sarcoma with cells showing grooved and indented nuclei, indistinct cytoplasmic borders, and a reticular framework that is easily seen even with this hematoxylin and eosin stain (×650).

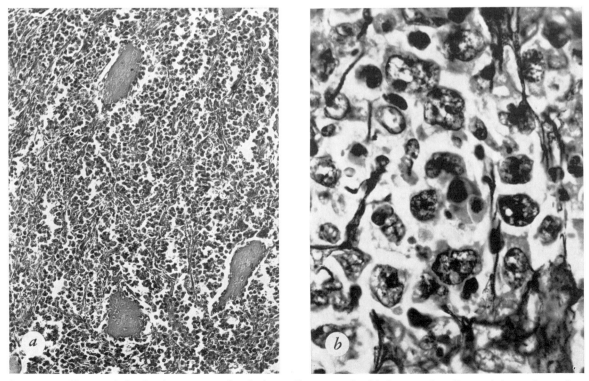

Fig. 15-9. a. Characteristic alveolar pattern of reticulum cell sarcoma, in this instance invading and destroying trabeculae of normal bone (×125). b. Higher magnification to show nuclear detail and strands of reticulin (reticulin stain; ×800). (Reproduced with permission from: Ivins, J. C., and Dahlin, D. C.: J. Bone & Joint Surg., 35A:835-842, 1953.)

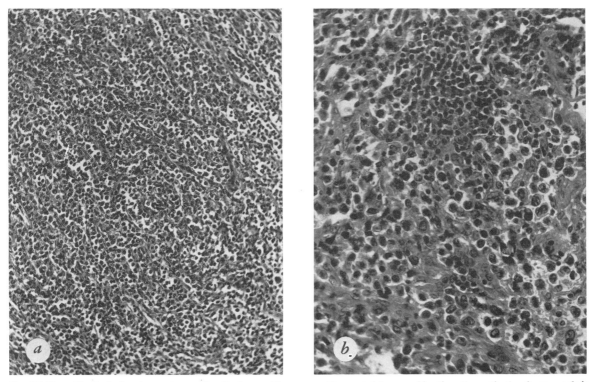

Fig. 15-10. *a.* Typical alveolar pattern of reticulum cell sarcoma. Even at this magnification the reticular framework is visible (×115). *b.* In this field are seen lymphoblasts and lymphocytes, cells commonly found in malignant lymphomas primary in bone (×300).

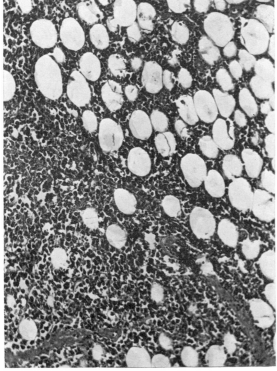

Fig. 15-11. Reticulum cell sarcoma with invasion into the adjacent fat, a feature that accounts for the poorly defined border ordinarily seen on gross inspection of one of these lesions (×150). (Reproduced with permission from: McCormack, L. J., Ivins, J. C., Dahlin, D. C., and Johnson, E. W., Jr.: *Cancer, 5*:1182-1192, 1952.)

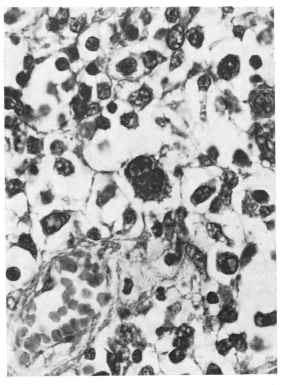

Fig. 15-12. Hodgkin's type of malignant lymphoma manifesting itself first as a destructive tumor of the sternum with invasion of structures behind and in front of the manubrium. Note centrally located Reed-Sternberg cell (×700).

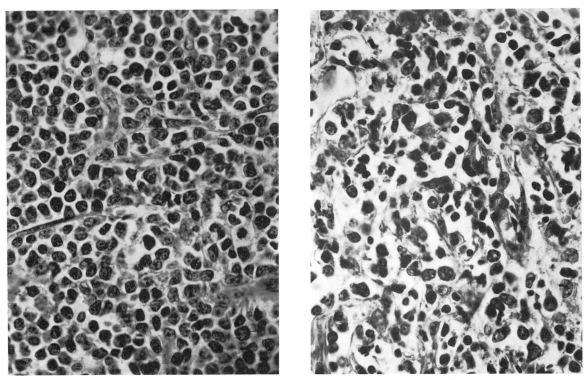

FIG. 15-13. *Left.* Lymphoblastic differentiation is prominent in this lymphoma (×600). *Right.* Lymphoma showing alveolar grouping and variation in size and shape of cells (×425).

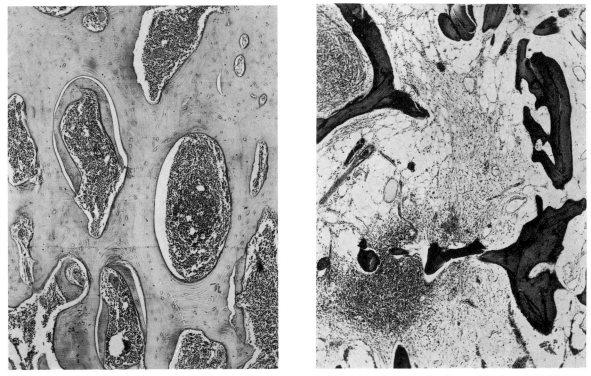

FIG. 15-14. Sclerotic reaction to lymphoma manifested by layers of new bone on preexisting trabeculae. *Left.* Tumor permeating skull (×80). *Right.* Sclerosing reaction at and even beyond the peripheray of a lymphoma of the ilium (×60).

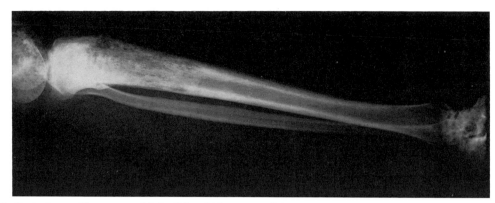

Fig. 15-15. Reticulum cell sarcoma of left tibia which appeared 3 years after amputation for the same type of tumor of the right tibia. See Figure 15-7. This case illustrates the unpredictability of these tumors.

Treatment

The accumulated experience with primary malignant lymphomas that are apparently solitary in bone does not yet allow one to be dogmatic regarding the treatment of choice. The consensus now favors irradiation for control of the primary lesion. Sometimes amputation becomes necessary because curative irradiation results in local necrosis that is disabling or because it fails to halt the growth of the primary tumor. These facts have made some feel that primary abaltive surgical procedures should be used, especially for tumors below the midfemur level. It is clear that the regional lymph nodes require attention, and radiation therapy is likely most efficacious for these. Irradiation is certainly indicated for those tumors not amenable to surgical removal. Chemotherapy with alkylating and other agents provides temporary subjective and objective relief for many patients with disseminated lymphoma; focal lesions in such patients may require radiation therapy.

Prognosis

Most reports indicate that reticulum cell sarcoma has the best prognosis of any of the primary malignant tumors of bone. Five-year survival rates of 40 to 50% and even higher have been reported. In the present series, slightly more than one third of the patients with primary lymphoma have survived 5 years. Many of these, unfortunately, succumb later. No rule applies in an individual case because of the well-known vagaries of the malignant lymphomas. Patients with one lesion adequately treated may have, in a period of months or many years, a tumor in another bone, in a distant lymph node, or in other soft tissue, or they subsequently may even have a leukemic blood picture, as developed in at least four patients in the present series.

The prognosis for the group with pure reticulum cell sarcoma was not unlike that for the much larger group with cytologically mixed lesions. The small groups with Hodgkin's and lymphocytic types appear to have a poorer outlook.

The majority of the small group of patients with mandibular tumors in the present series have become long-term survivors. The locally invasive and basically inoperable lymphomas of the maxillary region, not included in this series, can be cured in a gratifying percentage of cases by appropriate radiation therapy (Steg and co-workers, 1959).

Bibliography

1934 Craver, L. F., and Copeland, M. M.: Lymphosarcoma in Bone. *Arch. Surg., 28*:809-824.

1939 Parker, Frederic, Jr., and Jackson, Henry, Jr.: Primary Reticulum Cell Sarcoma of Bone. *Surg., Gynec. & Obst., 68*:45-53.

1942 Gall, E. A., and Mallory, T. B.: Malignant Lymphoma. A Clinico-Pathologic Survey of 618 Cases. *Am. J. Path., 18*:381-429.

1947 Sherman, R. S., and Snyder, R. E.: Roentgen Appearance of Primary Reticulum Cell Sarcoma of Bone. *Am. J. Roentgenol., 58*:291-306.

1947 Jackson, H., and Parker, F., Jr.: *Hodgkin's Disease and Allied Disorders.* New York, Oxford Univ. Press, pp. 1-177.

1949 Geschichkter, C. F., and Copeland, M. M.: *Tumors of Bone.* Philadelphia, J. B. Lippincott, pp. 537-579.

1950 Coley, B. L., Higinbotham, N. L., and Groesbeck, H. P.: Primary Reticulum-cell Sarcoma of Bone: Summary of 37 Cases. *Radiology, 55*:641-658.

1952 McCormack, L. J., Ivins, J. C., Dahlin, D. C., and Johnson, E. W., Jr.: Primary Reticulum-cell Sarcoma of Bone. *Cancer, 5*:1182-1192.

1952 Valls, J., Muscolo, D., and Schajowicz, F.: Reticulum-Cell Sarcoma of Bone. *J. Bone & Joint Surg., 34B*:588-598.

1954 Francis, K. C., Higinbotham, N. L., and Coley, B. L.: Primary Reticulum Cell Sarcoma of Bone; Report of 44 cases. *Surg. Gynec., & Obst., 99*:143-146.

1955 Bethge, J. F. J.: Die Ewingtumoren oder Omoblastome des Knochens. Differentialdiagnostische und kritische Erörterungen. *Ergebn. Chir. Orthop., 39*:327-425.

1955 Wilson, T. W., and Pugh, D. G.: Primary Reticulum-cell Sarcoma of Bone, With Emphasis on Roentgen Aspects. *Radiology, 65*:343-351.

1956 Medill, E. V.: Primary Reticulum-Cell Sarcoma of bone. *J. Fac. Radiologists, 8*:102-117.

1956 Magnus, H. A., and Wood, H. L.-C.: Primary Reticulo-Sarcoma of Bone. *J. Bone & Joint Surg., 38B*:258-278.

1958 Ullrich, D. P., and Bucy, P. C.: Primary Reticulum Cell Sarcoma of the Skull. *Am. J. Roentgenol., 79*:653-657.

1959 Steg, R. F., Dahlin, D. C., and Gores, R. J.: Malignant Lymphoma of the Mandible and Maxillary Region. *Oral Surg., 12*:128-141.

1961 Thomas, L. B., Forkner, C. E., Jr., Frei, E., III, Besse, B. E., Jr., and Stabenau, J. R.: The Skeletal Lesions of Acute Leukemia. *Cancer, 14*:608-621.

1973 Ivins, J. C., and Dahlin, D. C.: Malignant Lymphoma (Reticulum Cell Sarcoma) of Bone. *Proc. Staff Meet., Mayo Clin., 38*:375-385.

1963 Silverstein, M. N., and Kelly, P. J.: Leukemia with Osteoarticular Symptoms and Signs. *Ann. Int. Med., 59*:637-645.

Chapter 16

Chondrosarcoma (Primary, Secondary, and Mesenchymal)

CHONDROSARCOMA should be separated from osteogenic sarcoma because of basic pathologic differences which are reflected in vastly differing clinical, therapeutic, and prognostic features. The exact origin of chondrosarcomas is obscure but the salient pathologic fact is that their basic proliferating tissue is cartilaginous throughout. Large portions of these tumors may become myxomatous, or calcified or even ossified. Sometimes fibrosarcoma-like spindling of the cells is seen at the peripheries of the lobules of the tumor. Osseous trabeculae, when present, result from differentiation of chondroid substance. When, however, the malignant cells produce an osteoid lacework or osteoid trabeculae directly, even in small foci, the neoplasm has the clinical characteristics of osteogenic sarcoma and belongs in that category.

Chondrosarcoma usually has a slow clinical evolution. Metastasis is relatively rare and often late in appearance. Therefore, unlike osteogenic sarcoma, in which prompt ablative surgical treatment is imperative because of early hematogenous dissemination, the basic therapeutic problem is prevention of recurrence by adequate control of the lesion locally. Attainment of this goal demands adequate, frequently radical, early surgical treatment.

Chondrosarcomas can arise de novo in extraskeletal tissues or in teratomas and other mixed tumors. Their general characteristics are like those of the skeletal examples.

Secondary Chondrosarcoma

Secondary chondrosarcomas most commonly arise in osteochondromas (osteocartilaginous exostoses), especially in the multiple, familial type. In my experience it is extremely unusual to have a chondrosarcoma develop from an enchondroma that was originally clearly benign on critical analysis. In the Mayo Clinic series of 35 definitely secondary chondrosarcomas, 17 occurred in patients with multiple osteochondromas, 13 arose in solitary osteochondromas, and 5 developed in patients with multiple chondromas. Some of the details concerning these secondary chondrosarcomas are given in chapters 2 and 3.

Mesenchymal Chondrosarcoma

This rare, but histologically distinctive, tumor has clinical characteristics, including a marked potential for metastasizing, that justify its being separated from the ordinary chondrosarcomas.

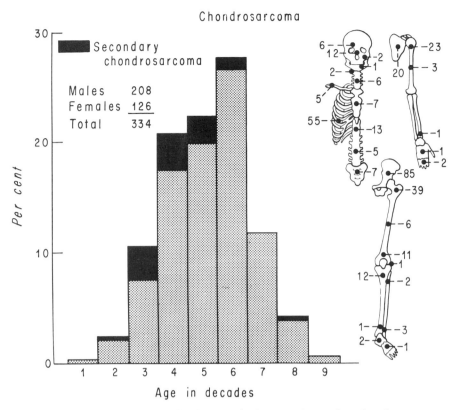

Fig. 16-1. Skeletal, age, and sex distribution of primary and secondary chondrosarcoma.

Incidence

Chondrosarcoma constituted slightly more than 11% of the malignant tumors in this series, and 90% of these were of the primary type. Osteogenic sarcoma was nearly twice as common.

Sex

Slightly more than 62% were males.

Age

This tumor is primarily one of adulthood and old age. Secondary chondrosarcomas occurred in a younger group on the average. The second decade of life, in which the peak incidence of osteogenic sarcoma occurs, contributed only 2.4% of the total. The one patient in the first decade was 9 years old.

Localization

More than three fourths of the tumors were in the trunk (including the shoulder girdle) and the upper ends of the femora and humeri. The majority in the maxillary region appeared to arise from the cartilage of the walls of the nasal cavity. Two developed from the hyoid bone. One was primary in the synovium and capsule of the knee joint; there was no histologic evidence of pre-existing benign synovial chondromatosis. The remarkable rarity of chondrosarcoma in the distal portions of the extremities, with only six of them occurring distal to the ankle and wrist joints, is noteworthy. Localization data concerning the secondary chondrosarcomas are given in Table 4.

TABLE 4

ANATOMIC LOCATION OF 35 SECONDARY CHONDROSARCOMAS ACCORDING TO PRIMARY CONDITION

	Multiple exostoses	Solitary exostoses	Multiple chondromas	Total
Innominate bone	9	5		14
Tibia	1		3	4
Humerus	1	1	1	3
Scapula	1	2		3
Vertebra		3		3
Fibula	3			3
Femur	1		1	2
Clavicle		1		1
Sacrum		1		1
Rib	1			1
Total	17	13	5	35

As indicated previously, the 17 patients with chondrosarcomas complicating multiple exostoses derived from a total of 67 patients who required operation for the latter condition. Of 427 patients requiring operation for solitary exostoses, only 13 had complicating chondrosarcomas. Five of 24 patients operated upon for multiple chondromas of the skeleton (Ollier's disease) had secondary malignant tumor. One of these five had chondromas in only one bone, the femur. These data should not be construed to represent the expected incidence of sarcomatous degeneration in the three conditions. Continued follow-up of the total groups will alter the data, and factors of selection probably increase the likelihood that the patient with sarcoma will gravitate to a large medical center.

Symptoms (All Chondrosarcomas)

Local swelling and pain, alone or in combination, are the significant presenting symptoms. Pain strongly suggests active growth of a central cartilaginous tumor. Except for some of the tumors of the pelvic girdle or spinal column, where referred pain may precede local pain or discernible physical or roentgenographic findings, localization of these tumors is easy. As in other tumors of bone, the characteristics of the pain or swelling offer little differential diagnostic aid. The prolonged clinical course so often observed affords a clue. A gradually enlarging tumor for periods ranging from 1 to 2 decades, or even more, may have been noted by those patients who have had an osteochondroma that undergoes malignant transformation. Such transformation often produces pain and rapid increase in size of a tumor of long duration. Patients with primary chondrosarcoma may also have had symptoms for several years before coming to definitive therapy. Inadequately treated tumors produce a typical history of many recurrences and, finally, of inoperable extension or metastasis that leads to death of the host. A few chondrosarcomas run a rapid clinical course because of a higher degree of malignancy initially or because of increased activity with recurrence.

The slow clinical evolution of chondrosarcoma is emphasized by the fact that approximately 10% of those that produced recurrence in this series had intervals of from 5 to 10 years between treatment and recurrence. Since recurrence may be so delayed, it is obvious that conclusions regarding efficacy of any form of treatment must be based not only on a sizable series of cases but also on such a series followed for a period of at least 10 years.

Physical Findings

Many chondrosarcomas produce a mass that can be palpated, but a sizable number of those affecting the trunk, or even the long bones of the extremities if they have not breached the cortex, will cause pain alone to indicate the presence of a lesion. When a mass is palpable, it is characteristically hard and may be painful. When no mass can be palpated, the diagnosis may be difficult. This is especially true of those chondrosarcomas of the innominate bone that have not produced definite roentgenologic changes. The region of the acetabulum, where many of the chondrosarcomas originate, is notorious for such "hidden" malignant tumors.

Roentgenologic Features

The roentgenogram is nearly always helpful and often affords almost pathognomonic evidence of chondrosarcoma. Osseous destruction in the lesional area combined with mottled densities owing to calcification and ossification is the usual finding. Central chondrosarcomas of long bones often produce fusiform expansion of the shaft associated with thickening of the cortex. Cortical destruction allows extraosseous extension of lesions that begin in the medulla. Those that do not involve the medullary cavity may show little or no cortical destruction but they usually contain minute or massive telltale calcific masses.

Chondrosarcoma of the innominate bone, especially near the acetabulum, may produce no discernible roentgenographic findings early. This is especially true of those that are completely lytic. Even large destructive lesions are quite nonspecific roentgenologically when they do not manifest mottling due to calcification or ossification.

The roentgenogram of an osteochondroma that has undergone malignant transformation may be similar to that of the benign lesion from which it originated, but the surface will ordinarily be indistinct and fuzzy and the clear demarcation from the adjacent soft tissue may be lost. A large mass, if associated with irregular shadows of bone or calcification, is especially characteristic. Sometimes the chondrosarcoma destroys and obscures the exostosis from which it arose. In the author's series, 17 of 35 patients with secondary chondrosarcoma had multiple exostoses, and the genesis of the malignant tumor from a benign osteochondroma could logically be assumed in these individuals even in the face of obscure evidence in the region of the chondrosarcoma.

141

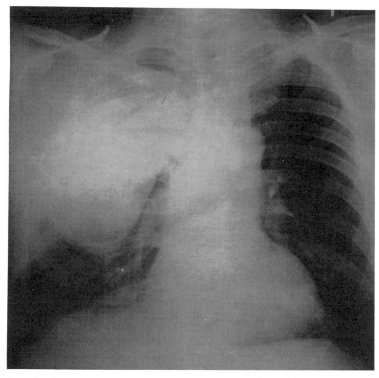

FIG. 16.2. Chondrosarcoma arising from an upper right rib of a 64-year-old man. His only symptom was local swelling of 1½ years' duration.

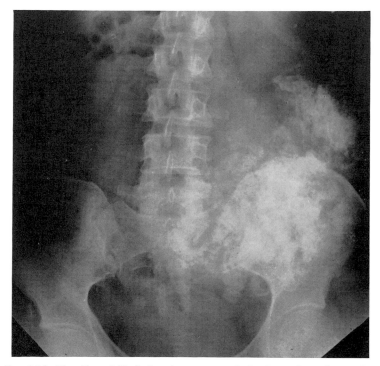

FIG. 16-3. Heavily calcified chondrosarcoma of the innominate bone of a 38-year-old woman. This tumor had produced pain for 4 years. (Reproduced with permission from: Dahlin, D. C., and Henderson, E. D.: *J. Bone & Joint Surg., 38A*:1025-1038, 1956).

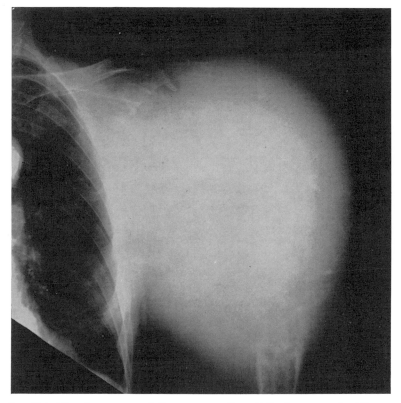

FIG. 16-4. Chondrosarcoma of the upper portion of the humerus of a 70-year-old man. He had had local pain and increasing swelling for 18 months.

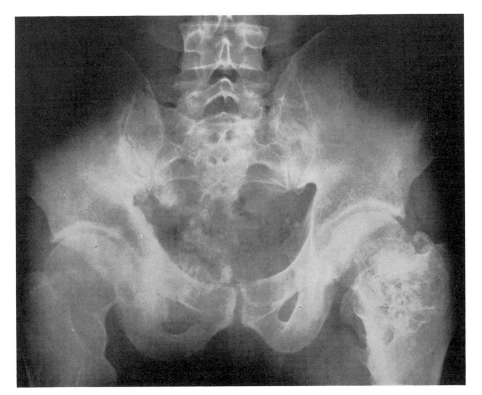

FIG. 16-5. Chondrosarcoma of the right innominate bone in a 36-year-old man who, as is seen in the roentgenogram, had multiple osteochondromas.

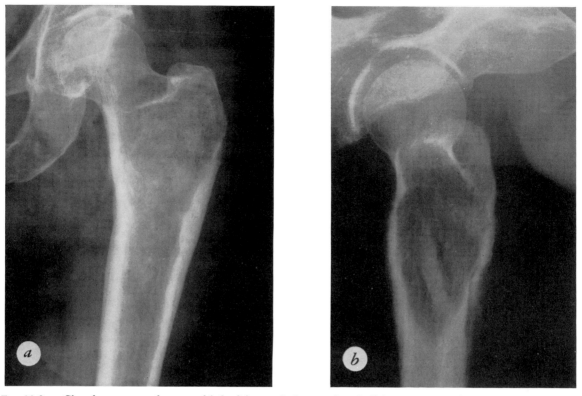

FIG. 16-6. *a.* Chondrosarcoma of upper third of femur. It has produced slight expansion of the shaft and thickening of the cortex. A small amount of calcification is present in the tumor. *b.* Another chondrosarcoma in this location. As can be seen from the roentgenogram, this tumor has broken through the cortex. The extraosseous mass had the pathologic features of grade 3 fibroblastic osteogenic sarcoma, although the intramedullary portion was typically grade 1 chondrosarcoma. (Figure 16-6*a* reproduced with permission from: Dahlin, D. C., and Henderson, E. D.: *J. Bone & Joint Surg., 38A:*1025-1038, 1956.)

Gross Pathology

Chondrosarcomas may be divided into central and peripheral types. In the examples in long bones, such a separation is usually obvious, with the rare peripheral sarcoma arising either on an osteochondroma or directly from the surface of a bone. In the case of an exostosis, a cartilaginous cap, irregularly thickened to more than 1 cm, must be viewed with suspicion; cartilaginous masses measuring 3 to 4 cm usually indicate chondrosarcoma. In the case of thin or flat bones such as in the pelvic girdle or thoracic cage, landmarks are so destroyed by the time the average tumor comes to attention that the exact site of origin can only be surmised, but most of them apparently begin centrally. As seen in roentgenograms, central chondrosarcomas often produce expansion and concomitant thickening of the cortex of long bones. In such cases the region of involved marrow is distinctly demarcated. The thickened cortex is invaded by tumor, and eventually break-through occurs.

These tumors are characteristically composed of lobules that vary from a few millimeters to several centimeters in diameter. Except at the tumor's periphery these lobules are more or less completely coalesced. The centers of the lobules often become necrotic, liquefied, and cystic. Necrotic foci often calcify in an irregular fashion. Some of the calcific zones observed grossly are actually osseous masses.

Chondrosarcomas produce a matrix substance that varies in consistency from that of firm hyaline cartilage to that of mucus. A myxoid quality is an ominous sign, strongly suggestive of malignancy. Sometimes the periphery or the recurrent form of a cartilaginous tumor is opaque and fibrous, resembling a fibrosarcoma or even an osteogenic sarcoma grossly and microscopically.

Metastasis to regional nodes is distinctly rare. Hematogenous dissemination to the lungs and elsewhere is uncommon when one compares chondrosarcoma to osteogenic or fibrosarcoma.

Chondrosarcoma has a marked propensity for local recurrence even when the surgeon "has gotten well around" the tumor.

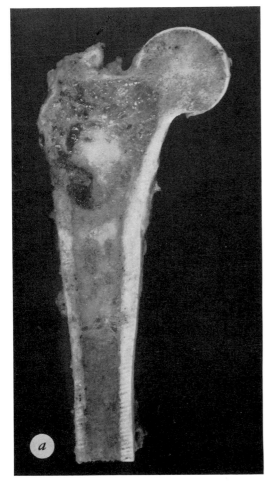
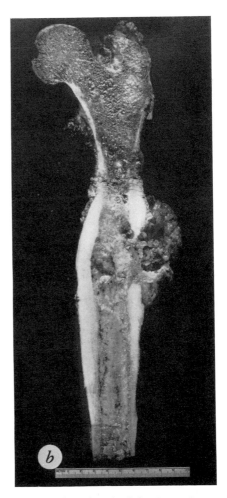

Fig. 16-7. *a.* Gross specimen of the case illustrated in Figure 16-6*a.* Note the rather sharply defined margins of this tumor which extends into the femoral neck and has produced thickening of the expanded cortex, especially on the medial side. *b.* Chondrosarcoma of the midfemur that has broken out into the periosseous tissues after having produced expansion of the bone and thickening of the cortex. (Reproduced with permission from: Dahlin, D. C., and Henderson, E. D.: *J. Bone & Joint Surg., 38A:*1025-1038, 1956.)

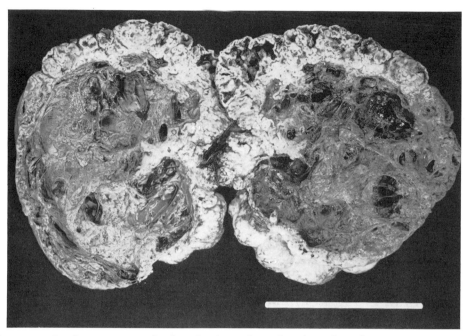

Fig. 16-8. Recurrent chondrosarcomatous implant in the peritoneal cavity. The primary tumor involved the right ilium. Note the lobulation, cyst formation, and extensive central zone of necrosis. The scale in the right lower corner of the picture is 15 cm long.

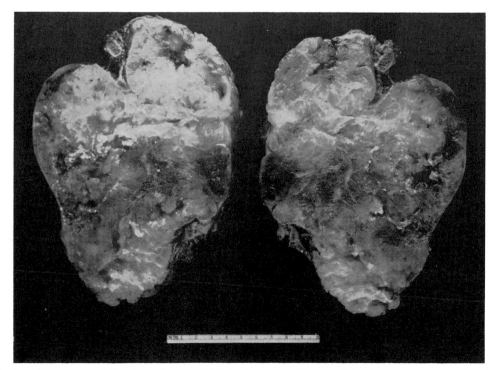

Fig. 16-9. Chondrosarcoma of the thoracic cage. This is the tumor illustrated in the roentgenogram in Figure 16-2.

146

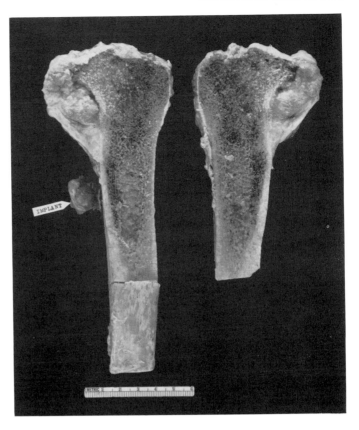

FIG. 16-10. Recurrent chondrosarcoma of the upper end of the tibia posteriorly. The original tumor had been exised by curettage 1 year previously. This recurrent tumor (Figure 16-16) was much more anaplastic than the original. In spite of amputation, pulmonary metastases developed and death occurred. Note the chondrosarcomatous implant in the original surgical scar. (Reproduced with permission from: Dahlin, D. C., and Henderson, E. D.: *J. Bone & Joint Surg., 38A*:1025-1038, 1956.)

Histopathology

Without question, chondrosarcoma is the most difficult of the malignant tumors of bone from the standpoint of the histopathologist. The highly malignant ones with numerous normal and pathologic mitotic figures and obvious anaplasia offer no problem. The criteria that separate a low-grade chondrosarcoma from a chondroma, however, are very subtle, and experience with these tumors is necessary for accurate appraisal. Cellularity correlates poorly with malignant potential, as emphasized by the highly cellular but benign chondromas of the hand. The features proposed by Lichtenstein and Jaffe are very helpful. These include, when one studies viable fields, (1) many cells with plump nuclei, (2) more than an occasional cell with two such nuclei, and especially (3) giant cartilage cells with large single or multiple nuclei or with clumps of chromatin. Correct diagnosis depends upon accurate interpretation of these subtle qualitative characteristics. When one remembers, furthermore, that manifestly malignant foci may be overshadowed by regions that are necrotic or by zones with insufficient cytologic evidence for diagnosis of sarcoma, the pathologist's task is placed in proper perspective.

It is obvious that generous material for biopsy is mandatory and that the crutches of clinical and roentgenologic evidence are extremely helpful. One cannot make a microscopic diagnosis on the basis of the clinical and roentgenologic evidence, but such evidence will guide one in the search for pathognomonic microscopic fields.

Using Broders' method of numerical grading, in which 1 signifies the least and 4 the most undifferentiated, no tumor in the Mayo Clinic series seemed to qualify for grade 4. The distribution was grade 3, 6%; grade 2, 37%; grade 1, 55%; and considered "borderline" for evidence of malignancy, 2%.

As indicated previously, chondrosarcoma secondary to proved solitary benign enchondroma was not found in this series. In recurrent cases, study of the original specimens, which included all those that had been removed at the Mayo Clinic and many of those that had been removed elsewhere, revealed cytologic evidence sufficient for the prediction of a malignant clinical course in each case. Retrospection makes analysis easier, and, with due allowance for this fact, it must be admitted that in a few instances the primary tissue was sufficiently "borderline" that one might well have hesitated to recommend extensive ablative surgical treatment.

The older literature is replete with descriptions of chondrosarcomas that were presumably secondary to benign central cartilaginous tumors, and many early cases in the present series had been similarly interpreted. Misinterpretation of the original tissue sections, insufficient microscopic sampling of the surgical material, or incomplete removal of the primary tumor can lead to underdiagnosis and the erroneous impression that malignant transformation caused the subsequent recurrence. Calcification results from degeneration of these tumors, but mature bone appears to develop by ossification of the hyaline cartilage

An additional histopathologic feature of chondrosarcoma requires comment. In approximately 10% of these tumors that are allowed to recur, there is an increase in degree of malignancy. Sometimes this is in the form of a more active pure chondrosarcoma; at other times the recurrence is in the form of highly malignant fibrosarcoma or osteogenic sarcoma. I have seen several instances of similar transformation of chondrosarcomas in the absence of surgical intervention.

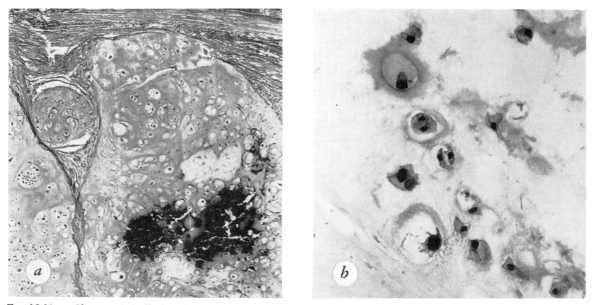

FIG. 16-11. *a.* Characteristically lobulated periphery of a chondrosarcoma, in this instance a grade 1 lesion. The black zones represent calcification secondary to necrosis (×40). *b.* Definite cytologic evidence of malignancy includes cells with large, dark, and sometimes multiple nucli ×(300). (Reproduced with permission from: Dahlin, D. C., and Henderson, E. D.: *J. Bone & Joint Surg., 38A*:1025-1038, 1956.)

The histopathologist should employ ancillary evidences to support the diagnosis of chondrosarcoma. These include large size, pain, invasiveness, extraosseous extension, myxoid quality, roentgenographic signs of aggressiveness, and rapid growth. Cartilaginous tumors in the distal parts of the skeleton, in a circumscribed subperiosteal location, or in the lining or capsule of joints are almost certain to be clinically benign.

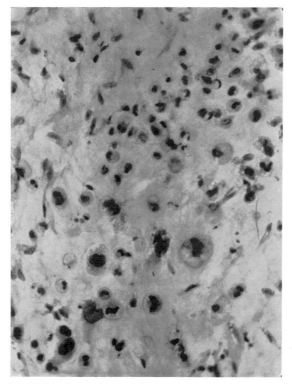

FIG. 16-12. Zone of grade 3 chondrosarcoma. Here the nuclear abnormalities and mitotic activity make the diagnosis of sarcoma an obvious one (×195).

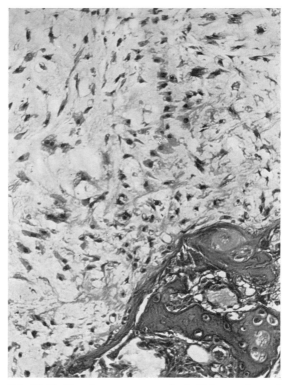

FIG. 16-13. Chondrosarcoma, grade 1. Fair numbers of binucleated cells are present and the ground substance is myxomatous. The cartilage is differentiating into mature bone (×180).

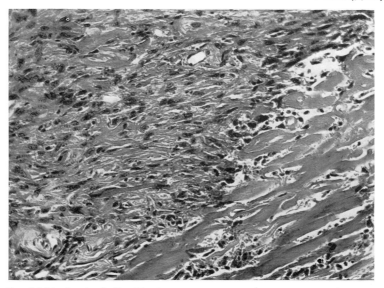

FIG. 16-14. Grade 3 fibroblastic osteogenic sarcoma (×160). This highly malignant tumor developed in the scar after amputation for a grade 2 chondrosarcoma that had fibrosarcoma-like elements at the periphery of the chondroid lobules. (Reproduced with permission from: Dahlin, D. C., and Henderson, E. D.: J. Bone &Joint Surg., 38A:1025-1038, 1956.)

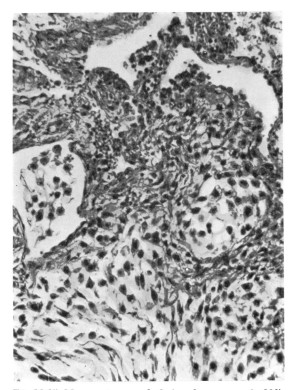

FIG. 16-15. Myxomatous grade 2 chondrosarcoma (×200). This is from a pulmonary nodule removed by segmental excision 16 months after a leg had been amputated for the primary tumor. The patient was alive and well 12 years after excision of the metastatic nodule.

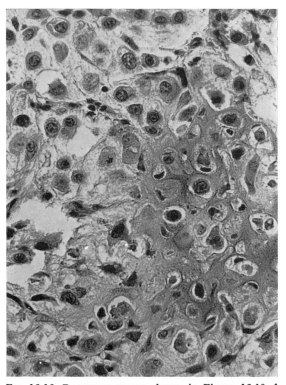

FIG. 16-16. Recurrent tumor shown in Figure 16-10, 1 year after curettage of grade 1 chondrosarcoma. This recurrent lesion has features of osteogenic sarcomas, grade 2, as shown here (×300). Death with pulmonary metastases occurred in less than a year after amputation for this recurrent lesion.

Treatment

Surgery is the mainstay in therapy of this radioresistant tumor. Irradiation will serve, at best, as palliation for those tumors not amenable to surgical removal. Surgeons with wide experience in the treatment of bone tumors have learned that the optimal treatment for chondrosarcoma is early radical removal with as wide a margin of uninvolved tissue as possible. Certain of these tumors in the region of the iliac crests can be radically excised with preservation of the lower extremity. Most chondrosarcomas that involve the innominate bone or the upper end of the femur require hindquarter amputation for adequate removal. Those that are in the thoracic cage should be excised widely with an adequate margin of uninvolved tissue. Chondrosarcoma of the clavicle or scapula can often be treated by wide local removal, but a similar tumor in the upper end of the humerus, unless small and confined to the bone, is probably best treated by forequarter amputation. For those chondrosarcomas of the major tubular bones that are away from the trunk, wide local excision with bone grafting as necessary is sometimes feasible. In such instances, recurrent tumors are often amenable to more radical treatment. Our experience indicates that wide local excision is apt to succeed for chondrosarcomas secondary to exostoses. Equivocal pathologic or roentgenographic evidence is indication for a conservative attitude.

Ideally, as with any of the surgical malignant tumors of bone, the definitive treatment should be carried out at the time of biopsy, but delay is doubtless of less importance in therapy of chondrosarcoma than of more anaplastic sarcomas. The roentgenogram may indicate the most aggressive and infiltrative portion of the tumor which is the best region for biopsy. The biopsy wound should be planned so that the definitive operation can include it as part of the tissue to be completely removed or ablated because of the notorious capability of chondrosarcomas to produce recurrence by implantation. The tumor itself should be completely excised with an adequate zone of surrounding tissue so that he surgeon does not break into or see the tumor at any time. An occasional recurrent lesion is much more anaplastic than the original tumor and may have features of osteogenic or fibrosarcoma, which is another reason for adequate primary surgical treatment.

Prognosis

The fact that recurrences of chondrosarcoma are not uncommon after 5 years and sometimes are encountered even after 10 years makes it obvious that 5-year survival is not very significant as a criterion of cure. Actually, because of the common error of underdiagnosis and consequent inadequate treatment in the earlier part of the present series, the overall rate of cure for chondrosarcoma was less than for osteogenic sarcoma in those years. Thoracic surgeons learned 4 decades ago that wide local excision was mandatory if one were to expect cure in the treatment of malignant cartilaginous tumors in the thoracic cage. Accordingly, many of the long-term survivors in the Mayo Clinic series are patients who had chondrosarcoma in this location. But in the last 25 years, when radical amputation has become common therapy for tumors in the pelvic and shoulder girdles, the upper part of the humerus, and the upper part of the femur, an increasing number of patients with chondrosarcoma in these locations are being cured. Long-term survival can be obtained in more than half the cases if adequate surgery is employed.

Mesenchymal Chondrosarcoma

This lesion was described by Lichtenstein and Bernstein in 1959. I had tentatively labeled as mesenchymomas a group of 10 strikingly similar tumors that fit their description exactly. Other cases have been documented by Benedetti (1961), Gilmer and associates (1963), and Dowling (1964). The other unusual chondroid tumors described by Lichtenstein and Bernstein do not have counterparts I have recognized in the material available for study. If any are present they have been classed with chondrosarcoma, chondromyxoid fibroma, and chondroblastoma.

Mesenchymal chondrosarcoma shows the paradoxical histologic combination of highly cellular zones composed of anaplastic small cells and islands of relatively benign-appearing chondroid substance which may be calcified and even ossified. The chondroid islands vary in size and number from one tumor to another and even in different regions in a neoplasm. The small cells which shade into the cells of the chondroid islands are usually somewhat spindle-shaped but may simulate reticulum cells and are sometimes related to blood vessels reminding one of hemangiopericytoma.

CHONDROSARCOMA

The 10 cases in this series comprise 0.3% of the malignant tumors. Including 6 tumors I have seen in consultation and others from the literature, a total of 22 tumors have been in patients whose ages varied from 5 to 58 years. Sexes have been equally affected. Vertebrae have accounted for six tumors, the jaws for five, the skull and ribs for three each, the ilium for two, and the scapula, femur, and metatarsal for one each. Roentgenologically they produce varying degrees of destruction and radiopacity. Grossly they are apt to appear cartilaginous, and they may be heavily mineralized. There have appeared to be multicentric skeletal foci in some cases. Hematogenous metastasis, which may be long delayed, has been common. Those patients who have been adequately followed have all died. It seems that early radical surgical therapy should be employed for this tumor.

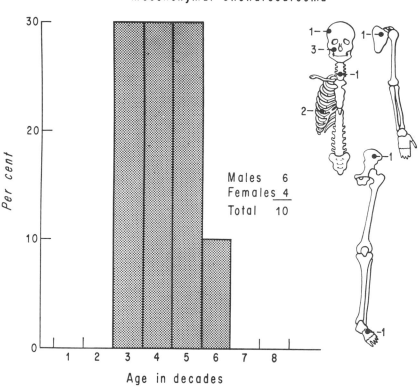

Fig. 16-17. Skeletal, age and sex distribution of mesenchymal chondrosarcoma.

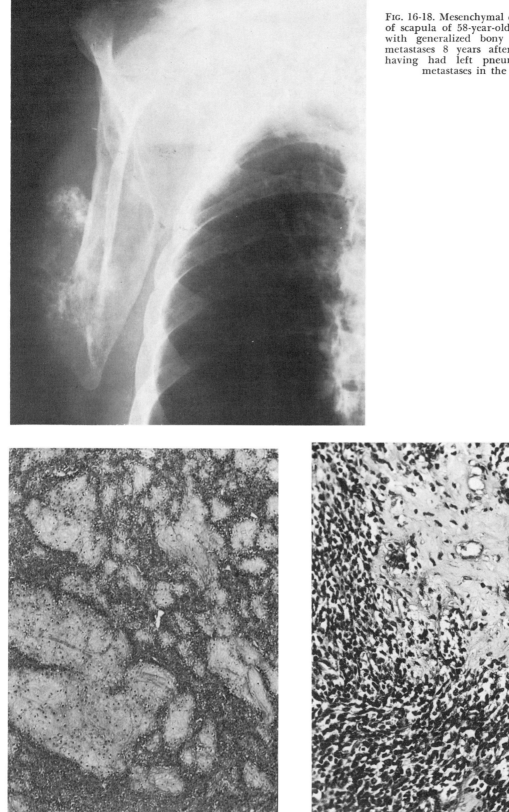

FIG. 16-18. Mesenchymal chondrosarcoma of scapula of 58-year-old man. He died with generalized bony and soft-tissue metastases 8 years after scapulectomy, having had left pneumonectomy for metastases in the interim.

FIG. 16-19. *Left.* Characteristic mesenchymal chondrosarcoma with numerus chondroid islands of varying size and a stroma of small cells with spindling nuclei. Note small size of nuclei within lacunae (×95). *Right.* A characteristic zone with slightly more than usual spindling of nuclei (×200).

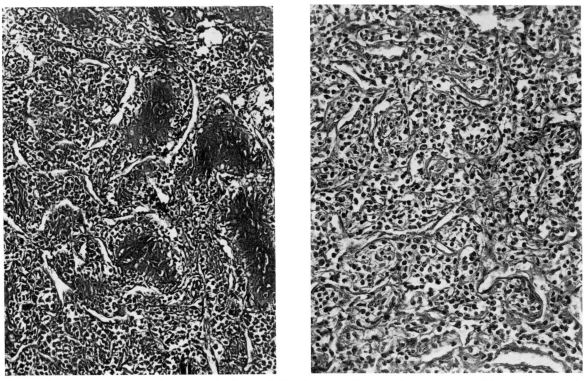

FIG. 16-20. *Left.* Zone showing clustering of cells in relation to thin-walled vessels, a pattern reminiscent of hemangiopericytoma. Note mineralization of chondroid foci ($\times$170). *Right.* Another instance of clustering of cells of mesenchymal chondrosarcoma. Note some resemblance to both reticulum cell sarcoma and hemangiopericytoma ($\times$245).

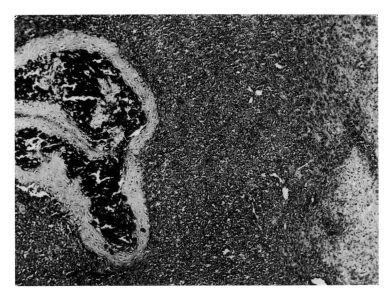

FIG. 16-21. Commonly observed calcification within a chondroid island. Sometimes ossification occurs in such zones ($\times$90). (Figures 16-18, 19, 20, and 21 reproduced with permission from: Dahlin, D. C., and Henderson, E. D.: *Cancer,* *15*:410-417 1962.)

Bibliography

1927 Harrington, S. W.: Surgical Treatment of Intrathoracic Tumors and Tumors of the Chest Wall. *Arch. Surg., 14:*406-431.

1943 Lichtenstein, Louis, and Jaffe, H. L.: Chondrosarcoma of Bone. *Am. J. Path., 19:*553-589.

1952 O'Neal, L. W., and Ackerman, L. V.: Chondrosarcoma of Bone. *Cancer, 5:*551-577.

1958 Lansche, W. E., and Spjut, H. J.: Chondrosarcoma of the Small Bones of the Hand. *J. Bone & Joint Surg., 40A:*1139-1145.

1959 Lichtenstein, L., and Bernstein, D.: Unsual Benign and Malignant Chondroid Tumors of Bone. *Cancer, 12:*1142-1157.

1960 Kragh, L. V., Dahlin, D. C., and Erich, J. B.: Cartilaginous Tumors of the Jaws and Facial Regions. *Am. J. Surg., 99:*852-856.

1961 Benedetti, G. B.: Tumore Condroblastico Della Mandibola A Caratteri Istologici Peculiari. *Chir. org. movimento, 50:*135-144.

1961 Lindbom, A., Söderberg, G., and Spjut, H. J.: Primary Chondrosarcoma of Bone. Acta radiol., *55:*81-96.

1962 Murphy, F. P., Dahlin, D. C., and Sullivan, C. R.: Articular Synovial Chondromatosis. *J. Bone & Joint Surg., 44A:*77-86.

1962 Dahlin, D. C., and Henderson, E. D.: Mesenchymal Chondrosarcoma: Further Observations on a New Entity. *Cancer, 15:*410-417.

1963 Goethals, P. L., Dahlin, D. C., and Devine, K. D.: Cartilaginous Tumors of the Larynx. *Surg., Gynec., & Obst., 117:*77-82.

1963 Gilmer, W. S., Jr., Kilgore, W., and Smith, H.: Central Cartilage Tumors of Bone. *Clin. Orthop., 26:*81-103.

1963 Henderson, E. D., and Dahlin, D. C.: Chondrosarcoma of Bone—A Study of Two Hundred and Eighty-eight Cases. *J. Bone & Joint Surg., 45A:*1450-1458.

1963 Gilmer, W. S., Jr., Higley, G. B., and Kilgore, W. E.: *Atlas of Bone Tumors.* Saint Louis, The C. V. Mosby Co., pp. 84-93.

1964 Dowling, E. A.: Mesenchymal Chondrosarcoma. *J. Bone & Joint Surg., 46A:*747-754.

1964 Phelan, J. T., and Cabrera, A.: Chondrosarcoma of Bone. *Surg., Gynec., & Obst., 119:*42-46.

1964 Pachter, M. R., and Alpert, M.: Chondrosarcoma of the Foot Skeleton. *J. Bone & Joint Surg., 46A:*601-607.

Chapter 17

Osteogenic Sarcoma

To QUALIFY in this category, the proliferating malignant cells of the neoplasm must produce osteoid substance or material histologically indistinguishable from it in at least small foci. A qualifying tumor, when sampled throughout, may show a predominance of elements with osteoid, chondroid, or fibromatoid differentiation. Accordingly, this series of osteogenic sarcomas is divided into osteoblastic, chondroblastic, and fibroblastic types, depending on the dominating element. This classification may be confusing until one realizes that its function is merely to indicate that wide variation is seen in the histopathology of osteogenic sarcoma. All of these tumors, however, have similar characteristics as regards bones of predilection, age of affected patients, marked tendency to early hematogenous dissemination, and necessity for prompt ablative surgical therapy. Malignant fibroblastic tumors with no definite osteoid production by neoplastic cells, regardless of their degree of anaplasia, are classed as fibrosarcomas. Similarly, those chondroblastic malignant tumors with no definite direct production of osteoid are designated as chondrosarcomas. Sometimes exact designation is difficult and must be arbitrary since there is no special stain for osteoid and its qualities merge with those of collagen and cartilaginous matrix.

It has not seemed practical to divide the osteogenic sarcomas into a variety of gross types as has been done in the past. Whether the tumor is "periosteal," "sclerotic," "lytic," "central," "telangiectatic," and so forth makes little difference if it is a bona fide osteogenic sarcoma.

Although the great majority of these tumors are of unknown cause, Paget's disease is a precursor of some sarcomas, especially in older people. Twenty of 650 osteogenic sarcomas in the present series arose in Paget's bone, as did 2 fibrosarcomas and 1 giant cell tumor.

An increasing number of sarcomas following in the wake of radiation therapy to bone are being recorded. There were 23 postirradiation osteogenic sarcomas in this series. Eighteen fibrosarcomas, one chondrosarcoma, and one Ewing's tumor also arose in previously irradiated bone.

The occasional chondrosarcoma which, after a characteristic indolent clinical course, develops a complicating anaplastic osteogenic or fibrosarcoma has been included in the overall data and discussion of chondrosarcoma in chapter 16.

A special type of osteogenic sarcoma which grows slowly, metastasizes late if at all, and is characteristically juxtacortical or parosteal in location is known as parosteal osteogenic sarcoma. This is discussed in the next chapter.

The rare extraskeletal osteogenic sarcomas (Fine and Stout, 1956) are very prone to metastasize and require aggressive therapy but must be carefully differentiated from benign heterotopic ossification.

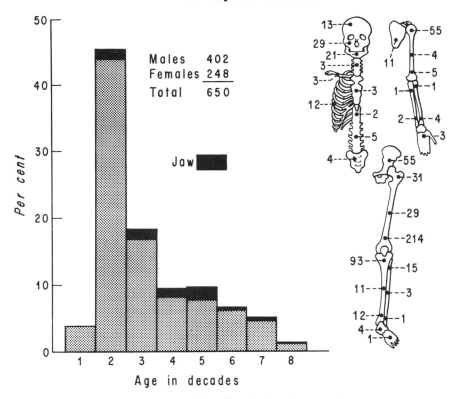

FIG. 17-1. Skeletal, age, and sex distribution of osteogenic sarcoma.

Incidence

The 650 osteogenic sarcomas (excluding the parosteal variety) comprised 21.9% of the total sarcomas in this series. Execpt for myeloma it was the commonest primary bone tumor.

Sex

Males contributed nearly 62% of all osteogenic sarcomas and 58% of those in the jawbones.

Age

Although there are a few osteogenic sarcomas in the first decade of life, the peak incidence is in the second decade and there is a steady, gradual decrease thereafter. The youngest of 650 patients with osteogenic sarcoma was 4 years old. Osteogenic sarcomas of the jaws occur in an older age group on the average; this is not related to the fact that 7 of the 50 were postirradiation sarcomas.

Localization

The metaphyseal part of the long bones is the site of predilection, and the region of the knee accounted for nearly half of the total number of osteogenic sarcomas in this series. Of the total number of osteogenic sarcomas, only eight were distal to the ankle and wrist joints. Those sarcomas that did not extend to within 5 cm of an articular surface of a long bone are indicated as being in its mid-portion in the illustration above.

Skeletal, Age, and Sex Distribution

Comparison of the detailed data shown in Tables 1, 2, and 3 in chapter 1 emphasizes the basic kinship of the osteoblastic, chondroblastic, and fibroblastic types of osteogenic sarcoma. Males predominate in all types. All three types have a predilection for the metaphyseal region of the long tubular bones, but chondroblastic osteogenic sarcoma has a greater tendency to involve the trunk than do the other two types.

The age distributions were similar for all three types and, contrary to some observations in the literature, no secondary peak was found in the older age groups. This secondary peak of incidence has been blamed on the influx of sarcomas secondary to Paget's disease in older people.

Data compiled on our first 469 osteogenic sarcomas and 218 chondrosarcomas are shown in Figure 17-2. They indicate the similarity of the distribution by age of the osteogenic sarcomas and its contrast with that of chondrosarcoma.

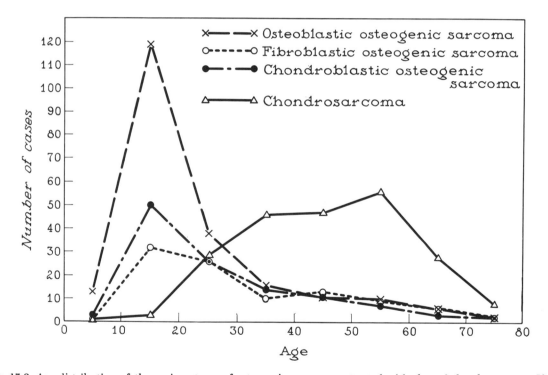

FIG. 17-2. Age distribution of the various types of osteogenic sarcoma contrasted with that of chondrosarcoma. If the data for osteogenic sarcoma had been expressed in percentages rather than in numbers of cases, the lines representing the three types would have been practically superimposed. Note that there are practically no chondrosarcomas in the second decade, the age of peak incidence of all histologic types of osteogenic sarcoma. In middle and old age, when chondrosarcoma is common, the osteogenic sarcomas become increasingly rare.

Symptoms

Pain, which may be intermittent at first, and swelling are again the cardinal symptoms. They are, obviously, nonspecific and for this reason one should not ignore the possibly serious nature of these complaints, especially when they occur in childhood, adolescence, or young adulthood. Pathologic fracture is uncommon.

The duration of symptoms prior to definitive therapy varies from a few weeks to several months. A history of trouble for more than 1 year is uncommon in patients with ordinary osteogenic sarcoma. Increasing pain or swelling is suggestive of malignant change in Paget's disease. Likewise a flare-up of symptoms in a patient who has had irradiation for a benign condition of bone should arouse suspicion.

Physical Findings

A painful mass in the affected region is usually apparent. Sometimes the mass is very large and then it may be associated with overlying engorged veins and even edema distal to the lesion. Physical examination is noncontributory in the case of some of the tumors that are covered by a thick layer of tissues. Evidence of pathologic fracture is distinctly uncommon.

Roentgenologic Features

Depending on the amount of ossification and calcification found in osteogenic sarcoma, there is great variation in the roentgenographic shadows produced. Tumors may be completely lytic or predominantly sclerotic, but they usually exhibit a combination of these features. The destructive process may be limited to the medulla but usually involves the cortex as well, since it is nearly always perforated by the growing tumor. There is a gradual transition from zones of marked lysis to zones of uninvolved bone, making the borders of the lesion indistinct. Non-neoplastic bone is deposited, sometimes in layers, when the periosteum is elevated by the perforating tumor. With continued development of the neoplasm one frequently sees a large soft-tissue mass contiguous to the bone.

Varying degrees of density are seen within the affected portion of bone when the osteogenic sarcoma produces calcifying and ossifying osteoid substance. These densities often extend into the contiguous soft tissues. The proliferated bone produced by the neoplastic cells characteristically has a streaked texture and ill-defined margins. The roentgenologic diagnosis is usually easily made in the case of those tumors that show a combination of destruction of bone and proliferation of new bone, but definitive therapy should never be recommended without confirmation by biopsy.

Osteoid substance, even if present in large amounts in an osteoblastic osteogenic sarcoma, produces no radiopacity if it is completely uncalcified.

Pulmonary metastases are rarely demonstrable when the patient first seeks medical advice. The question of the advisability of roentgenographic skeletal survey searching for other foci before doing ablative therapy is unsettled.

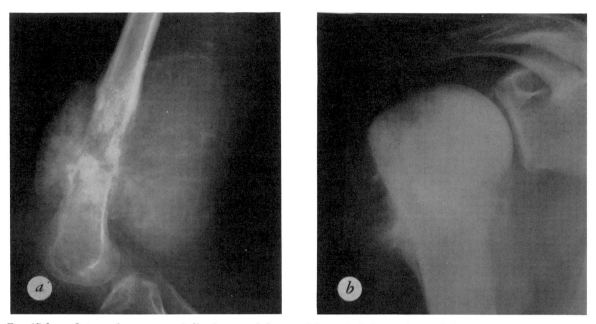

FIG. 17-3. *a*. Osteogenic sarcoma of distal part of femur with cortical destruction sufficient to produce pathologic fracture. *b*. Sclerosing osteogenic sarcoma of upper part of humerus, one of the more common sites for this tumor. Note "sunburst effect."

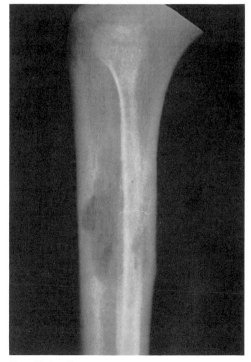

FIG. 17-4. Almost completely lytic, fibroblastic osteogenic sarcoma of upper, central portion of tibia.

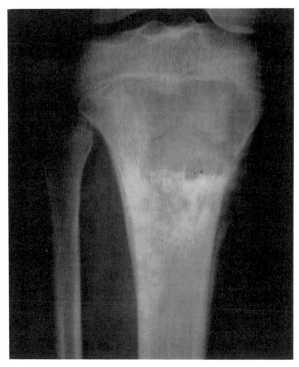

FIG. 17-5. Lytic and sclerotic sarcoma of upper part of metaphysis of tibia, the second commonest site of origin of osteogenic sarcoma.

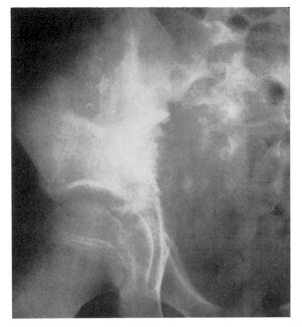

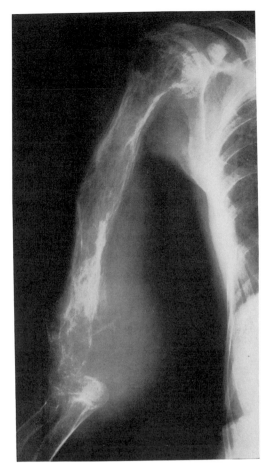

FIG. 17-6. *Above*. Chondroblastic osteogenic sarcoma of right ilium causing sclerosis. Note intrapelvic extension.

FIG. 17-7. *Right*. Lytic, but osteoblastic osteogenic sarcoma of distal portion of right humerus. The entire bone shows severe changes of Paget's disease.

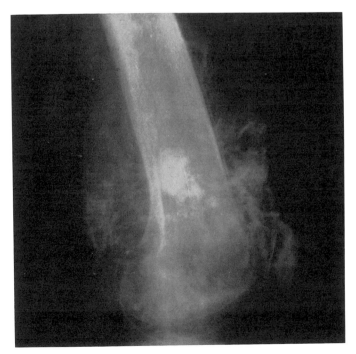

FIG. 17-8. Osteogenic sarcoma of distal portion of femur. Note destruction, sclerosis, and "sunburst" effect.

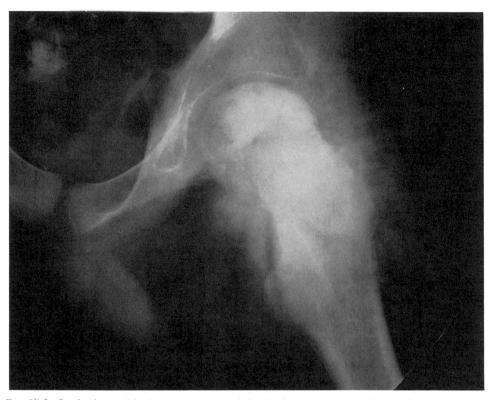

FIG. 17-9. Grade 4 osteoblastic sarcoma treated by hindquarter amputation. This operation has effected a survival of more than 18 years to the present time. (Reproduced with permission from: Coventry, M. B., and Dahlin, D. C.: *J. Bone & Joint Surg., 39A:*741-757, 1957.)

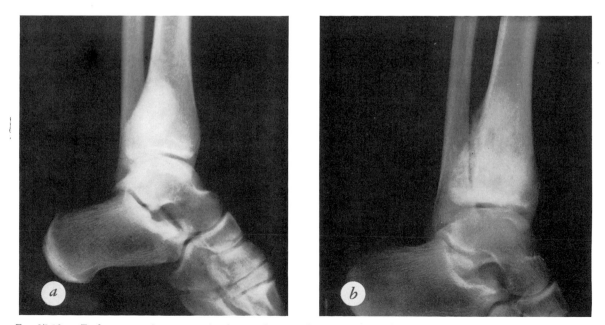

FIG. 17-10. *a.* Early osteogenic sarcoma, inadvertently treated conservatively. *b.* Five and a half months later the tumor has produced obvious cortical perforation and other signs indicative of malignancy. In spite of the delay in therapy the patient has survived 10 years since amputation.

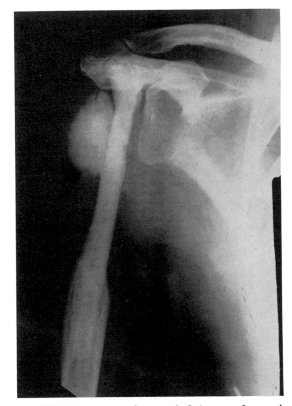

FIG. 17-11. Recurrence along graft 3½ years after excision of upper end of humerus for a grade 1 osteosarcoma that was basically central and presumably made the patient an ideal candidate for conservative therapy. Despite forequarter amputation, recurrence developed in the thoracic wall.

Gross Pathology

By the time an osteogenic sarcoma receives definitive therapy it has breached the cortex, in the average case. The extraosseous mass may even completely encircle the bone. The periosteum presents a barrier that often has become greatly distended before it is perforated. Slight to complete cortical destruction is found in the site of perforation.

Some of these tumors spread in the marrow cavity for surprising distances, not infrequently beyond that visible in the roentgenogram, and this must be reckoned with during therapy. In nearly all instances the extent of the marrow involvement is readily apparent grossly when one saws the bone longitudinally, and most tumors do not spread in the marrow beyond their gross extraosseous limits. Skip areas of medullary involvement are extremely rare.

Nearly all osteogenic sarcomas have such a prominent central component that a central origin is logically assumed. Rarely, however, a highly malignant one is outside the bone and involves only the outer portion of the cortex, suggesting a periosteal origin.

As suggested by the roentgenogram, these tumors vary from extremely soft, friable and granular masses through a variety that is firm and fibrous with foci of irregular ossification and variable amounts of chondroid material, to the densely sclerotic ones. Sclerosis, when present, is invariably most pronounced in the central regions. Nearly all osteogenic sarcomas, however sclerotic, have soft peripheral zones that can be sectioned without preliminary decalcification. Areas of necrosis, cyst formation, telangiectasis, and hemorrhage are most likely to occur in the soft tumors.

Metastasis is predominantly hematogenous, with the production of pulmonary deposits. Metastasis to other bones may be early and widespread suggesting multifocal origin of sarcoma, or delayed and localized suggesting that a new tumor has developed. Seven patients in this series had at least two major amputations because such presumably new osteogenic sarcomas appeared. One patient survived 26 years after the first and 12 years after the second amputation. Lymphatic metastasis was rare in our material, but the vast majority of patients died at home and were not subjected to necropsy.

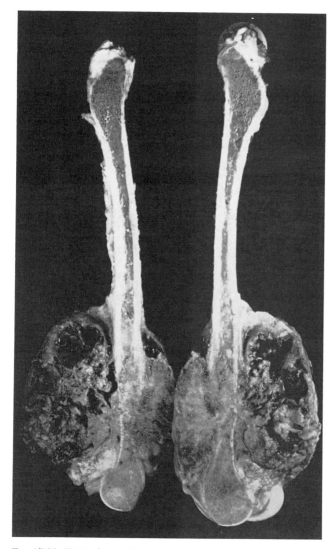

FIG. 17-12. Typical osteoblastic osteogenic sarcoma of lower portion of femur. Hemorrhage and degeneration but practically no intramedullary spread are seen. The roentgenogram of this tumor is shown in Figure 17-3.

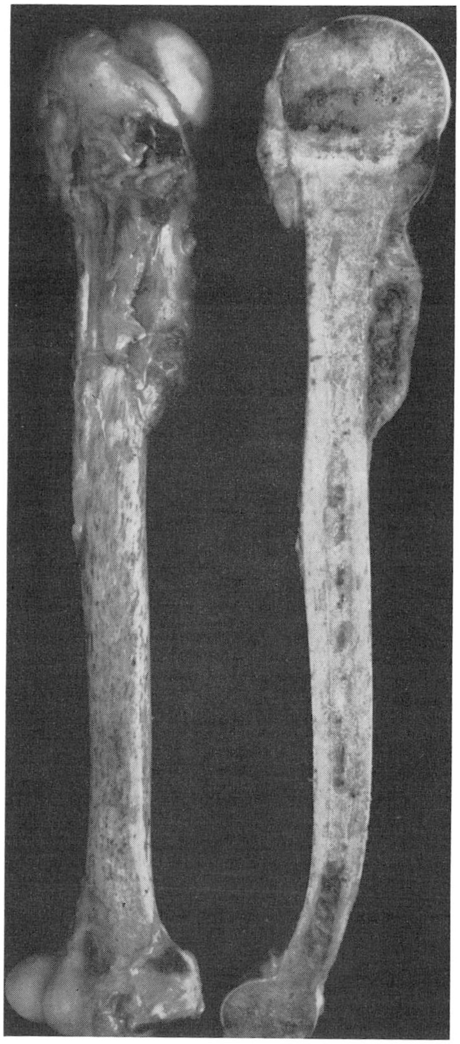

FIG. 17-13. Densely sclerotic osteosarcoma of upper part of humerus. Intramedullary spread nearly to the elbow has occurred.

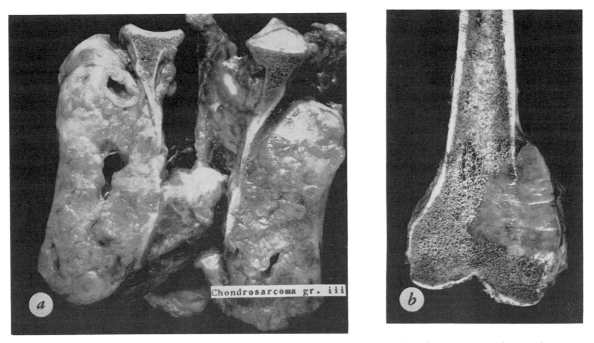

FIG. 17-14. *a.* Chondroblastic osteogenic sarcoma with areas of practically pure chondrosarcoma. This scapular tumor occurred in a 51-year-old woman. *b.* Fibroblastic osteosarcoma of distal part of femur. Note cortical perforation, periosteal elevation, and typical metaphyseal location.

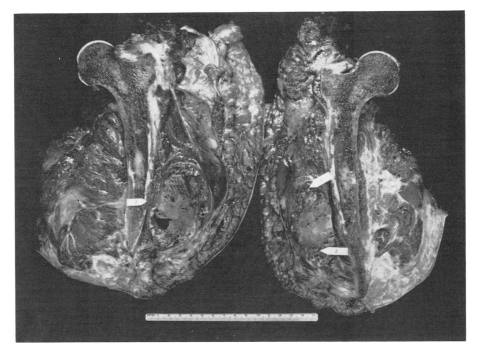

FIG. 17-15. An unusual finding—recurrence in the stump after high amputation through the thigh for an osteogenic sarcoma of the lower end of the femur. This may have been the result of implantation of tumor cells, if proper precautions were not observed, since the biopsy immediately preceded the amputation. The primary tumor, in this case was in the distal 8 cm of the femur and there was no intramedullary spread.

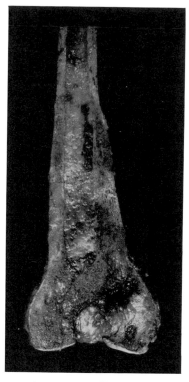

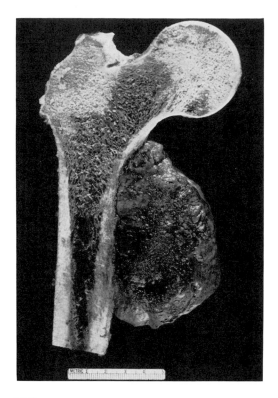

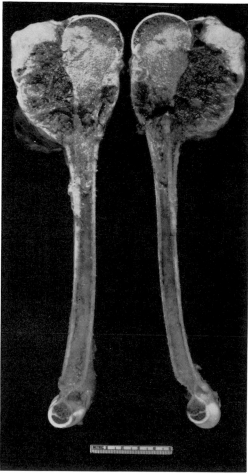

FIG. 17-16. Paget's disease of lower third of femur. It has produced thickening of the cortex and widening of the shaft. There is a secondary grade 4 fibroblastic osteogenic sarcoma in the medial condyle.

FIG. 17-17. *Above, right.* Peripheral or "periosteal" highly anaplastic osteosarcoma. There is some erosion of the cortex, but no intramedullary involvement. The high grade takes this lesion out of the parosteal osteogenic sarcoma class.

FIG. 17-18. *Right.* Predominantly cartilaginous (chondroblastic) osteogenic sarcoma of upper end of humerus. Medullary spread extends 5 cm below the external bulge of the tumor, and a distinct "Codman's angle" has been produced by elevation of periosteum.

166

Histopathology

A great variability in the histopathology of osteogenic sarcoma exists, as previously indicated. Lichtenstein has tersely stated the essential criteria as: "(1) the presence of a frankly sarcomatous stroma and (2) the direct formation of tumor osteoid and bone by this malignant connective tissue."

Although these sarcomas rather conveniently fall into the osteoblastic, chondroblastic, and fibroblastic groups, depending on the dominating histologic pattern, it is necessary to be arbitrary in some cases. One occasionally encounters a highly anaplastic tumor that contains no osteoid but is otherwise so similar in histologic appearance to osteoid-producing tumors that it logically must be classified as osteoblastic sarcoma unless one wishes to create a new group. Some tumors that appear as nearly pure fibrosarcomas contain foci of homogeneous, afibrillar, eosinophilic material that resembles hyalinized collagen. When such foci cannot be differentiated with certainty from osteoid tissue, tumors containing them are best classed as fibroblastic osteogenic sarcoma. The usual member of this group, however, contains obvious osteoid material. One must be similarly arbitrary in the case of occasional chondroblastic osteogenic sarcomas in which osteoid production directly by malignant cells is debatable, but, with few exceptions, it is possible to make a clear-cut differentiation of these lesions from chondrosarcoma.

According to the predominant differentiation, more than half (343) of these 650 tumors were osteoblastic, 155 chondroblastic, and 152 fibroblastic. Grading osteogenic sarcomas by the method of Broders is difficult, and most of them are in the anaplastic high grades. In this series, 85% were of grades 3 and 4, and only five were judged to be of grade 1. These latter sarcomas are differeniated from benign conditions such as fibrous dysplasia with difficulty. The roentgenogram or, as a last resort, the clinical course may resolve the problem.

The original osseous trabeculae are destroyed to a variable extent in the lesional zone. Frequently, however, especially in the more sclerotic tumors, residual trabeculae are seen being enveloped by the advancing neoplasm. The central portions of osteoblastic tumors are routinely the most sclerotic, and in practically every case there are peripheral lobules that are nonossified. The latter zones are the most satisfactory for histologic diagnosis because of the tendency for the cells to become small and less ominous in appearance when surrounded by sclerosing matrix. Some of the highly malignant, cellular tumors contain extensive zones of necrosis and hemorrhage.

Benign multinucleated cells in variable numbers are seen in a minority of osteogenic sarcomas, thus introducing the possibility of confusion with benign giant cell tumor of bone. The problem is especially difficult in the case of those sarcomas with relatively small cells. In these the subtle evidences of nuclear anaplasia are fortified by a malignant appearance in the roentgenogram which also usually reveals a metaphyseal epicenter for the tumor.

Exuberant callus, especially in some patients with fractures secondary to osteogenesis imperfecta, has been mistaken for sarcoma. This error can be avoided if one insists on cytologic evidence of malignancy in the diagnosis of sarcoma. It should be remembered, also, that the reactive subperiosteal new bone in "Codman's angle" is non-neoplastic and worthless for biopsy.

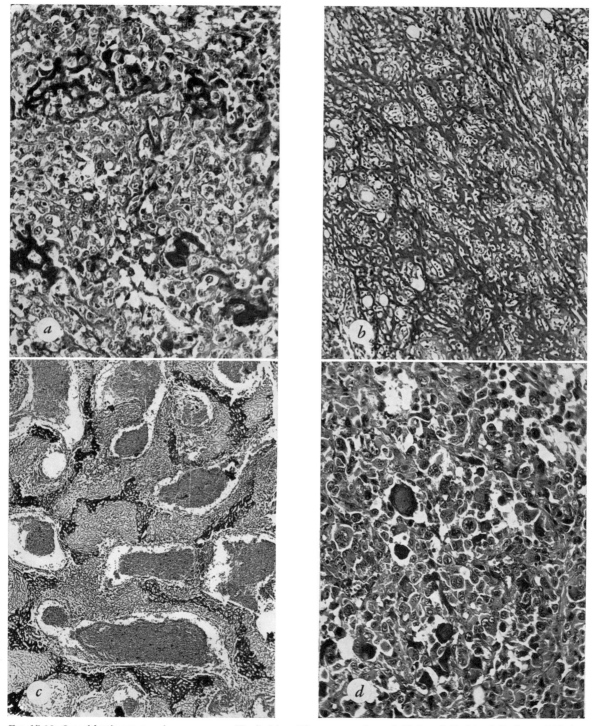

Fig. 17-19. Osteoblastic osteogenic sarcomas. *a.* Typical lace-like pattern of uncalcified and (dark) calcified osteoid being produced by highly anaplastic cells (×200). *b.* Densely sclerotic zone with shriveled cells compressed by osteoid (×100). *c.* Large pools of blood in a hemorrhagic "telangiectatic" lesion (×35). *d.* Extremely anaplastic osteogenic sarcoma with no osteoid production in this field (×165). (Figure 17-21*a* reproduced with permission from: Coventry, M. B., and Dahlin, D. C.: *J. Bone & Joint Surg., 39A:*741-757, 1957.)

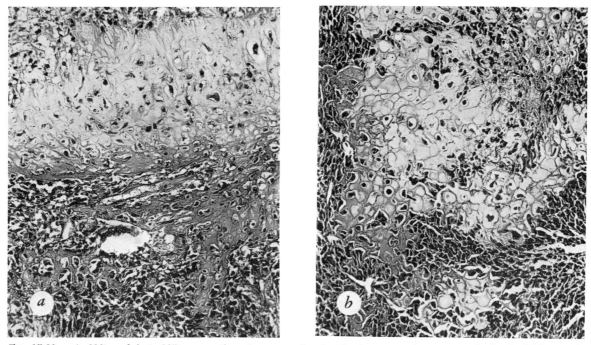

FIG. 17-20. *a* (×110) and *b* (×115) are sections from two chondroblastic osteogenic sarcomas, both of which contain dominating chondroid substance, but both also contain distinct, fine, darker-staining osteoid trabeculae that are derived from neoplastic cells near the bottom of each picture. (Figure 17-22a reproduced with permission from: Coventry, M. B., and Dahlin, D. C.: *J. Bone & Joint Surg., 39A:*741-757, 1957.)

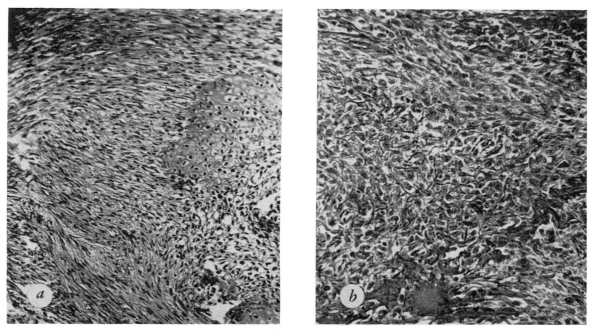

FIG. 17-21. *a.* Fibroblastic osteogenic sarcoma, grade 2, showing a focus of chondrosarcoma in this field (×100). *b.* Another basically fibroblastic tumor which, however, is producing "tumor" osteoid in the lower portion of the picture (×185). (Figure 17-23 *b* reproduced with permission from: Coventry, M. B., and Dahlin, D. C.: *J. Bone & Joint Surg., 39A:*741-757, 1957.)

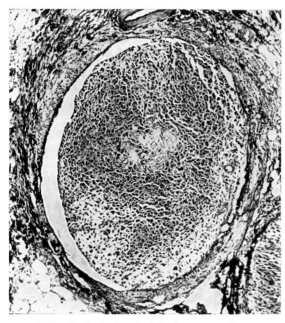

FIG. 17-22. Grade 3 chondroblastic osteogenic sarcoma of the upper end of the humerus, here shown in the lumen of a small regional vein (×70).

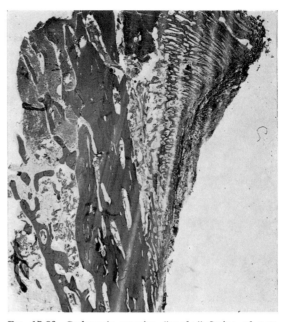

FIG. 17-23. Codman's reactive "angle." Striae of non-neoplastic bone are seen at right angles to the almost vertical broad trabeculae of the invaded cortical bone (×5).

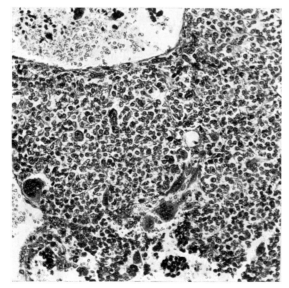

FIG. 17-24. Grade 4 osteogenic sarcoma. In this zone the cells are so small they resemble those of Ewing's tumor, and benign giant cells are present to confuse the issue further (×150).

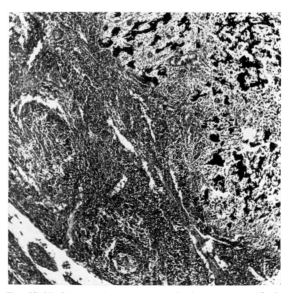

FIG. 17-25. Osteogenic sarcoma producing irregular black masses of osteoid in a lymph node. Lymph nodal metastasis was conspicuously rare in our material (×65).

Postirradiation Sarcoma

Forty-three sarcomas in this total series arose in bones that had received prior irradiation. Twenty-one of these have been reported previously. The interval between irradiation and the diagnosis of sarcoma varied from 3 to 42 years. In 36 cases, the interval was at least 5 years, in 20 at least 10 years, and in 10 at least 20 years. Of the 43 tumors, 23 were osteogenic sarcomas, 18 fibrosarcomas, 1 a chondrosarcoma, and 1 a Ewing tumor. Other unusual tumors following irradiation have been reported. Eighteen of the sarcomas affected major long bones, 9 the jaws, 3 the skull, and the remainder a variety of bones. The reasons for the radiation therapy are listed in Table 5.

TABLE 5

Conditions for Which Irradiation Was Given

Condition	Cases
Giant cell tumor of bone	9
Unverified osseous "lesion"	9
Fibrous dysplasia	6
Aneurysmal bone cyst	3
Benign osteoblastoma	1
Giant cell reparative granuloma	1
Miscellaneous nonosseous lesions	6
Carcinoma of the breast	3
Carcinoma of the uterus	3
Unverified brain tumor	2
Total	43

The miscellaneous nonosseous lesions included three benign cutaneous conditions, one hemangiopericytoma of the orbit, one chemodectoma of the temporal bone, and one instance of indeterminate pain in the shoulder. The nine verified giant cell tumors provided the largest definitive group. Four of the unverified osseous "lesions" were probably giant cell tumors also. The only examples of malignant transformation of fibrous dysplasia in our files are the six tabulated above. Fibrous dysplasia practically never becomes malignant unless irradiated. The three aneurysmal bone cysts that became sarcomatous introduce a note of caution for those who advocate irradiation for this disease. The same applies in the case of benign osteoblastoma, especially with regard to vertebral examples. Sarcoma following irradiation for uterine carcinoma has been reported very few times. An occasional sarcoma of the skull follows irradiation.

These sarcomas were treated as radically as the location of the tumor and the condition of the patient permitted but only four patients remained free of disease for long periods (ranging from 10 to 32 years) after therapy.

This group of cases emphasizes the folly of using radiation therapy in benign conditions for which it has no proved value. A cause-and-effect relationship cannot be established unequivocally in any of these 43 cases, but overwhelming experimental and clinical evidence indicates that one exists. When a patient in the older age group develops osteogenic or fibrosarcoma he should be suspected of having precursors such as Paget's disease or prior irradiation.

OSTEOGENIC SARCOMA

Osteogenic Sarcoma in Paget's Disease

Twenty (3.1%) of the 650 osteogenic sarcomas were complications of Paget's disease. The humerus appears to have a predilection for this problem, and in this series five of nine osteogenic sarcomas of the middle and lower portions of the humerus arose at sites of Paget's disease. The ilium contributed seven cases, the femur five, the tibia two, and the skull 1. In only 2 of the 20 was there a suggestion of multicentric origin of sarcoma. Eleven of the patients were in the seventh decade of life or older, and only 2 were less than 50 years old. Long-term survival for this type of sarcoma is rare but one patient in this series with sarcoma of the femoral head is living 12 years after hindquarter amputation, another with sarcoma of the lower part of the humerus is living 7 years after disarticulation at the shoulder, and a third is living 7 years after biopsy and cobalt-60 irradiation for an 8 by 6 cm lytic sarcoma in an ilium affected by Paget's disease.

Although patients with severe osteitis deformans have perhaps a 10% chance of developing sarcoma, the figure for all patients with Paget's disease is only about 1%. Fibrosarcoma, chondrosarcoma, and even giant cell tumor can complicate Paget's disease, and our series included 2 fibrosarcomas, 1 chondrosarcoma, and 1 giant cell tumor plus the 20 osteogenic sarcomas.

Osteogenic Sarcoma of the Jaws

Several peculiarities of osteogenic sarcoma of jawbones deserve special comment. The average age of the patients is significantly greater than that for conventional sites. This is true regardless of the dominant histologic pattern. Chondroid differentiation is more common; 23 of the 50 tumors in this series were judged to be chondroblastic, 15 osteoblastic, and 12 fibroblastic. Osteoid production may be minimal and difficult to recognize. In fact, some observers believe that some members of the chondroblastic group in this series should be called chondrosarcomas. This is a disagreement of academic interest primarily, as evidenced by observations of Scofield and Garrington who obviously regarded them as chondrosarcomas and found that osteogenic and chondrosarcomas of jaws affected patients of the same ages and gave practically identical 5-year survival rates. Long-term survival was poorer in their chondrosarcoma group. Chondrosarcoma of classic type, as seen in other portions of the skeleton, has been extremely uncommon in my experience.

Grading by the Broders method indicates an appreciably less degree of anaplasia in the osteogenic sarcomas of the jaws. One result is that occasional tumors are differentiated from benign processes with difficulty. Regardless of relatively little anaplasia, chondroid differentiation in a lesion of the jaws should be viewed with alarm, because it is almost never found in a benign process, exclusive of callus, in these bones.

Hematogenous metastasis is much less frequently observed from osteogenic sarcoma of the jaws than from those in more usual sites. Accordingly, wide local excision provides a reasonable chance of curing patients with these tumors.

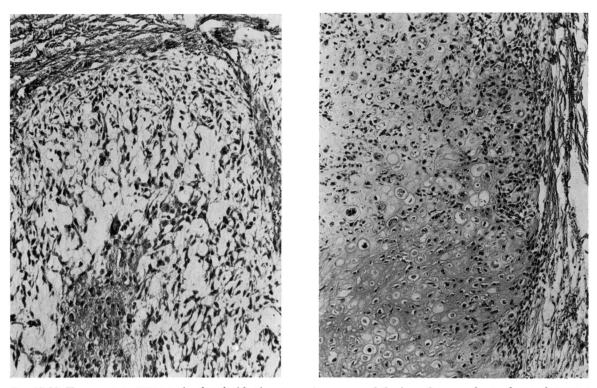

FIG. 17-26. Two common patterns in chondroblastic osteogenic sarcoma of the jaws. Some prefer to class such tumors with the chondrosarcomas. *Left*. Most of this tumor shows chondromyxoid differentiation, but near lower center, homogeneous acidophilic osteoid tissue is seen ($\times$100). *Right*. Despite predominant chondroblastic differentiation, tumors like this produce osteoid in their peripheral portions, such as that along the right side. Regardless of how these tumors are classified, they behave like the more conventional osteogenic sarcomas of the jaws.

Treatment (All Osteogenic Sarcomas)

Because osteogenic sarcoma is a radioresistant neoplasm, ablative surgical treatment is the procedure of choice. Surgical treatment of cancer aimed at cure is based on the premise that the tumor should be removed from the patient before metastasis becomes established. Metastasis obviously must occur at some specific time in the evolution of a given sarcoma. Accordingly, some patients will pay with their lives when treatment is delayed unnecessarily. One must, of course, examine the patient, roentgenograms of his thorax, and possibly the remainder of his skeleton for evidence of metastasis before instituting therapy.

Nearly all osteogenic sarcomas contain small or large foci that require no decalcification prior to sectioning and these foci routinely have the best cytologic details for diagnosis. Good fresh frozen sections are adequate for definitive diagnosis by one familiar with the pathology of bone.

Ordinarily in suspected osteogenic sarcoma of the extremities two tourniquets are applied, one above the tumor and one above the proposed site of amputation, thereby precluding the possible dissemination of tumor emboli by the biopsy procedure. Amputation is performed between the tourniquets after diagnosis by examination of fresh frozen sections of biopsy material. Extreme care should be employed to prevent implantation of tumor cells at the definitive amputation level. Those averse to diagnosis by fresh frozen sections should have permanent sections of nearly all osteogenic sarcomas ready for diagnosis in 1 day's time. Detailed study of heavily ossified portions of the tumor or adjacent cortical bone is rarely necessary in establishing the correct diagnosis.

A good rule is to amputate through the bone above the affected bone, but it requires modification in the treatment of the common sarcomas of the distal portion of the femur. Data have not yet proved whether disarticulation at the hip is preferable to amputation through the upper part of the femur for these. Since a small percentage of osteogenic sarcomas show marked spread in the marrow, it is mandatory that the level of transection be checked to determine the adequacy of any amputation through the affected bone. Hindquarter amputations are necessary for tumors of the upper end of the femur and some of those in the innominate bone, and forequarter amputations for those of the upper part of the humerus. Lymph nodes are so rarely involved that dissection of nodes is probably not indicated unless they are enlarged.

Radical local excision should be employed whenever possible for those tumors not in the extremities. Local excision of osteogenic sarcoma in the extremities is rarely, if ever, indicated.

Radiation therapy is indicated for those tumors not amenable to ablative surgical treatment. Irradiation prior to amputation has been advocated recently, but whether such treatment will affect the cure rate favorably or unfavorably is as yet unknown.

A growing number of patients in whom a localized pulmonary metastatic growth develops after the primary one has been controlled have had pulmonary resection. The overall value of such resections for metastatic osteogenic sarcoma is not yet known, but some long-term survivals, including two in this series, have been effected.

Prognosis

The 5-year survival rate for 408 eligible patients in this series was 20.3% and the 10-year rate for 359 patients was 17.3%. More than 99% of patients in these groups had been traced. All patients who had no known metastasis and who had their definitive treatment at the Mayo Clinic are included in these survival data. Seven are known to have died of their sarcomas more than 5 years after therapy. For reasons unknown, tumors of the tibia were more favorable than those of the femur, the 5-year survival rates being 36.6 and 18.6% respectively. The 5-year survival rates for the osteoblastic, chondroblastic, and fibroblastic types were 17.1, 22.3, and 25.5% respectively. The highly undifferentiated sarcomas had but a slightly poorer prognosis than the better differentiated minority. Age did not have a significant bearing on prognosis. Three patients with sarcomas complicating Paget's disease survived, as did four who had irradiation alone, at least 5 years.

These relatively favorable data on a large series of patients should help dispel the unfounded notion held by some that the prognosis of osteogenic sarcoma is so poor that prompt and proper therapy is useless.

Bibliography

1955   Cade, Stanford: Osteogenic Sarcoma: A Study Based on 133 Patients. *J. Roy. Coll. Surgeons Edinburgh, 1:*79-111.

1956   Sabanas, A. O., Dahlin, D. C., Childs, D. S., Jr., and Ivins, J. C.: Postradiation Sarcoma of of Bone. *Cancer, 9:*528-542.

1956   Fine, G, and Stout, A. P.: Osteogenic Sarcoma of the Extraskeletal Soft Tissues. *Cancer, 9:*1027-1043.

1957   Coventry, M. B., and Dahlin, D. C.: Osteogenic Sarcoma: Critical Analysis of 430 Cases. *J. Bone & Joint Surg., 39A:*741-757.

1957   Porretta, C. A., Dahlin, D. C., and Janes, J. M.: Sarcoma in Paget's Disease of Bone. *J. Bone & Joint Surg., 39A:*1314-1329.

1958   Kragh, L. V., Dahlin, D. C., and Erich, J. B.: Osteogenic Sarcoma of the Jaws and Facial Bones. *Am. J. Surg., 96:*496-505.

1961   Bacon, G. A., and Moe, J. H.: Primary Bone Tumor Study 1940-1956. *Univ. Minnesota M. Bull., 32:*312-319.

1961   Tanner, H. C., Dahlin, D. C., and Childs, D. S.: Sarcoma Complicating Fibrous Dysplasia. *Oral Surg., 14:*837-846.

1961   Lindbom, Å., Söderberg, G., and Spjut, H. J.: Osteosarcoma. A Review of 96 Cases. *Acta radiol., 56:*1-19.

1962   Platt, Sir H.: Survival in Bone Sarcoma. *Acta Orthop. scandinav., 32:*267-280.

1962   Wende, S.: Sarkom der Schädelkalotte nach Röntgentherapie. *Fortschr. Geb. Röntgenstrahlen, 96:*278-282.

1962   Ackerman, L. V., and Spjut, H. J.: *Tumors of Bone and Cartilage.* Atlas of Tumor Pathology, Section II, Fascicle 4, Armed Forces Institute of Pathology, Washington, D.C., National Research Council, pp. 82-97.

1963   Aegerter, E., and Kirkpatrick, J. A.: *Orthopedic Diseases,* Ed. 2, *Philadelphia,* W. B. Saunders Co., pp. 554-560.

1963   Brody, G. L., and Fry, L. R.: Osteogenic Sarcoma: Experience at The University of Michigan. *Univ. Michigan M. Bull., 29:*80-87.

1964   McKenna, R. J., Schwinn, C. P., Soong, K. Y., and Higinbotham, N. L.: Osteogenic Sarcoma Arising in Paget's Disease. *Cancer, 17:*42-66.

1964   Lee, E. S., and MacKenzie, D. H.: Osteosarcoma: A Study of the Value of Preoperative Megavoltage Radiotherapy. *Brit. J. Surg., 51:*252-274.

1965   Steiner, G. C.: Postradiation Sarcoma of Bone. *Cancer, 18:*603-612.

1965   Lichtenstein, L.: *Bone Tumors,* Ed. 3, St. Louis, The C. V. Mosby Company, pp. 202-228.

1965   Scofield, H. H., and Garrington, G. E.: *Osteogenic Sarcoma and Chondrosarcoma of the Jaws.* Exhibit at the annual Meeting of the American Society of Clinical Pathologists, October.

1966   McKenna, R. J., Schwinn, C. P., Soong, K. Y., and Higinbotham, N. L.: Sarcomata of the Osteogenic Series (Osteosarcoma, Fibrosarcoma, Chondrosarcoma, Parosteal Osteogenic Sarcoma, and Sarcomata Arising in Abnormal Bone): An Analysis of 552 Cases. *J. Bone & Joint Surg., 48A:*1-26.

Chapter 18

Parosteal Osteogenic Sarcoma (Juxtacortical Osteogenic Sarcoma)

This tumor is considered separately from the remainder of the osteogenic sarcomas because it is distinctly less malignant and, therefore, has a vastly different clinical behavior. As the name implies, this tumor is on the outer surface of the cortex of a bone, and some prefer to call it a juxtacortical sarcoma.

The rarity of this lesion, comprising less than 4% of osteogenic sarcomas, has delayed its general recognition. Although occasional typical cases were documented in the literature, it was not until the description of a collected series by Geschickter and Copeland in 1951 that the entity was established. There are gradations from the even more uncommon, completely benign parosteal osteoma, through the lesion with minimal evidence of malignancy to the frankly malignant, though fairly well-differentiated, parosteal tumor. It is obvious that when the diagnosis of sarcoma depends on such subtle changes as are found in some of these tumors the problem is often a difficult one.

Osteogenic tumors of a high degree of malignancy histologically (that is, of high grade by the method of Broders) are occasionally seen predominantly on the surface of a bone but they do not belong in the category under discussion. Inclusion of tumors that are histologically like the ordinary osteogenic sarcoma or fibrosarcoma will decrease the usefulness of the term "parosteal osteogenic sarcoma."

Although there is a rare benign counterpart of parosteal osteogenic sarcoma (Figures 6-4, 5, and 6), our series suggests that the usual tumor of this type is an indolent malignant growth from its inception and the dense basal region of the tumor results from progressive ossification of this older portion.

There are very rare, extremely well-differentiated osteogenic sarcomas that begin within bone. Reference to the roentgenogram or to the gross specimen may be required in differentiating them from parosteal osteogenic sarcoma. Correct diagnosis and proper management of patients with these tumors is heavily dependent on judgment based on experience with them.

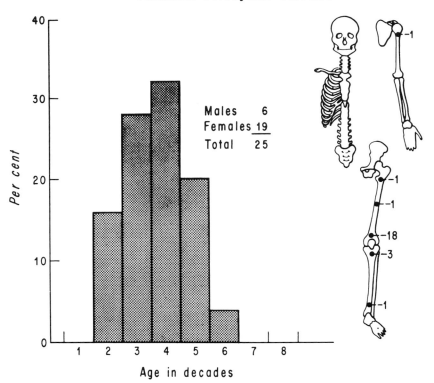

FIG. 18-1. Skeletal, age, and sex distribution of parosteal osteogenic sarcoma.

Incidence

Parosteal sarcoma is a distinctly rare neoplasm. It comprised less than 1% of the Mayo Clinic series of malignant tumors primary in bone.

Sex

Females constituted 76% of the patients in this series, but males have predominated in some series. Two tumors of the humerus in males, from our earlier group, have been deleted, one because it contained no definitely malignant zones and the other because it is now considered to be an ossified subperiosteal hematoma.

Age

The average age of patients with this tumor is greater than that of those with ordinary osteogenic sarcoma, a difference that can be explained at least in part by its slow growth.

Localization

Practically all of the recorded parosteal osteogenic sarcomas have involved the femur, humerus, and tibia, in that order of frequency. Other bones may, however, be affected. By far the most common site for its development is the distal portion of the shaft of the femur posteriorly. In common with the ordinary osteogenic sarcoma, this lesion most often affects the metaphyseal region.

177

PAROSTEAL OSTEOGENIC SARCOMA

Symptoms

Swelling is the most important symptom. Because of the inherent slow growth of the tumor, the swelling is often of several years' duration. Sometimes the patient has noted swelling for only a few days or weeks, when it is obvious from the roentgenograms and the pathologic characteristics that the lesion has been present for much longer. The tumor may be painful.

A common and practically pathognomonic history is as follows: Several years previously the patient underwent excision of a tumor that had been considered to be an atypical osteochondroma roentgenologically. The pathologist regarded it as an unusual osteochondroma, and perhaps described it as cellular. In the interim, the tumor may or may not have required repeated excision because of recurrence. When seen now, there is a recurrent, ossified juxtacortical mass in one of the sites of predilection.

Physical Findings

A mass at the lesional site, which is sometimes painful to pressure, is the only significant physical finding. The mass may be of enormous size.

Roentgenologic Features

The tumor is seen to be juxtacortical and usually has a remarkable tendency to encircle the shaft. This is best demonstrated by stereoscopic roentgenograms. It is seen to be firmly attached to the cortex along a part of its broad base, but it tends to grow peripherally in mushroom fashion to lie in proximity to, but not necessarily attached to, the remainder of the underlying shaft which it encircles. In most cases, therefore, there is a partially free space of varying length and 1 to 3 mm in thickness between the tumor and the underlying bone. Ordinarily the tumor is lobular in outline, but sometimes angular projections extend into the soft tissues. From 75 to 90% of the tumor's bulk shows a variable, usually marked, degree of ossification. The periphery of the tumor is typically less ossified than its base. Numerous poorly defined and irregular radiolucent defects are ordinarily seen in the substance of the tumor because of zones of irregular fibrous or cartilaginous tissue. Ordinarily the osseous mass is amorphous, but occasionally true osseous trabeculation may be observed. Periosteal elevation at the edge of the tumor and consequently Codman's angle are conspicuously absent. Medullary involvement ordinarily does not occur except in extremely long-standing tumors or especially in tumors that have been previously treated unsuccessfully. Even recurrent tumors, however, are usually still juxtacortical.

The roentgenogram is important in the differential diagnosis. The heterotopic bone seen in myositis ossificans usually shows a well-organized and clear-cut trabecular pattern in contrast to what is seen in parosteal osteogenic sarcoma. Although the lesion of myositis ossificans may abut on a bone and especially overlap it when seen on only one roentgenographic projection, careful study will show that it does not have the characteristic broad base of parosteal osteogenic sarcoma.

Osteochondroma (osteocartilaginous exostosis) can ordinarily be differentiated with assurance from parosteal osteogenic sarcoma from the roentgenographic standpoint. The continuity of the bony cortex with the pedunculated or sessile base of an osteochondroma as well as the continuity of the cancellous bone with the core of an osteochondroma is absent in parosteal osteogenic sarcoma. Evidence of cortical destruction, extensive medullary involvement, Codman's reactive angle, and an ill-defined border differentiate ordinary osteogenic sarcoma from parosteal osteogenic sarcoma. Occasional benign parosteal osteomas, which in the author's experience are much less common than the malignant counterpart under discussion may be impossible to differentiate on a roentgenographic basis. This fact is not surprising when one realizes the differentiation is so subtle that it can sometimes be made with no real assurance even by the histopathologist.

The roentgenogram is usually so characteristic that the correct diagnosis of parosteal osteogenic sarcoma, especially in advanced cases, is practically certain on this basis alone.

Gross Pathology

Although these tumors merge with the cortex of the affected bone, they do not disrupt it until late, and ordinarily only after one or more recurrences following inadequate therapy. Accordingly, medullary involvement is a late phenomenon if it occurs at all.

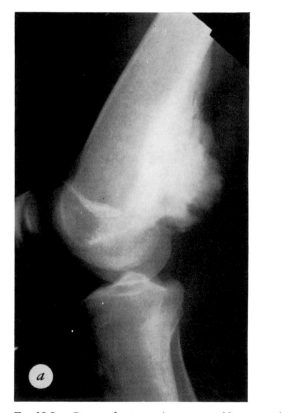 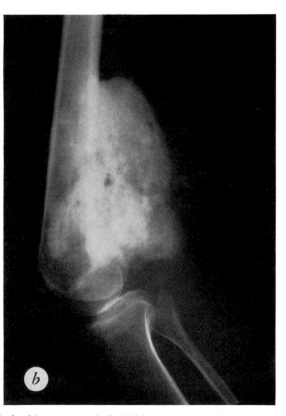

FIG. 18-2. *a.* Parosteal osteogenic sarcoma of lower portion of shaft of femur posteriorly. Without stereoscopic views, the absence of medullary involvement is not apparent. This tumor recurred within a year after local excision. *b.* This tumor of the femur had been present for 7 years. At the time of biopsy and amputation, zones of grade 2 sarcoma were present, but there was still no medullary involvement. The patient died with pulmonary metastases 6 years after amputation. (Reproduced with permission from: Dwinnell, L. A., Dahlin, D. C., and Ghormley, R. K.: *J. Bone & Joint Surg., 36A:*732-744, 1954.)

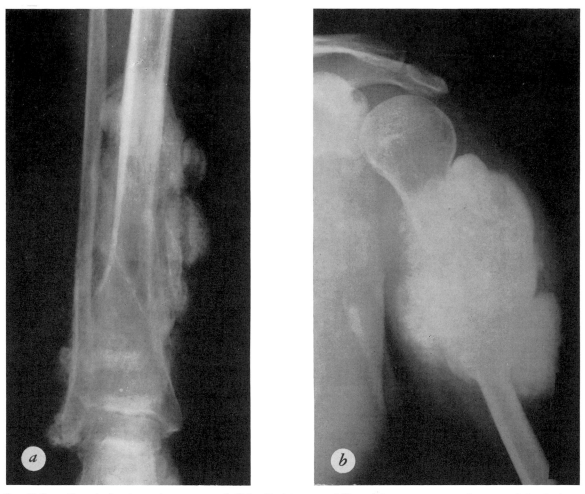

Fig. 18-3. *a.* Parosteal osteogenic sarcoma of tibia. Excision was followed by recurrence and eventual death from metastasis. *b.* This parosteal sarcoma encased the upper portion of the shaft of the humerus. Local removal was unsuccessful in controlling the lesion. (Reproduced with permission from: Dwinnell, L. A., Dahlin, D. C., and Ghormley, R. K.: *J. Bone & Joint Surg., 36A:732-744,* 1954.)

As indicated by the roentgenograms, these tumors are predominantly ossified. Ordinarily, however, there are softer, fibrous foci, especially near or at the periphery of the neoplasms. These zones are the ones most likely to afford histologic evidence of malignancy. Small or prominent chondroid foci are often found in these lesions.

Recurrent tumors of this type, especially when they show an increased degree of malignancy histologically, may be only slightly sclerotic if at all. In fact, such lesions may simulate closely the appearance of ordinary osteogenic sarcomas.

Myositis ossificans, which must be considered in the differential diagnosis, is often completely separated from the bone. When it does abut on bone it rarely coapts itself to the cortex so as to produce an extensive broad base such as that seen in parosteal osteogenic sarcoma. Another important differential feature is the maturation and ossification usually found first in the peripheral portion of a mass of benign heterotopic ossification, whereas the advancing edge of these sarcomas is nearly always the least mature and the least ossified part.

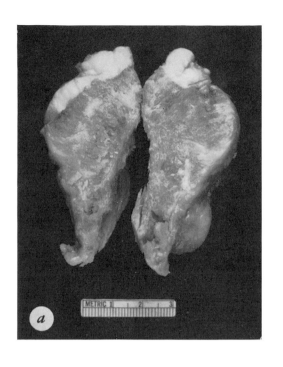
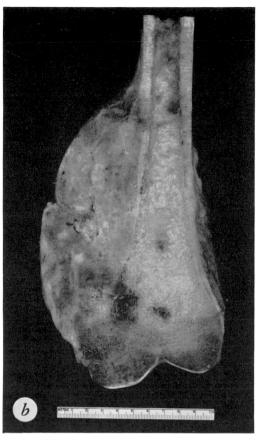

FIG. 18-4. *a*. Cut surface of parosteal osteogenic sarcoma illustrated in Figure 18-2*a*. Local excision was followed by recurrence within a year, and amputation was performed. *b*. Gross specimen of the lesion shown in Figure 18-2*b*. Although this tumor had been present for 7 years, there was no medullary involvement. (Reproduced with permission from: Dwinnell, L. A., Dahlin, D. C., and Ghormley, R. K.: *J. Bone & Joint Surg.*, *36A*:732-744, 1954.)

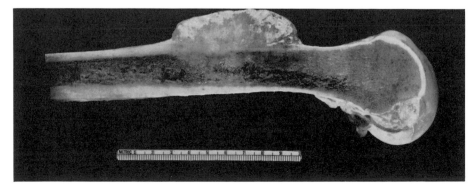

FIG. 18-5. Although this tumor resembles a parosteal osteogenic sarcoma of the ordinary type, it is actually a high-grade osteogenic sarcoma and does not belong in the indolent pathologic variety under discussion.

Histopathology

The most prominent feature of parosteal osteogenic sarcoma is its component of rather regularly arranged osseous trabeculae. Apparently the more immature trabeculae undergo maturation in this slowly developing tumor and become "normalized." Between these more or less normal trabeculae are atypical, proliferating, spindle-shaped or polyhedral cells in which one finds occasional or sometimes fairly numerous mitotic figures. The spaces between the trabeculae are not filled with fat or hematopoietic cells as in osteochondroma. This fact alone serves clearly to differentiate osteocartilaginous exostosis from parosteal osteogenic sarcoma. The same atypical spindle cell elements alluded to make up the purely fibrous zones of these tumors. Evidence of malignancy may be found only in small foci, making it necessary to study multiple sections for accurate appraisal. Variable amounts of osteoid are found deposited in the proliferating spindle cell stroma, apparently owing to metaplasia of the basically fibroblastic cells into a type capable of producing osteoid. This osteoid matures into the bony trabeculae. Islands of chondrosarcoma are commonly seen in these tumors.

Occasional tumors in this group show an increase in histologic activity with recurrence.

The majority of parosteal osteogenic sarcomas reveal, at their peripheries, an intermixing with muscle and fat cells. This finding has added to the confusion that exists in the differentiation of this malignant tumor from myositis ossificans, and pathologically suggests a kinship with desmoid tumors of the soft tissues of the extremities.

Differentiation of this malignant tumor from myositis ossificans histologically depends on the lack of true anaplasia in the proliferating cells of the latter lesion. Gross and roentgenographic guidance should direct one's suspicion, as indicated above. Similar criteria aid in the recognition of benign heterotopic ossification of other kinds including that resulting from avulsion of periosteum from any cause. Cytologic evidences of activity, including numerous mitotic figures, may be found in these benign conditions.

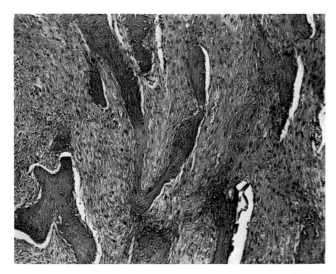

FIG. 18-6. Typical microscopic field from a parosteal osteogenic sarcoma. Note well-formed osseous trabeculae separated by actively proliferating fibroblastic tissue that is undergoing metaplasia to a type capable of producing osteoid substance and bone ($\times$100).

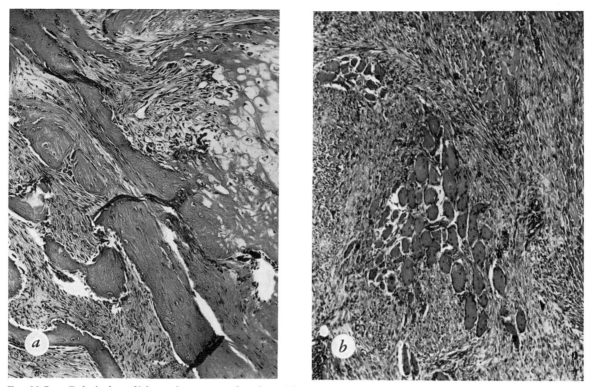

FIG. 18-7. *a.* Relatively well-formed osseous trabeculae with intervening fibroblastic tissue and chondroid zone (×100). *b.* Periphery of parosteal osteogenic sarcoma showing invasion of striated muscle, large fibers of which are here shown in cross section (×80). (Reproduced with permission from: Dwinnell, L. A., Dahlin, D. C., and Ghormley, R. K.: *J. Bone & Joint Surg., 36A:732-744, 1954.*)

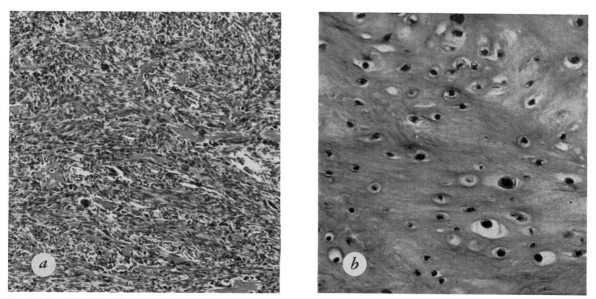

FIG. 18-8. *a.* Peripheral zone of grade 2 fibrosarcoma in tumor illustrated in Figures 18-2*b* and 18-4*b. b.* Island of chondrosarcoma from one of these tumors (×200). (Reproduced with permission from: Dwinnell, L. A., Dahlin, D. C., and Ghormley, R. K.: *J. Bone & Joint Surg., 36A:732-744, 1954.*)

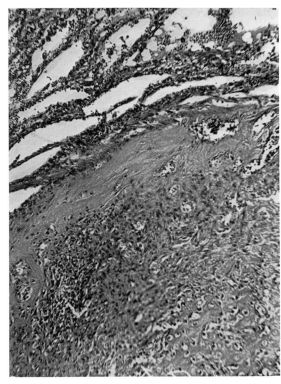

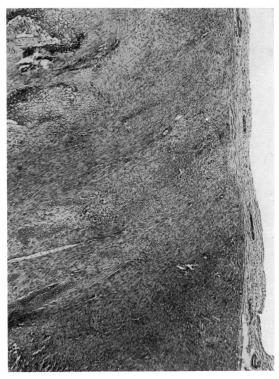

FIG. 18-9. Nodule of metastatic parosteal sarcoma in lung ($\times$100). Death from metastasis occurred 20 years after the first surgical treatment for a lesion of the distal portion of the femur and 6 years after amputation.

FIG. 18-10. Typical cellular fibroblastic advancing edge of parosteal osteogenic sarcoma ($\times$35).

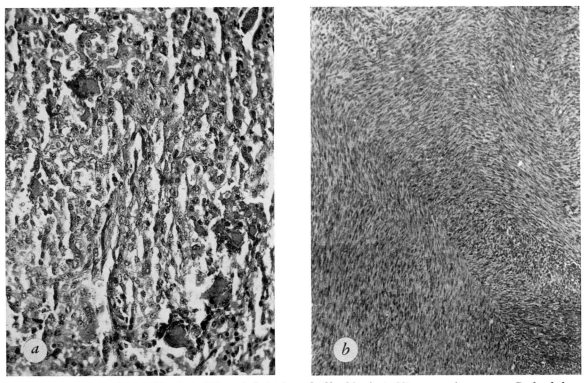

FIG. 18-11. *a*. High-grade osteoblastic ($\times$200) and, *b*, high-grade fibroblastic ($\times$80) osetogenic sarcomas. Both of these were found in recurrent tumors that followed local excision for parosteal osteogenic sarcoma. (Figure 18-11*b* reproduced with permission from: Dwinnell, L. A., Dahlin, D. C., and Ghormley, R. K.: *J. Bone & Joint Surg., 36A:*732-744, 1954.)

Treatment

Studies of several series now reported support the following conclusions. Simple excision practically inevitably leads to recurrence. If the tumor has indisputable, albeit minimal, histologic evidence of malignancy, amputation is the treatment of choice for those tumors that are large or recurrent. For small, nonrecurrent parosteal osteogenic sarcomas it may be feasible to employ resection, but the surgeon must be able to encompass the tumor widely, getting well into normal bone and uninvolved soft tissues.

If critical analysis, which may require study of the entire tumor, fails to uncover proof that the tumor is malignant, wide local excision and careful follow-up studies are indicated.

A factor of importance in contemplating conservative management is that these tumors may increase in histologic activity with recurrence, and some become highly malignant, rapidly metastasizing sarcomas.

Prognosis

Six of our 25 patients have died with metastases; all but one of these had local excision as their primary treatment and had at least one recurrence before amputation was performed.

The indolent behavior of parosteal osteogenic sarcoma is emphasized by one of the fatal cases. A recurring tumor of the lower end of the femur was subjected to six excisions during a 14-year period. Then amputation was performed but the patient succumbed, with proved pulmonary metastasis, 6 years after amputation and 20 years after the first excision.

Early adequate treatment should cure the majority of patients.

Bibliography

1951   Geschickter, C. F., and Copeland, M. M.: Parosteal Osteoma of Bone: A New Entity. *Ann. Surg., 133:*790-806.

1954   Dwinnell, L. A., Dahlin, D. C., and Ghormley, R. K.: Parosteal (Juxtacortical) Osteogenic Sarcoma. *J. Bone & Joint Surg., 36A:*732-744.

1957   Stevens, G. M., Pugh, D. G., and Dahlin, D. C.: Roentgenographic Recognition and Differentiation of Parosteal Osteogenic Sarcoma. *Am. J. Roentgenol., 78:*1-12.

1959   D'Aubigné, R. M., Meary, R., and Mazabrand, A.: Sarcome Ostéogénique Juxtacortical. *Rev. chir. orthop., 45:*873-884.

1959   Copeland, M. M., and Geschickter, C. F.: The Treatment of Parosteal Osteoma of Bone. *Surg., Gynec., & Obst., 108:*537-548.

1962   Scaglietti, O., and Calandriello, B.: Ossifying Parosteal Sarcoma: Parosteal Osteoma or Juxtacortical Osteogenic Sarcoma. *J. Bone & Joint Surg., 44A:*635-647.

Chapter 19

Ewing's Tumor

Ewing's tumor is a distinctive, small round cell sarcoma that is the most lethal of the bone tumors. It is the subject of controversy in the literature because of the somewhat nonspecific histologic characteristics of the tumor, which is composed of solidly packed, small cells. Until recently some of the small cell osteogenic sarcomas, most of the reticulum cell sarcomas, and even benign conditions such as eosinophilic granuloma were at times classified with Ewing's tumor.

A practical working definition is to regard as Ewing's tumors those highly anaplastic, small round to oval cell sarcomas that have the clinical and radiologic characteristics of a primary osseous lesion. Inherent in this concept is the exclusion of cytologically incompatible lesions such as myeloma, malignant lymphoma, and histiocytosis X. Production of a chondroid or osteoid matrix by the neoplastic cells likewise excludes Ewing's sarcoma. It is sometimes impossible to differentiate a biopsy specimen of a metastatic malignant tumor such as neuroblastoma, small cell cancer of the lung, or even leukemic infiltrate from a specimen of Ewing's tumor even after critical histologic study according to modern concepts. From the practical standpoint, however, when the physician, after careful study of the patient, is confronted with what is clinically a primary lesion in bone that is typical of Ewing's tumor, he is obliged to treat it as such and he will rarely make a significant error. Armchair meditations regarding whether the tumor being appraised may possibly be a metastatic lesion from an undisclosed primary tumor can usually be verified only after studies at necropsy.

Speculation regarding the possible origin of the cells that comprise Ewing's tumor has been fruitless, and it seems best to regard them as arising from undifferentiated mesenchyme.

Although Ewing's tumor and reticulum cell sarcoma can be distinguished histologically in the majority of cases, occasional tumors appear to fall midway between them. In the present series there were tumors which contained cells that were larger and somewhat more irregular than those of classic Ewing's tumor. Their clinical characteristics and prognosis made it seem most practical to include them with Ewing's tumors rather than to attempt to segregate a new tumor type.

A soft tissue counterpart of Ewing's sarcoma is occasionally encountered.

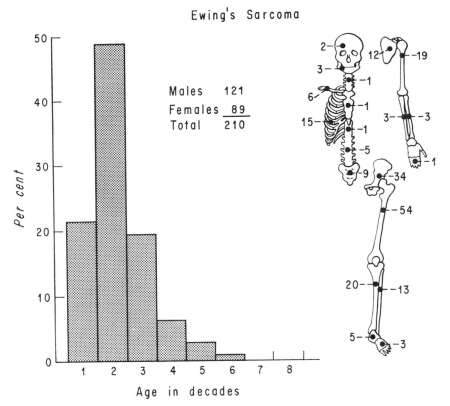

FIG. 19-1. Skeletal, age, and sex distribution of Ewing's tumor.

Incidence

Ewing's tumor comprised slightly more than 7% of the total malignant tumors in the Mayo Clinic series.

Sex

Ewing's tumor has a distinct predilection for males.

Age

The persons affected by this tumor are, on the average, younger than those affected by any other primary malignant tumor of bone. The youngest patient in the present series was 18 months of age; two others were less than 5 years old. When confronted with the problem of Ewing's tumor in patients who are past the third decade of life, one must be especially careful to exclude metastatic carcinoma. In the very young, metastatic neuroblastoma and even acute leukemia must be considered.

Localization

A majority of Ewing's tumors are in the extremities, but any bone of the body may be involved. Any portion of a long tubular bone may be affected. The lower extremities and pelvic girdle accounted for 61.4% of the tumors in this series. Sixteen involved the spinal column, including the sacrum, and the fibula accounted for 13 cases. Three were in metatarsals and one in the proximal phalanx of a finger.

187

EWING'S TUMOR

Symptoms

Pain and swelling are the commonest symptoms of Ewing's tumor. Pain is the first symptom in well over half the cases. It may be intermittent at first, and it tends to increase in severity with time. Although swelling in the region of the tumor is common by the time the patient seeks medical advice, it is rarely the first symptom. Pathologic fracture is unusual. The average patient has had symptoms for several months before he seeks medical care.

Physical and Laboratory Findings

The majority of patients have a palpable tender mass and some have dilated veins over the tumor. The patient should be thoroughly examined, searching for evidence of a primary tumor, or for indications of metastatic disease, elsewhere.

Patients with Ewing's tumor sometimes have an elevated temperature, often associated with some secondary anemia and sometimes with leukocytosis. These findings may suggest that the osseous lesion is inflammatory in origin. It has been found that Ewing's tumor, when associated with these systemic features, has a prognosis that is even worse than average.

Roentgenologic Features

Ewing's tumor tends to be extensive, sometimes involving the entire shaft of a long bone. Even so, more of the bone will be found involved pathologically than was obvious from the roentgenogram, in the average case. Lytic destruction is the most common finding but there may be regions of density owing to stimulation of new bone formation. As the tumor bursts through the cortex, which may show only minimal roentgenographic changes, it often elevates the periosteum in stages. This produces the characteristic multiple layers of subperiosteal reactive new bone which gives the "onionskin" appearance of Ewing's tumor. Radiating spicules from the cortex of an affected bone are not uncommon, a fact which complicates the differentiation from osteogenic sarcoma. When the initial roentgenogram shows extensive destruction of bone combined with a large extraosseous mass, the lesion is usually clearly malignant. Occasionally Ewing's tumor produces an expansion of the affected bone and may even superficially resemble a cyst.

Rare examples of Ewing's sarcoma have little or no medullary component. A few are almost completely in a juxtaosseous position and show but little cortical destruction of part of a bone's circumference.

Experienced observers have concluded that although Ewing's tumor can sometimes be diagnosed with a high degree of assurance from its roentgenologic features and although it very often produces features that are virtually pathognomonic of malignant bone tumor, there are a number of conditions that can produce a similar picture. Among these are acute or chronic osteomyelitis, eosinophilic granuloma, malignant lymphoma, metastatic malignant tumor, and even osteogenic sarcoma.

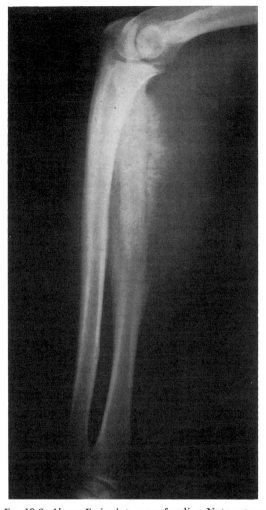

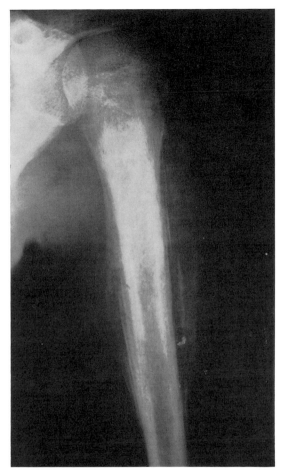

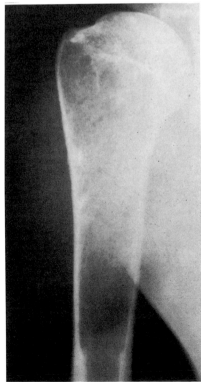

FIG. 19-2. *Above*. Ewing's tumor of radius. Note prominent radial spicules in periosseous tissues. (Reproduced with permission from: McCormack, L J., Dockerty, M. B., and Ghormley, R. K.: *Cancer, 5:*85-99, 1952.)

FIG. 19-3. *Above, right*. Ewing's tumor of humerus showing multiple layers of subperiosteal, reactive, new, non-neoplastic bone. (Reproduced with permission from McCormack, L. J., Dockerty, M B., and Ghormley, R. K.: *Cancer, 5:*85-99, 1952.)

FIG. 19-4. *Right*. Ewing's tumor producing cyst-like rarefaction of upper one third of humerus. There was no definite cortical breakthrough.

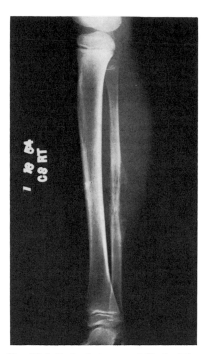

FIG. 19-5. Ewing's tumor of fibula. The gross lesion is shown in Figure 19-7, the histology in Figure 19-10.

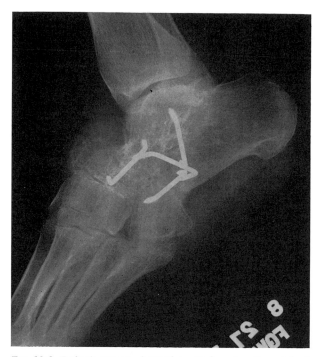

FIG. 19-6. Ewing's tumor of tarsal navicular. An attempt had been made to produce arthrodesis, pursuant to an erroneous diagnosis. The gross lesion is shown in Figure 19-8.

Gross Pathology

Solid masses of viable tumor are characteristically gray-white, moist, glistening, and somewhat translucent. They may be almost liquid in consistency. Tumor frequently invades bone beyond the limits suggested by the roentgenogram. Zones of necrosis, hemorrhage, and even cyst formation are common. The neoplastic tissue is often admixed with proliferating bony and fibrous tissue in the periosseous regions.

The medullary cavity appears to be the site of origin of nearly all of these tumors. Although they may affect any portion of a long bone and commonly involve a great length of it, the bulk of the tumor is frequently in the metaphyseal region.

Metastasis is characteristically to the lungs and to other bones. The latter feature is so prominent that some have suggested that Ewing's tumor may have a multicentric origin.

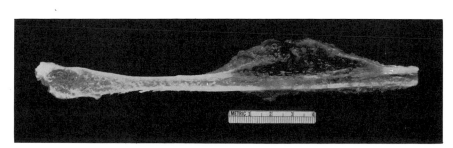

FIG. 19-7. Gross specimen from the case represented in Figure 19-5. The patient is alive and well 10 years after amputation above the knee.

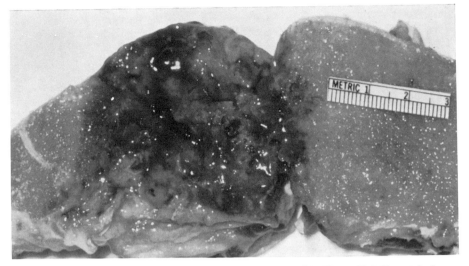

FIG. 19-8. Ewing's tumor of tarsus. This is the case represented in Figure 19-6. Note gelatinous, almost fluid consistency of the tumor. The patient is alive and well 10 years after amputation. The histology of this tumor is shown in Figures 19-11a and 19-12a.

Histopathology

Even with low-power magnification the microscopist observes that Ewing's tumor is remarkably cellular and that there is little intercellular stroma except for widely separated strands of fibrous tissue. These strands compartmentalize the cellular aggregates into zones that are sometimes larger than the area covered by a low-power microscopic field. The cells that lie in the compartments are noteworthy for their regularity when studied under higher magnification, and they have round to oval nuclei. The cytoplasm surrounding these nuclei is slightly granular and the cell outlines are indistinct. The nuclei themselves contain a rather finely dispersed chromatin that imparts a "ground-glass" appearance. Nucleoli may be present but they are inconspicuous. Mitotic figures are rarely numerous.

Special stains disclose that there is little stainable reticulin within the compartments described above. Minor variation in nuclear size from region to region in one of these tumors is often explained by the fact that some zones are undergoing necrosis and the nuclei are degenerating. The perithelial pattern that has led to the belief that this tumor arises from blood vascular endothelial cells is sometimes prominent. Collars of viable cells often surround small blood vessels, and beyond these viable collars the cells are necrotic, a histologic pattern that is best explained on a nutritional basis and one that seems unlikely to be explained on the basis of derivation of the tumor.

Occasionally one encounters a tumor the cells of which contain nuclei that are somewhat larger and less regular in shape than are those of an average Ewing tumor. The general histologic structure is otherwise like the remainder of the Ewing group. These larger-celled lesions do not have the specific cytologic features of the malignant lymphomas. Their prognosis is very poor and it seems appropriate to regard them as variants of Ewing's tumor.

The presence of reactive osseous and fibroblastic tissue resulting from periosteal elevation and

191

invasion of soft tissues as well as large zones of necrosis may complicate the histologic picture.

Schajowicz (1959) advocated the glycogen stain in the differentiation of Ewing's sarcoma from reticulum cell sarcoma, stating that the cells of the former tumor contain glycogen whereas those of the latter do not.

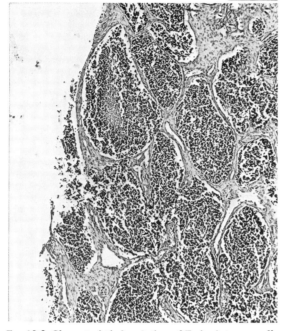

FIG. 19-9. Characteristic loculation of Ewing's tumor cells by septa of connective tissue that are widely separated (×50).

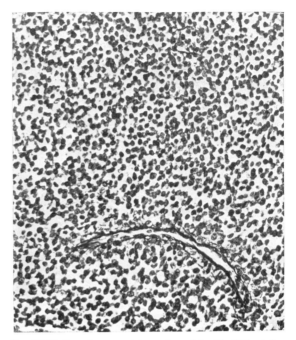

FIG. 19-10. Regular round to oval nuclei with little stainable reticulin are characteristic of Ewing's tumor (reticulin stain; ×250).

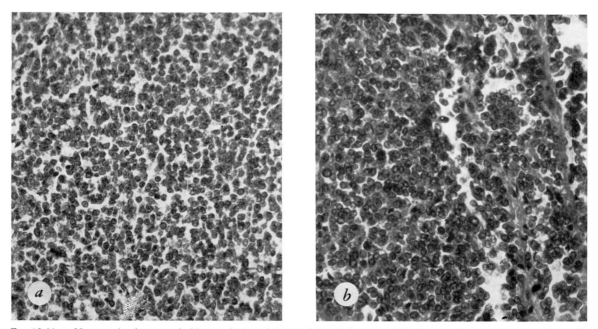

FIG. 19-11. *a*. Note again the remarkable regularity of the nuclei and the poor delimitation of the cytoplasm of the cells of these tumors. Practically no ground substance is present (×265). *b*. Another photomicrograph to emphasize the features already described (×285).

192

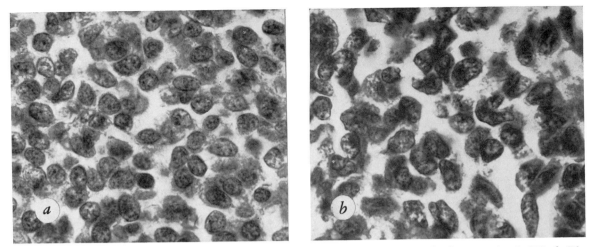

FIG. 19-12. *a.* Typical Ewing's tumor with round and oval nuclei, all of approximately the same size ($\times 800$). *b.* The larger-cell type of Ewing's tumor. Note that the nuclei are more irregular in shape ($\times 800$).

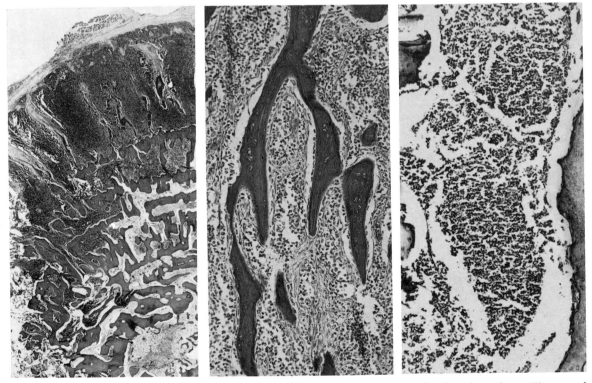

FIG. 19-13. *Left.* Ewing's tumor of fibula showing "onionskin" layers and vertical trabeculae of new bone. The central part of the tumor, at lower right, is necrotic ($\times 8$). *Center.* Ewing's tumor cells among trabeculae of new bone. Early reactive osteoid clumps like these may be confused with the osteoid produced by malignant cells ($\times 100$). *Right.* Infiltrate of acute leukemia in the femur of a 2-year-old. It was erroneously interpreted as Ewing's sarcoma prior to hematologic investigation ($\times 100$).

Treatment

Opinion is divided as to whether irradiation or ablative surgical treatment is best for Ewing's tumor. The rarity of the tumor and the low incidence of cure makes it difficult to procure convincing data on this point. Amputation has the advantage that it assures control of the local lesion. It sometimes becomes necessary as a palliative measure whether the primary tumor has been irradiated or not. Bhansali and Desai (1963) concluded, after reviewing the literature, that "surgery appears to be the superior treatment when feasible." Nevertheless, most authorities consider irradiation the mainstay of therapy for Ewing's tumor. My preference is to amputate for Ewing's sarcomas located below the midfemur. An increasing number of long-term survivors following irradiation of metastases are being documented. Chemotherapy for this tumor is being evaluated.

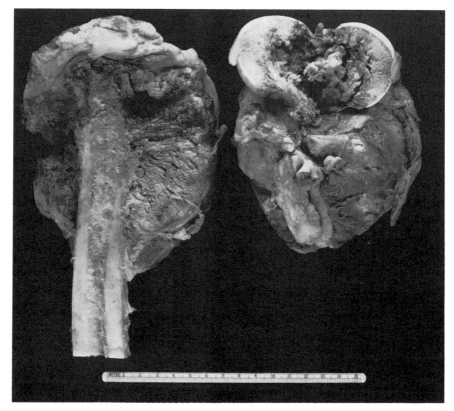

FIG. 19-14. Ewing's tumor from a long-term survivor. This recurrent lesion, 13 by 12 by 10 cm, of the upper portion of the femur in a 22-year-old man, was removed by hindquarter amputation after several courses of irradiation, the first of which had been given 4 years previously. Pulmonary metastases were demonstrated by roentgenogram and irradiated 4 months after the amputation. Eight years after amputation he was alive and well.

Prognosis

Careful study of the pathology and follow-up data on more than 98% of the patients with Ewing's sarcomas in the present series indicated the serious nature of this tumor, but there were some hopeful aspects. The 5-year survival rate was 15%; tumors in these survivors were not distinguishable from the remainder pathologically. Unfortunately, 6 of the 20 who had survived 5 years subsequently died of their tumors, one 12 years after the initial treatment. The 10-year survival rate was 10.7%. Details regarding these survivors were published in 1961. Our experience parallels that of several other series in that a number of the long-term survivors had radiation therapy for metastatic disease, most often in the lungs.

Apparently reliable reports in the literature give 5-year survival rates that vary down to zero. Our experience indicates, however, that patients with Ewing's tumor have a chance for survival if prompt adequate treatment is employed.

Bibliography

1921 Ewing, James: Diffuse Endothelioma of Bone. *Proc. New York Path. Soc. n.s., 21:*17-24.

1948 Uehlinger, E., Botsztejn, Ch., and Schinz, H. R.: Ewingsarkom und Knochenretikulosarkom: Klinik, Diagnose und Differentialdiagnose. *Oncologia, 1:*193-245.

1952 McCormack, L. J., Dockerty, M. B., and Ghormley, R. K.: Ewing's Sarcoma. *Cancer, 5:*85-99.

1953 Wang, C. C., and Schulz, M. D.: Ewing's Sarcoma: A Study of Fifty Cases Treated at the Massachusetts General Hospital, 1930-1952 Inclusive. *New England J. Med., 248:*571-576.

1955 Bethge, J. F. J.: Die Ewingtumoren oder Omoblastome des Knochens. Differentialdiagnostische und kritische Eröterungen. *Ergebn. Chir. Orthop., 39:*327-425.

1956 Lumb, George, and Mackenzie, D. H.: Round-cell Tumours of Bone. *Brit. J. Surg., 43:* 380-389.

1956 Sherman, R. S., and Soong, K. Y.: Ewing's Sarcoma: Its Roentgen Classification and Diagnosis. *Radiology, 66:*529-539.

1959 Schajowicz, F.: Ewing's Sarcoma and Reticulum Cell Sarcoma of Bone: With Special Reference to the Histochemical Demonstration of Glycogen as an Aid to Differential Diagnosis. *J. Bone & Joint Surg., 41A:*349-356.

1960 Willis, R. A.: *Pathology of Tumors.* Ed. 3, Washington D.C., Butterworth Inc., p. 691.

1961 Dahlin, D. C., Coventry, M. B., and Scanlon, P. W.: Ewing's Sarcoma. A Critical Analysis of 165 Cases. *J. Bone & Joint Surg., 43A:*185-192.

1963 Baird, R. J., and Krause, V. W.: Ewing's Tumor: A Review of 33 Cases. *Canad J. Surg., 6:*136-140.

1963 Bhansali, S. K., and Desai, P. B.: Ewing's Sarcoma: Observations on 107 Cases. *J. Bone & Joint Surg., 45A:*541-553.

1964 Phelan, J. T., and Cabrera, A.: Ewing's Sarcoma. *Surg., Gynec., & Obst., 118:*795-800.

Chapter 20

Malignant Giant Cell Tumor

To be certain of the diagnosis of malignant giant cell tumor, the pathologist must be able to demonstrate zones of typical benign giant cell tumor in the malignant neoplasm under appraisal or in previous tissue obtained from the same neoplasm. When confronted with an obviously malignant growth that contains a few or many benign, osteoclast-like giant cells one can prove a relationship to benign giant cell tumor in no other way. This is true because other neoplasms of bone including many of the osteogenic sarcomas contain a scattering or many of these benign giant cells. I have seen classic low-grade parosteal osteogenic sarcoma recur as a highly malignant sarcoma with such an abundance of benign giant cells that, without reference to the original neoplasm, one might make the mistake of regarding it as a malignant giant cell tumor. Some of the osteogenic sarcomas of soft-tissue origin also contain numerous benign giant cells but obviously bear no relationship to giant cell tumor of bone. The stromal cells, not the benign multinucleated cells, in any given neoplasm must determine its classification. Troup and co-workers (1960) have provided clinicopathologic correlations to support this point of view.

With this absolute type of definition of malignant giant cell tumor, 10 of the 14 such tumors in the present series followed treatment for typical benign giant cell tumors—tumors that contain no feature that distinguishes them from the remainder of the group of giant cell tumors. Nine of these 10 "secondary" malignant tumors followed histologically verified benign giant cell tumors at intervals that averaged 6 years from the time of treatment of the benign neoplasm—treatment that included irradiation in each instance. In these nine instances, the malignant tumor completely overran and destroyed any evidence of the original benign tumor. The tenth "secondary" malignant tumor developed 1½ years after simple curettage of the benign giant cell tumor, and remnants of it remained at the time of amputation. The remaining four tumors contained foci of sarcoma as detailed in chapter 9 under prognosis.

Increasing evidence is being accumulated that irradiation may be influential in triggering the malignant transformation of a variety of osseous lesions, especially giant cell tumor. In 5 of the 14 cases in this series, however, irradiation could not be incriminated. Recently, since the data for this book were compiled, the series accumulated another case in which fibrosarcoma developed at the site of a giant cell tumor which had been treated by curettage and bone grafting 22 years and again 15 years previously; no irradiation had been employed.

Analysis of the literature on malignant giant cell tumor is virtually impossible because of lack of strict definition of this entity. No attempt has been made to list all of the pertinent references. The subject is further clouded by the extremely rare "benign metastasizing" giant cell tumor. The single one among the 155 giant cell tumors in the present series is illustrated in Figure 9-16.

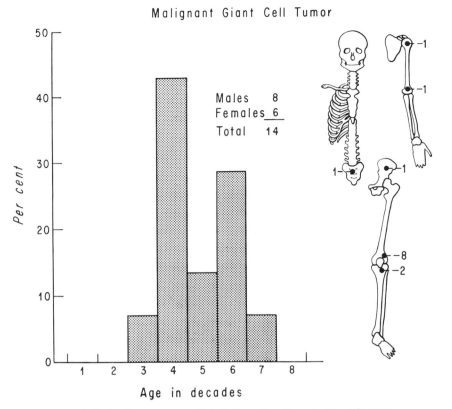

FIG. 20-1. Skeletal, age, and sex distribution of malignant giant cell tumor.

Incidence

The malignant giant cell tumors comprised less than 0.5% of the total group of malignant tumors and 9% of the giant cell tumors.

Sex

In this small group men and women were equally affected, whereas females represented 58% of the cases of benign giant cell tumor. The tumor in one of the women in the earlier series has been reclassified.

Age

These patients were somewhat older, on the average, than were those with benign giant cell tumor. This is at least partially explained by the fact that most of the tumors developed several years after treatment of their benign precursors.

Localization

The distribution of these tumors is not significantly different from that of those benign giant cell tumors that do not undergo malignant transformation. As may be seen above, 10 of them involved the region of the knee, 2 the humerus, and 1 each the ilium and the sacrum.

197

MALIGNANT GIANT CELL TUMOR

Symptoms

Most of these 14 patients had the symptoms of ordinary benign giant cell tumor at the outset. As mentioned, 9 of the 14 malignant tumors occurred an average of 6 years after the histologic diagnosis of benign giant cell tumor, and therapy included irradiation in each of these. The three patients whose giant cell tumors contained malignant foci at the original operation had had preoperative pain in the region for 1, 1, and 2 years respectively.

It should be stressed that when the originally benign giant cell tumors became sarcomas, the clinical features changed abruptly from those of slowly progressing or quiescent giant cell tumors to those of the rapidly-growing sarcomas they had become.

Physical Findings

The physical examination reveals the evidence likely to be presented by any malignant tumor of bone. Cutaneous changes from prior radiation are common and may alert the physician to elicit the history of such therapy.

Roentgenologic Features

Roentgenologic changes do not differ from those described for fibrosarcoma or osteogenic sarcoma except that in long bones the lesion is almost certain to be in the very end of the bone. The classic features of malignant destruction are present and usually the process is completely lytic. Earlier roentgenograms of the lesion ordinarily afford evidence of the preexisting benign giant cell tumor. Sometimes the malignant change is reflected in the roentgenogram considerably later than its occurrence had been suggested by the clinical history.

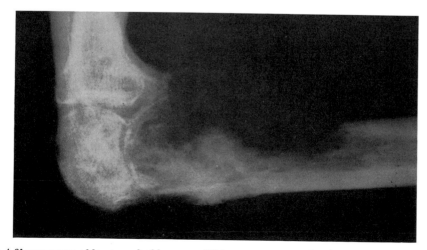

Fig. 20-2. Grade 4 fibrosarcoma of lower end of humerus. This tumor arose at the site of a benign giant cell tumor that had expanded the epiphyseal and adjacent metaphyseal region of the bone. It had been treated by curettage and irradiation 8 years before the above roentgenogram was made. Despite amputation, death occurred within 1 year.

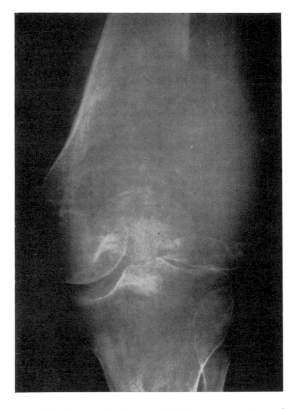

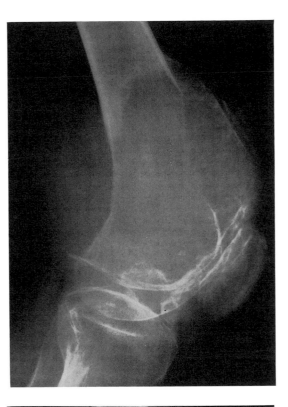

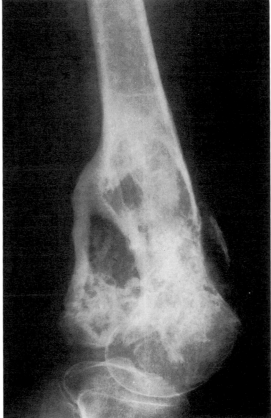

FIG. 20-3. *Above* and *Above, right.* Anteroposterior and lateral views of benign giant cell tumor of the lower end of the femur. It was treated by insertion of radium following curettage. *Right.* The same lesion 2 years after treatment. Two years after this roentgenogram was taken the leg was amputated for grade 3 fibrosarcoma which had completely replaced the original benign tumor.

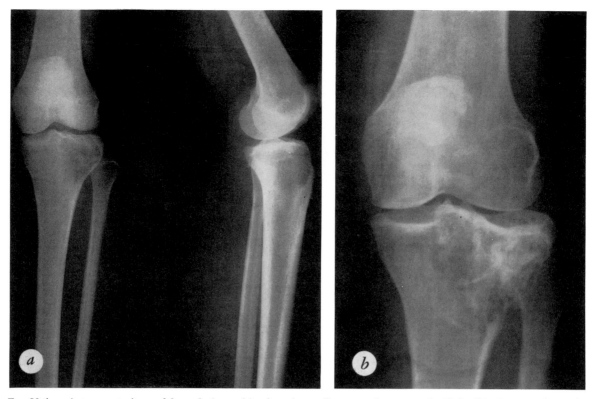

FIG. 20-4. *a.* Anteroposterior and lateral views of benign giant cell tumor of upper end of left tibia. It was curetted in 1943 and given roentgen therapy in 1944. *b.* The same lesion in 1948. By this time a grade 3 fibrosarcoma had replaced the benign tumor and, despite amputation, the patient died with pulmonary metastasis 3 years later. (Figure 20-4*a* reproduced with permission from: Sabanas, A. O., Dahlin, D. C., Childs, D. S., Jr., and Ivins, J. C.: *Cancer, 9:*528-542, 1956.)

Gross Pathology

The rare, malignant giant cell tumor that shows both benign and sarcomatous zones at the time of the first treatment is grossly indistinguishable from its benign counterpart. It produces variable degrees of expansion of the end of a bone, and it is ordinarily contained by the expanded periosteum. The commoner, secondarily malignant giant cell tumor exhibits characteristic evidence of sarcoma such as invasion of surrounding osseous and soft tissues, hemorrhage and necrosis, although the last two of these are by no means uncommon in genuine benign giant cell tumor. The gross appearance of these secondary sarcomas will often have been modified by previous treatment which commonly includes the incorporation of bone grafts into the defect that follows curettage. Such grafts will have been partially or completely dissolved.

In general, the gross features of malignant giant cell tumor are not specific, and frequently it requires multiple microscopic sections to establish that foci of sarcoma are present in a lesion that still contains benign regions.

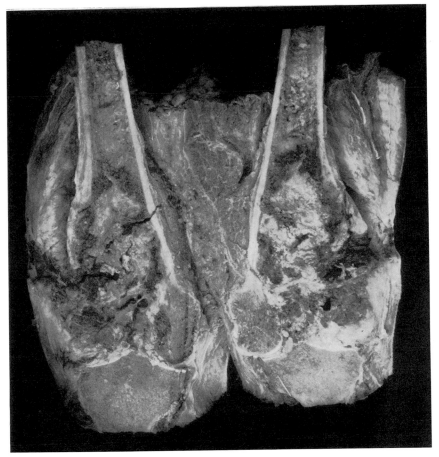

Fig. 20-5. Malignant giant cell tumor of lower end of femur. Roentgenograms of this lesion are shown in Figure 20-3.

Histopathology

In most cases, in my experience, when sarcomatous change has occurred, the preexisting benign giant cell tumor is no longer recognizable as such. The sarcoma that replaces it is ordinarily overtly malignant and presents no problem in diagnosis. In fact, in nine of these in this series that were originally completely benign, one could not have suspected a relationship to benign giant cell tumor from study of the subsequent sarcoma. Seven of these secondary tumors were pure fibrosarcomas and 2 were osteogenic sarcomas. In the 5 other tumors, 2 of which had had previous surgical therapy, there were foci of osteogenic or fibrosarcoma. These sarcomatous foci contrasted sharply with the zones of residual giant cell tumor. The sarcomas apparently arise from the stomal cells.

Careful review of the numerous tissue sections of the benign tumors in this series that subsequently underwent malignant change offered no histologic clue by which one might differentiate them from those that remained benign. Furthermore, the giant cell tumors that recurred after conventional therapy were not distinguishable from those that did not. Grading of bona fide giant cell tumors on a histologic basis has not been of value in my experience.

201

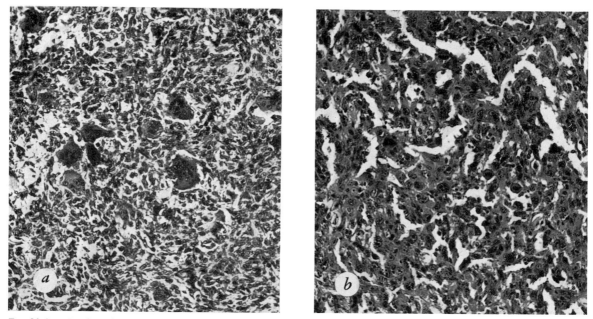

FIG. 20-6. *a*. Benign giant cell tumor of distal end of femur (×175). *b*. Recurrent tumor, 1½ years later, contained foci of sarcoma like that shown above, admixed with typically benign areas of giant cell tumor (×175).

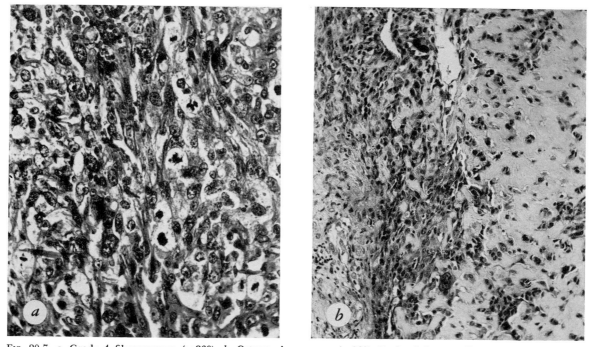

FIG. 20-7. *a*. Grade 4 fibrosarcoma (×260). *b*. Osteogenic sarcoma (×160). Both of these malignant tumors occurred at the sites of benign giant cell tumors that had been treated several years previously by a combination of surgery and irradiation. (Reproduced with permission from: Williams, R. R., Dahlin, D. C., and Ghormley, R. K.: *Cancer*, 7:764-773, 1954.)

Treatment

When indisputable evidence of malignant change is found in a giant cell tumor or in the zone previously occupied by one, ablative surgical treatment is the procedure of choice. The sarcoma that develops is characteristically radioresistant, being either fibrosarcoma or osteogenic sarcoma. The same principles outlined for the treatment of these sarcomas when they occur primarily should be followed. Irradiation, at least as a palliative measure, may be employed for tumors not amenable to ablation.

Prognosis

When frankly malignant transformation has occurred in a benign giant cell tumor, its prognosis is that of the sarcoma present. Eight of 10 patients with secondary malignancy have succumbed, and two have survived 21 and 32 years respectively after amputation. Two of the patients with tumors composed of mixed benign and malignant components at the time of the first operation were cured, one by amputation and one by an en bloc excision of the affected segment of bone. Two others with malignant and benign areas in the first tissue examined died in less than 2 years in spite of amputation.

Bibliography

1953 Jaffe, H. L.: Giant-cell Tumour (Osteoclastoma) of Bone: Its Pathologic Delimitation and the Inherent Clinical Implications. *Ann. Roy. Coll. Surgeons England, 13:*343-355.

1954 Williams, R. R., Dahlin, D. C., and Ghormley, R. K.: Giant-cell Tumor of Bone. *Cancer, 7:*764-773.

1956 Murphy, W. R., and Ackerman, L. V.: Benign and Malignant Giant-cell Tumors of Bone, *Cancer, 9:*317-339.

1956 Sabanas, A. O., Dahlin, D. C., Childs, D. S., Jr., and Ivins, J. C.: Postradiation Sarcoma of Bone. *Cancer, 9:*528-542.

1958 Coley, B. L., Higinbotham, N. L., and Kogure, T.: Giant Cell Tumor of Bone. *Am. J. Surg., 96:*479-491.

1960 Troup, J. B., Dahlin, D. C., and Coventry, M. B.: The Significance of Giant Cells in Osteogenic Sarcoma: Do They Indicate a Relationship Between Osteogenic Sarcoma and Giant Cell Tumor of Bone? *Proc. Staff Meet., Mayo Clin., 35:*179-186.

1962 Hutter, R. V. P., Worcester, J. N., Jr., Francis, K. C., Foote, F. W., Jr., and Stewart, F. W.: Benign and Malignant Giant Cell Tumors of Bone. A Clinicopathological Analysis of the Natural History of the Disease. *Cancer, 15:*653-690.

1963 Copeland, M. M., and Geschickter, C. F.: Malignant Bone Tumors: Primary and Metastatic. *CA, 13:*149-155, 187-196, 232-238.

Chapter 21

"Adamantinoma" of Long Bones

"Adamantinoma" of long bones is a peculiar neoplasm which on the basis of roentgenographic and pathologic features arises within the osseous substance. The origin of the epithelium-like islands in this tumor is unknown. Some have postulated traumatic implantation of epithelium, a concept that is favored by the fact that almost all reported "adamantinomas" have occurred in bones near the cutaneous surface. Others have expressed the belief that congenital rests of epithelium may be the source of these tumors. Still others have stated the view that the so-called adamantinoma of long bones is not epithelial at all but represents rather an unusual manifestation of some sarcoma, especially synovial sarcoma.

Perhaps the most acceptable view, advanced by Changus, Speed, and Stewart in 1957, is that the tumor is angioblastic in origin. Many of the pertinent cases available for my review strongly favor this concept.

Despite this controversial literature, the fact remains that "adamantinoma" of long bones comprises a small group of distinctive tumors that present as primary lesions of bone. It may be that several histogenetically different tumors can produce the picture of "adamantinoma." None of the proposed theories of origin explains its peculiar predilection for the tibia.

The name "adamantinoma" was given to these tumors because of their histologic resemblance to the common adamantinoma (ameloblastoma) of the jawbones. These odontogenic tumors of the jaws and the histologically related tumor that arises from Rathke's pouch are obviously not related and are excluded from the discussion that follows.

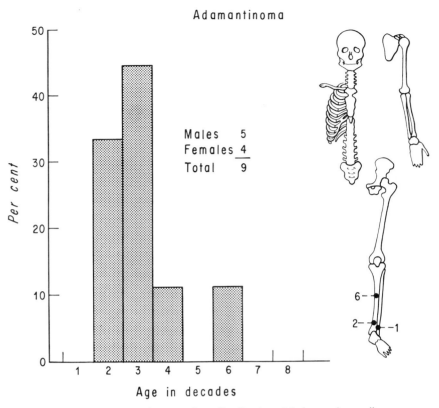

FIG. 21-1. Skeletal, age, and sex distribution of "adamantinoma."

Incidence

Somewhat more than 50 examples of adamantinoma of long bones have been recorded in the literature. The nine cases in the Mayo Clinic series comprised less than one third of 1% of the malignant primary tumors of bone.

Sex

No distinct sex predilection has become apparent.

Age

Patients with this tumor have varied from 10 to 74 years of age (Gloor, 1963). More than half have been in the second and third decades of life.

Localization

Approximately 90% of all reported adamantinomas of long bones have involved the tibia, but examples have been described in the humerus, ulna, femur, and fibula. Most of these tumors have been in the middle portion of the affected bone.

Symptoms

The prolonged clinical course of many patients with this tumor indicates its slow rate of growth in the average case. Pain is the most common initial symptom, whereas local tumefaction is the

205

first complaint in a minority of cases. The duration of symptoms prior to diagnosis has varied from a few months up to 17 years.

Physical Examination

A mass which may be painful is the only physical finding of consequence.

Roentgenologic Features

In most cases, the tumor appears as a well-defined, sometimes trabeculated central area of rarefaction in the shaft of the tibia near its midportion. Long-standing tumors may attain great size and produce considerable expansion of the contour of the bone. Cortical breakthrough is distinctly unusual in patients that have not been treated, and reactive periosteal formation of new bone is rarely observed. Occasional "adamantinomas" have been eccentric, eroding one side of the cortex and bulging the overlying periosteum.

Rarefied areas that resemble those of fibrous dysplasia histologically have been seen in the tibia distal to the neoplasm. These were present in three cases in this series and also in the tibia of the patient with "adamantinoma" of the fibula. In two instances of tibial "adamantinoma," similar foci were found in the adjacent fibula. These fibrous zones presented most often as subperiosteal punctate osteolytic foci having a narrow rim of surrounding, sclerotic bone, rather than as the well-circumscribed central areas of rarefaction producing thinning and expansion of the overlying cortex which is more typical of classic fibrous dysplasia.

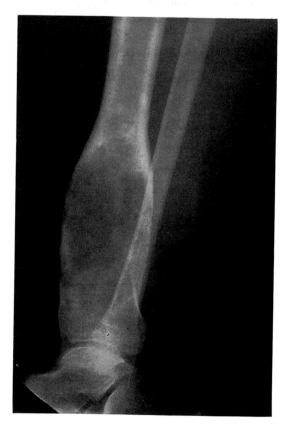

FIG. 21-2. "Adamantinoma" of tibia of 27-year-old woman. She had noted swelling for 8 years. The lesion was removed by curettage, but despite initial improvement amputation became necessary 16 years later. The nature of the lesion at the time of amputation is not known.

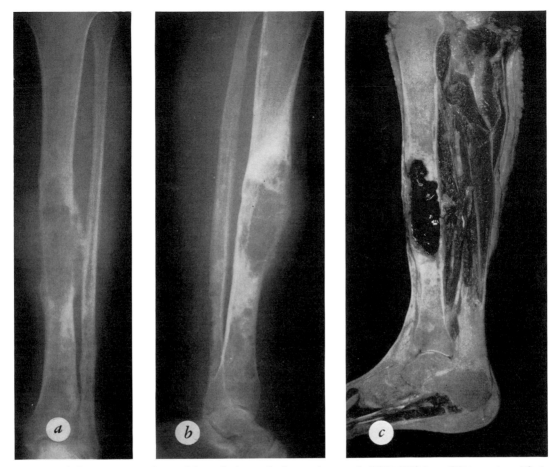

FIG. 21-3. *a* and *b*. Anteroposterior and lateral views of adamantinoma of tibia of 24-year-old man. A surgical procedure had been performed elsewhere 15 months previously. The defects seen in the fibula and in the lower portion of the tibia were composed of fibrous tissue. *c*. Amputated specimen showing defect produced by curettage that had been performed 9 days previously. (Reproduced with permission from Dockerty, M. B., and Meyerding, H. W.: *J.A.M.A., 119:*932-937, 1942.)

Gross Pathology

Ordinarily "adamantinomas" are clearly delimited peripherally as indicated by the roentgenograms. Their contour is often somewhat lobulated. Most of the tumors are gray or white and they vary in consistency from firm and fibrous to soft and brain-like. They may contain spicules of bone and calcareous material. Cystic cavities which may contain blood or straw-colored fluid are sometimes encountered. Some of the tumors burst through the overlying cortex, but this is unusual in patients that have not been subjected to surgical therapy. As previously mentioned, a few "adamantinomas" have been distinctly eccentric, not involving the medulla.

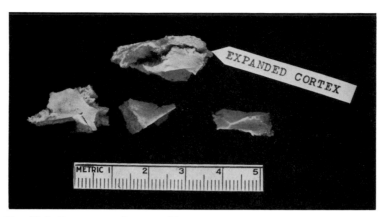

FIG. 21-4. Fragments of tumor illustrated in Figure 21-2. Note that the tissue is firm and fibrous and the cortex is expanded, although it was intact.

Histopathology

A variety of histologic patterns have been described, but all of them have an epithelial quality. There is variation from tumor to tumor and even within different fields of the same tumor. A common pattern consists of neoplastic islands in which the peripheral cells, often columnar, are arranged in palisaded fashion. In the centers of some of these islands, a stellate reticulum-like appearance is observed. Even cyst formation may occur within these islands, and this basic pattern has prompted use of the term "adamantinoma." A second pattern consists of islands of cells that resemble cutaneous basal cells. As in the preceding type, these cellular aggregates often show peripheral palisading of nuclei, and they are ordinarily disposed in a fibrous stroma. The appearance of this second type is very similar to that of basal cell carcinoma of the skin. Additional variation in the histopathologic appearance is afforded by fields that closely resemble squamous cell carcinoma and other fields that mimic ordinary adenocarcinoma.

It is obvious that the problem of differentiating adamantinoma from metastatic carcinoma may be difficult, especially if one considers only the histopathologic features.

The vascular origin of "adamantinoma" of long bones was strongly supported in the evidence presented by Changus and co-workers in 1957. They pointed out the histologic similarity of the proliferating cells of these tumors to the angioblasts in the embryologic formation of normal blood vessels. The angioblastic character of the cells was further supported by histochemical studies. The tumors in the present series have features in accord with their views.

The relationship of the fibrous dysplasia-like lesions, separate from but in the vicinity of these "adamantinomas," to the neoplasm is still obscure. When present, however, they afford the roentgenologist additional evidence that the principal lesion is an "adamantinoma."

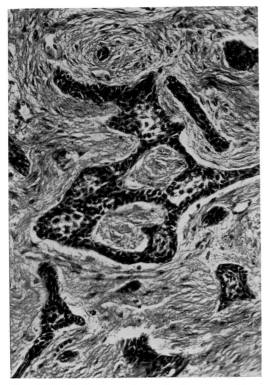

FIG. 21-5. Multiple sections of the tumor illustrated in Figures 21-2 and 21-4 showed the pattern above (×200).

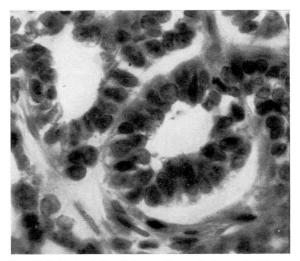

FIG. 21-6. Part of the "adamantinoma" shown in Figure 21-3 had a glandular pattern, as shown above, whereas other zones resembled squamous cell carcinoma (×600). (Reproduced with permission from: Dockerty, M. B., and Meyerding, H. W.: *J.A.M.A., 119*:932-937, 1942.)

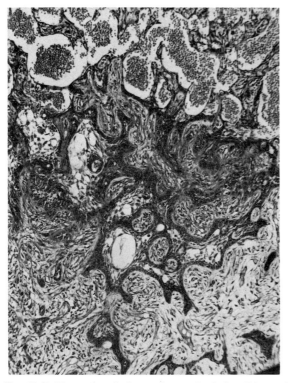

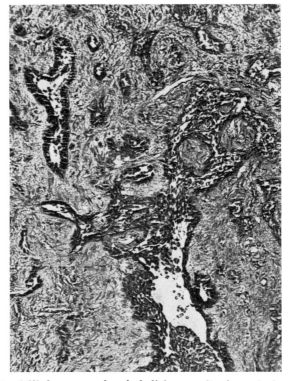

FIG. 21-7. Two other "adamantinomas" of the tibia. *Left.* Blood-filled spaces and endothelial-type cells above shade into the classic "adamantinoma" pattern below (×125). *Right.* Here the glandular pattern has become prominent (×175).

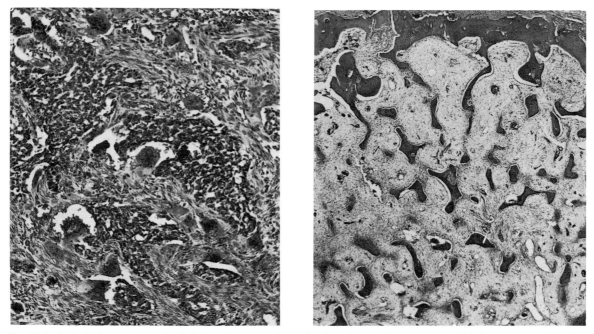

FIG. 21-8. *Left.* "Adamantinoma" of tibia with a prominent benign giant cell component. This is an unusual finding (×115). *Right.* One of the fibrous zones near a tibial "adamantinoma." Such zones we have studied have not contained recognizable neoplasm (×22).

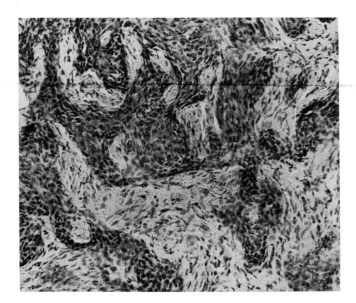

FIG. 21-9. *Left.* The markedly squamous appearance seen in some of these tumors (×100).

Treatment

After carefully reviewing all the recorded cases and amplifying the available information by sending questionnaires to the authors who reported the cases, Baker and his associates came to the conclusion that amputation is the treatment of choice. This conclusion was based upon the fact that in two thirds of the cases recurrence was known to have followed local excision, and recurrence was followed by death in eight instances.

One might be justifiably tempted to employ wide block excision of the involved segment of bone if the lesion is small and well located. This less radical approach for selected lesions has been recommended by a number of authors.

Prognosis

Early radical therapy should effect a high proportion of cures. It is known, however, that temporizing with inadequate attempts at local excision has produced death in a number of patients, owing to metastasis. Although the average "adamantinoma" runs an indolent course, some otherwise typical examples metastasize early. Metastasis may be by either the hematogenous or the lymphatic route.

Bibliography

1913 Fischer, B.: Über ein primäres Adamantinom der Tibia. *Frankfurt. Ztschv. Path.*, *12*:422-441.

1930 Richter, C. S.: Ein Fall von adamantinomartiger Geschwulst des Scheinbeins. *Ztschr. Krebsforsch.*, *32*:273-279.

1940 Hebbel, R.: Adamantinoma of the Tibia. *Surgery*, *7*:860-868.

1942 Dockerty, M. B., and Meyerding, H. W.: Adamantinoma of the Tibia: Report of Two New Cases. *J.A.M.A.*, *119*:932-937.

1954 Baker, P. L., Dockerty, M. B., and Coventry, M. B.: Adamantinoma (So-called) of the Long Bones: Review of the Literature and a Report of Three New Cases. *J. Bone & Joint Surg.*, *36A*:704-720.

1954 Lederer, H., and Sinclair, A. J.: Malignant Synovioma Simulating "Adamantinoma of the Tibia." *J. Path. & Bact.*, *67*:163-168.

1954 Hicks, J. D.: Synovial Sarcoma of the Tibia. *J. Path. & Bact.*, *67*:151-161.

1957 Changus, G. W., Speed, J. S., and Stewart, F. W.: Malignant Angioblastoma of Bone. A Reappraisal of Adamantinoma of Long Bone. *Cancer*, *10*:540-559.

1960 D'Aubigne, R. M.: Adamantinome Du Tibia. *Rev. chir. orthop.*, *46*:92-96.

1962 Cohen, D. M., Dahlin, D. C., and Pugh, D. G.: Fibrous Dysplasia Associated with Adamantinoma of the Long Bones. *Cancer*, *15*:515-521.

1962 Elliott, G. B.: Malignant Angioblastoma of Long Bone, So-called "Tibial Adamantinoma." *J. Bone & Joint Surg.*, *44B*:25-33.

1963 Gloor, F.: Das sogenannte Adamantinom der langen Röhrenknochen. *Virchows Arch. path. Anat.*, *336*:489-502.

Chapter 22

Fibrosarcoma and Desmoplastic Fibroma

Fɪʙʀᴏsᴀʀᴄᴏᴍᴀ occurring in bone is defined as a malignant tumor of spindle-shaped cells which produce no osteoid material in the primary lesion or in secondary deposits. Collagen production varies from abundant to none, tending to be less in the highly anaplastic examples. Fibrosarcoma may be so well differentiated that it is difficult to distinguish from benign conditions such as fibrous dysplasia.

It is somewhat didactic to separate fibrosarcoma of bone from its close relative, fibroblastic osteogenic sarcoma. Relatively minor clinical features distinguish these two entities and both are best treated by ablative surgical means. Occasionally, one finds osteoid substance only after prolonged search through many sections of a tumor that is predominantly fibroblastic, indicating that the separation is an artificial one.

After exclusion of the tumors that merely abutted on bone, on the premise that they were very likely of soft-tissue origin, there remained in the Mayo Clinic series no distinct group of tumors that one might logically call "periosteal fibrosarcomas." This manner of selection perhaps excludes some sarcomas of periosteal origin. From the gross pathologic features, it is apparent that most fibrosarcomas of bone arise in the medullary or the cortical regions, although some undoubtedly begin in the periosteum.

"Secondary" fibrosarcoma accounted for 25% of the 100 in this series. Eighteen followed radiation for a variety of conditions, 3 developed in giant cell tumors that had had no irradiation, 2 occurred in Paget's disease, 1 in a focus of chronic osteomyelitis, and 1 in a long-standing bone lesion of unknown type. Fibrosarcoma has also been described arising in infarcts of bone.

Multicentric origin is suggested in some cases of fibrosarcoma of bone. I have seen several examples, especially in material sent in for consultation, in which two or more skeletal foci were present when the patient first sought medical care.

Myxosarcoma-like foci may be prominent in fibrosarcoma of bone. Rarely the entire tumor has an appearance that tempts one to designate it as a myxosarcoma. Transitional types between these and obvious fibrosarcomas make me prefer to include such lesions with the fibrosarcomas.

Desmoplastic Fibroma

This rare tumor was listed among the benign conditions in Tables 1, 2, and 3 in chapter 1. Its locally infiltrative quality puts it in a "borderline" position with regard to malignancy. Hence, the three examples in this total series of bone tumors are briefly described in this chapter.

212

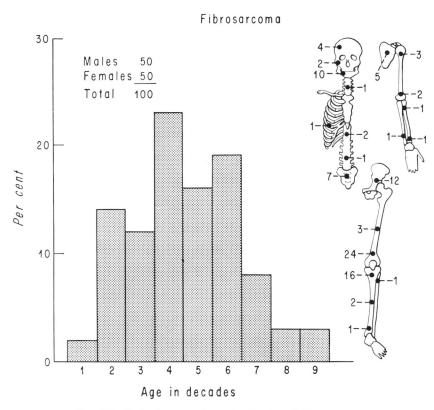

FIG. 22-1. Skeletal, age, and sex distribution of fibrosarcoma.

Incidence

The 100 fibrosarcomas in this series comprised 3.4% of the total primary malignant bone tumors. Fibrosarcoma was less than one sixth as common as osteogenic sarcoma.

Sex

Males and females were equally affected.

Age

The fibrosarcomas were rather evenly distributed among the second through the sixth decades of life. The tendency of fibrosarcoma to occur among older people as commonly as among the younger is the major clinical difference between it and osteogenic sarcoma. This tendency is partially explained by the 25 tumors which occurred as late complications of preexisting conditions.

Localization

The sites involved by fibrosarcoma do not differ remarkably from those involved by osteogenic sarcoma. The long bones, where the tumor is usually found in the metaphyseal region, contributed more than 50% of cases. Several tumors that affected the maxillary antrum, including its bony walls, were excluded for lack of evidence of osseous origin.

FIBROSARCOMA AND DESMOPLASTIC FIBROMA

Symptoms

Fibrosarcoma produces the ordinary symptoms of malignant tumor in bone, namely pain and swelling. In the average case, these are of short duration. Patients whose fibrosarcomas arise secondarily give an appropriate history of the original condition and often have had radiation therapy many years before the malignant tumor appears.

Physical Examination

Painful swelling in the region of the tumor is usually found unless the tumor is covered by a thick layer of uninvolved tissue. Spindle cell sarcoma and even carcinomas with spindle-shaped cells may metastasize to the skeleton and mimic primary fibrosarcoma, so evidence for such hidden lesions should be sought.

Roentgenologic Features

As Pugh (1954) has so aptly stated, there are no roentgenologic features that distinguish fibrosarcoma of bone from osteolytic osteogenic sarcoma. The essential destructive characteristics of the latter tumor have been described previously. Periosteal, reactive new bone formation may be seen. There are no pathognomonic features of fibrosarcoma of bone, but in the average case the diagnosis of malignant tumor can be made with reasonable assurance. The neoplastic tissue often permeates the affected bone well beyond the lytic zone seen in the roentgenogram.

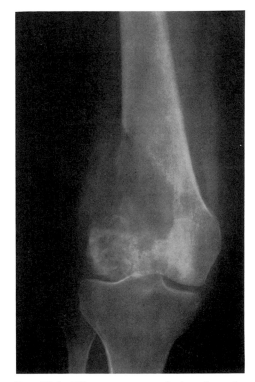

FIG. 22-2. Fibrosarcoma producing irregular destruction of lower portion of femur.

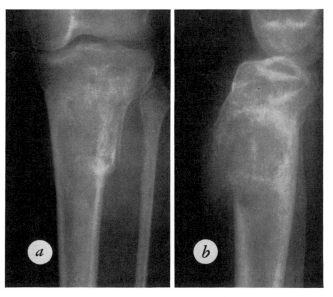

FIG. 22-3. Anteroposterior (a) and lateral (b) views of fibrosarcoma of upper metaphyseal portion of tibia. Note cortical destruction, especially anteriorly.

Gross Pathology

Fibrosarcoma of bone may be composed of a firm, fibrous mass of tissue or of soft, fleshy, friable, and sometimes even myxoid tissue which invades the bone in an irregular fashion. Some tumors of this type, however, are reasonably well circumscribed and can be shelled out of the bone of origin rather readily. Areas of necrosis and hemorrhage may be present. Almost all of the fibrosarcomas of central origin will have broken through the cortex and will present with a large or small extraosseous component. Permeation of bone and invasion through the cortex help differentiate these tumors from benign fibrous conditions. The average tumor of this type has its longest axis parallel to and within the bone or origin. Practically any bone and any portion of it can be affected by this neoplasm. In some instances the tumor is chiefly outside the bone and thus quite likely of periosteal origin.

Fibrosarcoma, like osteogenic sarcoma, metastasizes primarily by the hematogenous route, producing secondary deposits in the lung most commonly but also in various sites including other bones.

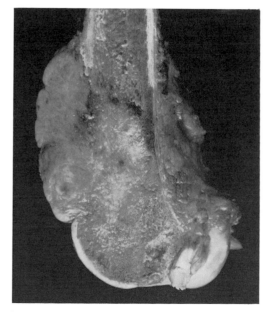

FIG. 22-4. Fibrosarcoma of lower portion of femur. This is the specimen from the case represented in Figure 22-2.

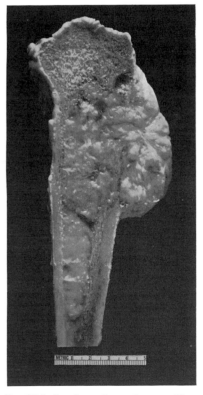

FIG. 22-5. Specimen from the case illustrated in Figure 22-3a and b.

FIBROSARCOMA AND DESMOPLASTIC FIBROMA

Histopathology

Fibrosarcoma in bone has the same histologic features as its soft-tissue counterpart. Sections may, however, reveal that it is invading and destroying bone, especially near the periphery of the tumor. There is wide variation in the degree of differentiation of the component fibroblasts and in the amount of collagen produced. The nuclei vary from long and slender to oval in shape. Nuclear irregularities and the number of mitotic figures are increased in the more anaplastic (higher-grade) tumors. The collagen is arranged in rather orderly bands and whorls in the lower-grade lesions. Some highly anaplastic spindle cell tumors produce no recognizable collagen, but such tumors are logically included among the fibrosarcomas because of their histologic kinship.

Benign multinucleated cells are sometimes found in fibrosarcomas, but they are more commonly seen among the malignant cells of osteogenic sarcomas.

A few fibrosarcomas are so low grade that the problem of differentiation from benign lesions arises. The benign conditions that may enter into the problem of differentiation include cellular lesions of fibrous dysplasia and nonosteogenic fibroma of bone. I have seen a number of cases in which the original specimen from a fibrosarcoma had been underdiagnosed as some benign condition. Attention to signs of aggressiveness as may be indicated in the roentgenogram or by permeation of tumor among preexisting trabeculae or destruction of the overlying bony cortex helps one avoid this error.

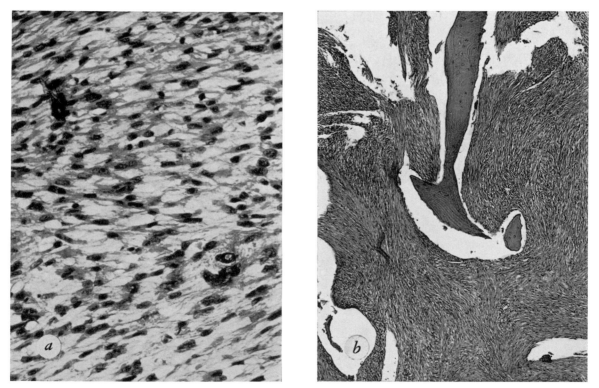

Fig. 22-6. *a.* Grade 2 fibrosarcoma (×200). This section, which shows only slight collagen production, came from the tumor illustrated in Figures 22-3 and 22-5. *b.* Periphery of fairly well-differentiated fibrosarcoma shown invading bone (×75). (Figures 22-2, 3, 4, 5, and 6 reproduced with permission from: McLeod, J. J., Dahlin, D. C., and Ivins, J. C.: *Am. J. Surg., 94*:431-437, 1957.)

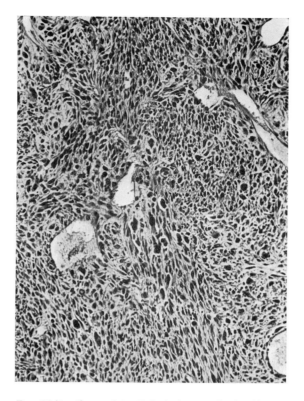

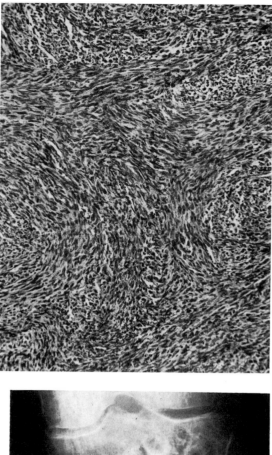

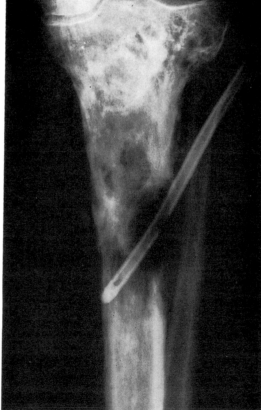

Fig. 22-7. *Above, left.* Relatively anaplastic fibrosarcoma with bizarre and irregular nuclei but with considerable collagen production (×100).

Fig. 22-8. *Above, right.* Fibrosarcoma with moderate differentiation and characteristic whorls of cells (×110).

Fig. 22-9. *Right.* Infected fibrosarcoma destroying junction of upper and middle thirds of tibia. This developed 28 years after irradiation of an aneurysmal bone cyst in this area.

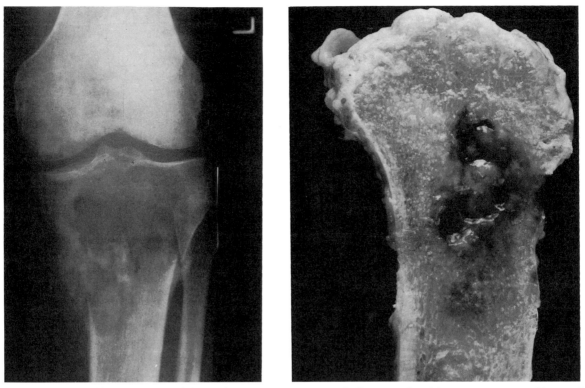

FIG. 22-10. *Left.* Fibrosarcoma of tibia. This lytic tumor was markedly myxoid. *Right.* A similar myxoidtype of fibrosarcoma. Although not grossly obvious, the tumor completely permeated the upper end of the tibia.

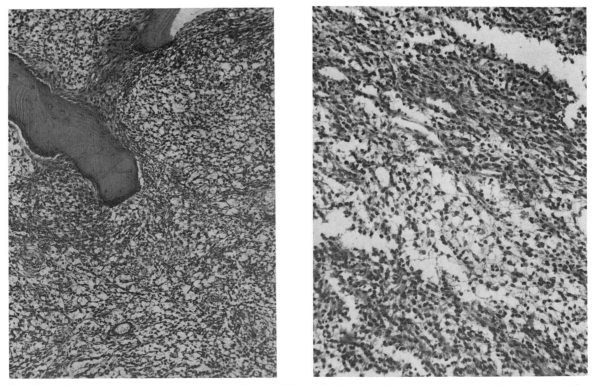

FIG. 22-11. *Left.* Section from tumor shown in Figure 22-10, *right.* Parts of this fibrosarcoma which is permeating the bone resemble myxoid liposarcoma but stains for fat were negative ($\times$100). *Right.* Another fibrosarcoma containing foci of loosely arranged myxoid-appearing cells ($\times$125).

Treatment

Ablative surgical treatment of the type used for osteogenic sarcoma is usually indicated for fibrosarcoma of bone. Details regarding management of tumors of various sites are given in chapter 17. Fibrosarcoma is radioresistant.

Some have made a convincing plea for conservative, block-excisional therapy for some of the well-localized fibrosarcomas of long bones on the premise that they are relatively benign. Experience at the Mayo Clinic indicates, however, that fibrosarcoma is practically as lethal as osteogenic sarcoma and demands prompt, adequate therapy.

Prognosis

Although 26.8% of the patients in our earlier series (McLeod and co-workers, 1957) survived 5 years, more than one fourth of these survivors subsequently succumbed to the effects of their tumors. Most authorities believe that the well-differentiated fibrosarcomas have a prognosis distinctly better than that of osteogenic sarcoma.

Desmoplastic Fibroma

Only some 12 cases of this tumor have been documented. It has been seen in patients from 8 to 40 years of age with the sexes about equally affected. Long tubular bones have been the sites of predilection but this lesion has also been found in various sites such at the ilium, os calcis, scapula, mandible, and vertebra. Roentgenologically, the rarefying defect is generally central and reasonably well demarcated, often having an irregular border which produces a "trabeculated" appearance. Grossly, there is a dense, tough rubbery, whorled mass of fibrous tissue which bears a remarkable similarity to desmoids of soft-tissue origin. Histologically, there are hypocellular bundles of collagenous tissue with sparse, small, slender, spindle-shaped nuclei. Mitotic activity is absent or practically so. The lack of giant cells and hypocellularity contrast with the findings in nonosteogenic fibroma. There is no osseous metaplasia as in fibrous dysplasia. Lack of nuclear anaplasia and of mitotic activity allows differentiation from fibrosarcoma. Complete resection is apparently the best therapy; sometimes this may entail segmental resection of the affected part of a bone.

The three desmoplastic fibromas in this series of 3,987 bone tumors attest to their rarity. One was in the os calcis of a 21-year-old woman, one in the radius of a 16-year-old man, and one in the mandible of a 25-year-old man. I have also seen material in consultation from an unreported desmoplastic fibroma of the skull and another of the radius.

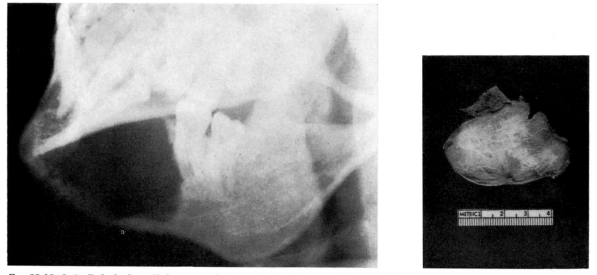

FIG. 22-12. *Left*. Relatively well-demarcated desmoplastic fibroma of the mandible in a 25-year-old man who had noted swelling in the region for 4 months. *Right*. Dense, whorled, fibrous mass that was removed by resection of the involved segment of the mandible.

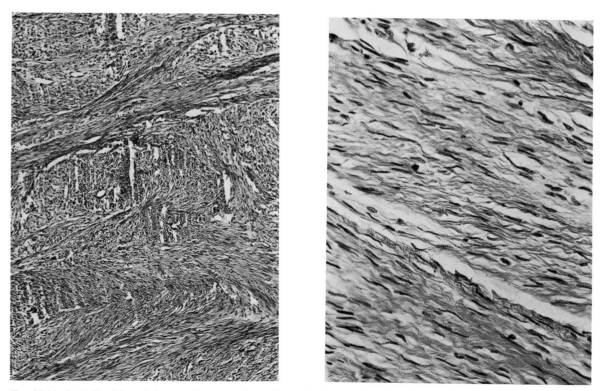

FIG. 22-13. *Left*. Fascicles of dense collagenous tissue from the desmoplastic fibroma illustrated in Figure 22-12 ($\times$65). Note marked similarity to desmoid tumors of soft-tissue origin. *Right*. Higher magnification to show nuclear details ($\times$250).

Bibliography

1944 Steiner, P. E.: Multiple Diffuse Fibrosarcoma of Bone. *Am. J. Path., 20:*877-893.

1948 Stout, A. P.: Fibrosarcoma: The Malignant Tumor of Fibroblasts. *Cancer, 1:*30-63.

1954 Pugh, D. G.: *Roentgenologic Diagnosis of Diseases of Bones.* Baltimore, Williams & Wilkins, p. 559AW.

1957 McLeod, J. J., Dahlin, D. C., and Ivins, J. C.: Fibrosarcoma of Bone. *Am. J. Surg., 94:*431-437.

1958 Goidanich, I. F., and Venturi, R.: I Fibrosarcomi Primitivi Dello Scheletro. *Chir. org. movimento, 46:*1-90.

1958 Jaffe, H. L.: *Tumors and Tumorous Conditions of the Bones and Joints.* Philadelphia, Lea & Febiger, pp. 298-313.

1958 Gilmer, W. S., Jr., and MacEwen, G. D.: Central (Medullary) Fibrosarcoma of Bone. *J. Bone & Joint Surg., 40A:*121-141.

1960 Furey, J. G., Ferrer-Torells, M., and Reagan, J. W.: Fibrosarcoma Arising at the Site of Bone Infarcts. A Report of 2 Cases. *J. Bone & Joint Surg., 42A:*802-810.

1960 Whitesides, T. E., Jr., and Ackerman, L. V.: Desmoplastic Fibroma. A Report of Three Cases. *J. Bone & Joint Surg., 42A:*1143-1150.

1961 Christensen, E., Hojgaard, K., and Winkel Smith, C. C.: Congenital Malignant Mesenchymal Tumors in a Two Month Old Child. *Acta path. et microbiol. scandinav., 53:*237-242.

1962 Nielsen, A. R., and Poulsen, H.: Multiple Diffuse Fibrosarcomata of the Bones. *Acta path. et microbiol. scandinav., 55:*265-272.

1964 Dahlin, D. C., and Hoover, N. W.: Desmoplastic Fibroma of Bone. Report of Two Cases. *J.A.M.A., 188:*685-687.

1965 Lichtenstein, L.: *Bone Tumors,* Ed. 3, St. Louis, The C. V. Mosby Co., pp. 229-240.

Chapter 23

Chordoma

CHORDOMA is a neoplasm that develops from remnants of the primitive notochord. It apparently can arise from normal products of the notochord, the nuclei pulposi, or from abnormal "rests" of notochordal tissue. It ordinarily grows slowly and is malignant because of local invasion, but metastasis is relatively uncommon.

Chordoma has a distinct predilection for the ends of the spinal column. Thus the sacrococcygeal region and the base of the skull in the vicinity of the spheno-occipital synchondrosis account for the great majority of cases. Small, non-neoplastic masses of vestigial notochordal tissue are not uncommonly found in the region of the spheno-occipital junction in the midline.

This tumor is relatively uncommon in the dorsal and lumbar portions of the vertebral column, which is strange in view of the fact that the largest masses of notochordal products, in the form of the nuclei pulposi, occur in these regions.

One might question whether chordoma is correctly classed among the neoplasms of bone. The intimate relationship of the notochord to the skeleton and the clinical and roentgenologic features of these tumors make the inclusion a logical one.

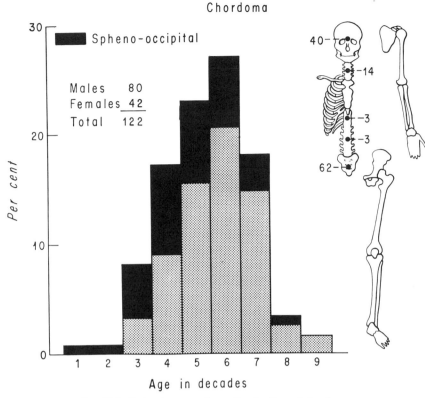

Fig. 23-1. Skeletal, age, and sex distribution of chordoma.

Incidence

Chordoma is usually referred to as a very rare neoplasm, but it accounted for more than 4% of the malignant tumors in this series. Possibly a selection factor operates in a series such as this which includes many referred patients.

Sex

Chordoma affects males approximately twice as commonly as females. Seventy-four per cent of the sacrococcygeal tumors were in males, whereas only 55% of the spheno-occipital ones were.

Age

As indicated in the illustration above, chordoma is distinctly uncommon in patients less than 30 years of age. There was one patient in each of the first 2 decades of life and 10 in the third. Spheno-occipital chordomas are recognized clinically approximately a decade earlier in life than those in the sacrococcygeal region.

Localization

Chordoma is so strictly localized to the midline regions of the body that this affords important diagnostic evidence. Half the tumors occurred in the sacrococcygeal region, and nearly one third at the base of the brain. Most of the remainder involved the cervical vertebrae. The dorsal and lumbar vertebral regions are rarely affected.

CHORDOMA

Symptoms

The duration of symptoms prior to the time the patient seeks medical care varies from months to several years. Pain is a practically constant feature of sacrococcygeal chordoma, and characteristically it is located at the tip of the spinal column. Constipation owing to the presence of the tumor, and complaints resulting from pressure on or destruction of nerves emerging from the distal portion of the spinal cord, may develop. In rare instances a sacrococcygeal chordoma produces a postsacral mass.

Spheno-occipital chordoma may cause symptoms referable to any of the cranial nerves, but those resulting from involvement of the nerves to the eye are by far the most common. This tumor may destroy the pituitary gland and produce evidence of its dysfunction, protrude laterally and give signs suggestive of a tumor of the cerebellopontine angle, or even erode inferiorly and obstruct the nasal passages. Large intracranial extension may evoke the general features of intracranial neoplasm.

Those chordomas that arise along the remainder of the spinal column frequently produce symptoms that result from compression of nerve roots or the spinal cord, or they produce a mass.

Physical Findings

Almost every sacrococcygeal chordoma has a presacral extension that may be detected on careful rectal examination. The mass is, of course, firm and fixed to the sacrum. Digital and proctoscopic examination discloses that it is extrarectal. Evidences of nerve dysfunction, such as "cord" bladder, anesthesias, and paresthesias, are relatively unusual and late features.

Those chordomas that arise at the base of the brain may, as already indicated, produce signs referable to any of the cranial nerves, or to involvement of the pituitary. Examination of the visual fields may disclose defects that suggest the correct diagnosis. Only rarely does a patient complain of nasal obstruction.

Since chordoma of the cervical, thoracic, and lumbar portions of the vertebral column may present posteriorly, laterally, or anteriorly, a great variety of symptoms may be produced. For example, one in the cervical region of the spinal column may give clinical features that suggest the diagnosis of chronic retropharyngeal abscess. Physical examination often discloses evidence of encroachment on the nerves or spinal cord.

Roentgenologic Features

Roentgenographic study reveals evidence of osseous involvement or a soft-tissue mass in more than 90% of cases. Seventy-five per cent of sacrococcygeal examples are characterized by an irregular zone of destruction which begins in the midline of the sacrum. Residual osseous trabeculae and amorphous masses of calcification may be seen in the lesion. The sacrum is often expanded owing to the slow growth of the neoplasm. A soft-tissue mass, almost always anterior, is usually visible.

Cranial chordoma nearly always produces roentgenographic changes but rarely contains radiopaque masses. Destruction of bone in the spheno-occipital or hypophyseal region is usually evident. Some portion of the sella turcica is affected in the majority of cases. Invasion and destruction of the sphenoid and petrous bones are occasionally seen. Ventriculography and cerebral angiography may aid in localizing the lesion.

The chordomas that involve the cervical, thoracic, and lumbar segments of the spinal column usually produce significant roentgenographic changes. Zones of bone destruction, sometimes containing dense foci, are seen involving one or more vertebrae. Some of these tumors, especially if they displace the pharynx or trachea, produce a significant soft-tissue mass.

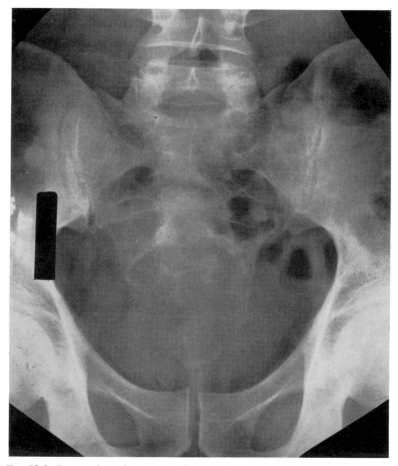

FIG. 23-2. Destruction of sacrum and coccyx by a chordoma that has also produced a large soft-tissue mass in the pelvis. (Reproduced with permission from: Utne, J. R., and Pugh, D. G.: *Am. J. Roentgenol.*, 74:593-608, 1955.)

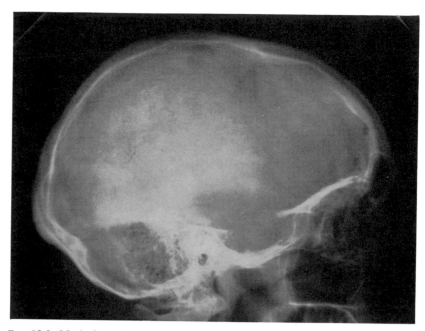

FIG. 23-3. Marked involvement in the region of the sella by a chordoma of the spheno-occipital zone. (Reproduced with permission from: Dahlin, D. C., and Mac-Carty, C. S.: *Cancer, 5*:1170-1178, 1952.)

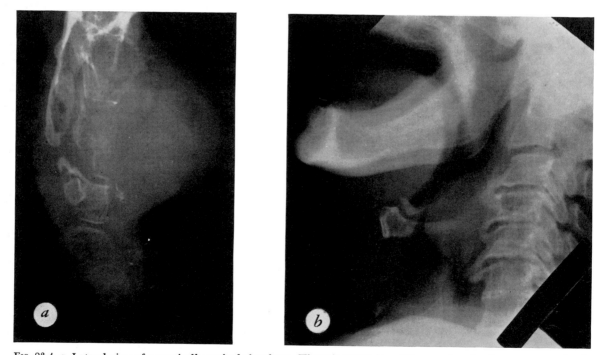

FIG. 23-4. *a*. Lateral view of a surgically excised chordoma. There is expansion of the sacral cortex by an antesacral soft-tissue mass. *b*. Lateral view of the cervical segment of the spinal column demonstrating the soft-tissue shadow of a cervical chordoma anterior to the third, fourth, and fifth cervical vertebrae. (Reproduced with permission from: Utne, J. R., and Pugh, D. G.: *Am. J. Roentgenol., 74*:593-608, 1955.)

Gross Pathology

A chordoma is a soft, lobulated, grayish tumor that is semitranslucent and resembles chondrosarcoma or even mucous adenocarcinoma. It is usually well encapsulated except in the region of bone invasion, where no distinct edge of the tumor may be delineated. Sacral chordoma practically always has a presacral extension that is usually covered by the elevated periosteum. It may extend into the spinal canal. A spheno-occipital chordoma almost always bulges into the cranial cavity and distorts or destroys structures at the base of the brain.

Sometimes chordoma at the base of the brain penetrates into and fills the sphenoid sinus or even the nasal or nasopharyngeal cavities.

An occasional chordoma contains focal calcification or ossification but such foci are rarely prominent. Like chondrosarcomas, some chordomas are relatively firm and others are extremely myxoid and semiliquid.

Perhaps 10% of chordomas metastasize, usually by the hematogenous route. Deposits may develop in unusual locations, including the skin. Recurrence often produces multiple nodules in the region of previous surgical excision.

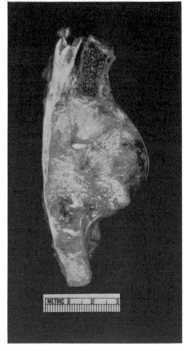

FIG. 23-5. Sacral chordoma with anterior extension. This is the smallest surgically excised tumor of this region in the present series. (Reproduced with permission from: Dahlin, D. C., and MacCarty, C. S.: *Cancer,* 5:1170-1178, 1952.)

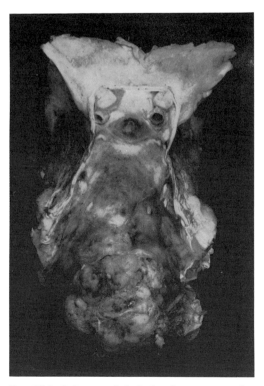

FIG. 23-6. Spheno-occipital chordoma removed at necropsy. Note the mass posterior to the region of the optic nerves, the carotid vessels, and the pituitary body.

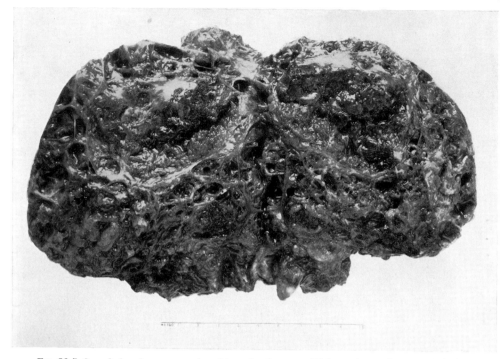

Fig. 23-7. Sacral chordoma more than 10 cm in diameter. This specimen shows the lobular feature of chordoma especially well.

Histopathology

Chordoma cells are characteristically disposed in lobules. Physaliferous cells that are vacuolated because of intracytoplasmic, mucous droplets are usually described as characteristic of chordoma, and they can be found in most of these tumors. Sometimes, however, they are present in only small numbers and constitute an insignificant portion of the histologic picture. The intracellular vacuoles, when they are present, vary in size from those that are barely visible to those that are several times the diameter of the cell's nucleus. Syncytial strands of cells lying in a mass of mucus that has no doubt been formed by the cells are almost as characteristic as are the physaliferous cells. Cell boundaries in these syncytial strands are indistinct.

Considerable variation of nuclear size and chromatin is seen in some of these tumors and mitotic figures may also be present. Such evidences of cellular activity did not alter the clinical course of the sacrococcygeal chordomas in the present series.

Chordoma cells often give a positive reaction to glycogen stains, but a similar type of reaction is observed in chondrosarcoma. Mucous stains are likewise of little value because the other differential diagnostic problem, mucous adenocarcinoma, as well as chordoma, produces mucicarmine-positive material.

Chordoma that arises in the spheno-occipital region is sometimes histologically very similar to chondrosarcoma. Three sarcococcygeal chordomas in the present series contained discrete foci of chondrosarcoma. One of these also contained islands of osteogenic and fibrosarcoma.

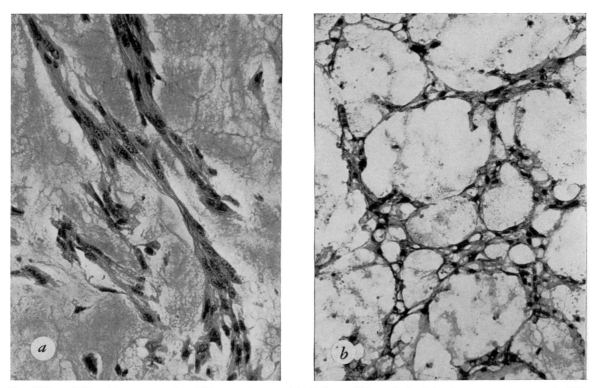

FIG. 23-8. *a*. Cells with scanty eosinophilic cytoplasm and indistinct cell boundaries lying in a mass of mucus (×325). This is a common finding in chordoma. *b*. Physaliferous cells arranged in strands separated by mucus (×205). This is another of the patterns produced in chordoma.

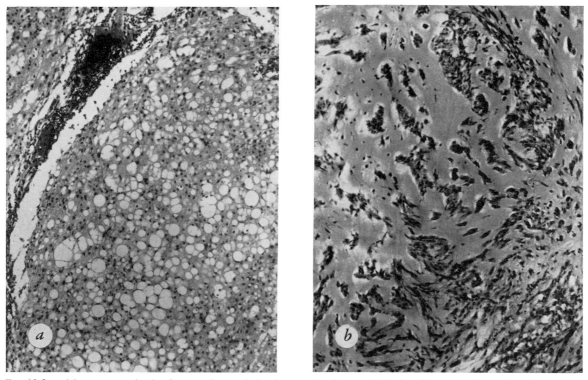

FIG. 23-9. *a*. Mucous vacuoles in the cytoplasm of chordoma cells, the so-called physaliferous cells (×100). *b*. Syncytial strands of cells in a sea of mucus, a very common pattern in chordoma (×100). Reproduced with permission from: Dahlin, D. C., and MacCarty, C. S.: *Cancer*, 5:1170-1178, 1952.)

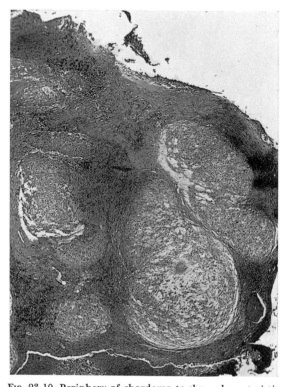

Fig. 23-10. Periphery of chordoma to show characteristic lobular pattern seen in these tumors (×30). (Reproduced with permission from: Dahlin, D. C., and Mac-Carty, C. S.: *Cancer, 5*:1170-1178, 1952.)

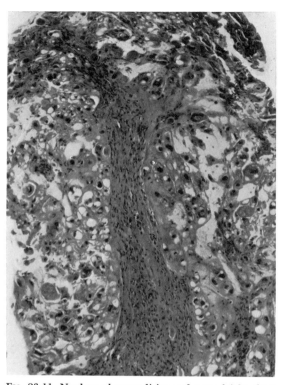

Fig. 23-11. Nuclear abnormalities and even fairly abundant mitotic figures are seen in a minority of chordomas (×100). (Reproduced with permission from: Dahlin, D. C., and MacCarty, C. S.: *Cancer, 5*:1170-1178, 1952.)

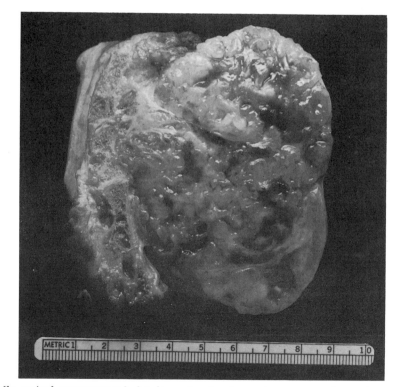

Fig. 23-12. Surgically excised sacrococcygeal chordoma showing tumor in sacrum and prominent presacral extension. Its histologic features are shown in Figure 23-13. This was one of three sacrococcygeal chordomas that contained foci indistinguishable from chondrosarcoma. The patient has survived more than 5 years since operation was performed.

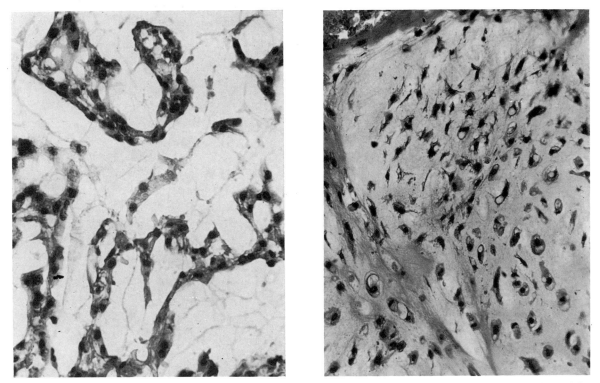

Fig. 23-13. *Left*. Chordoma illustrated in Figure 23-12. Typical cords of cells and intercellular mucus (×400). *Right*. Lobules of classic chondrosarcoma, as depicted here, were present in the same tumor and were indistinguishable grossly from the main mass of chordoma (×225).

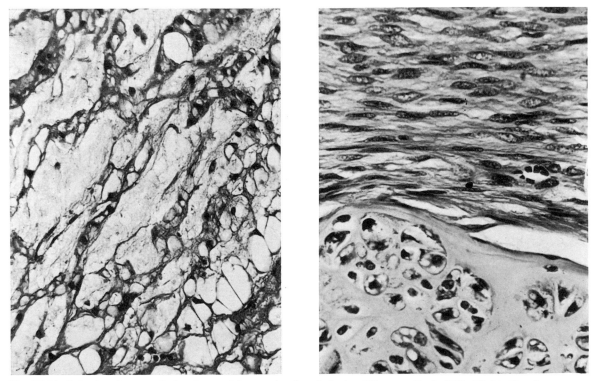

Fig. 23-14. *Left*. Another sacral chordoma with strands of typical physaliferous cells (×375). *Right*. Chondrosarcoma and fibrosarcoma in the same tumor as that shown at *left*. Foci of osteogenic sarcoma were also present, and metastasis developed promptly (×445).

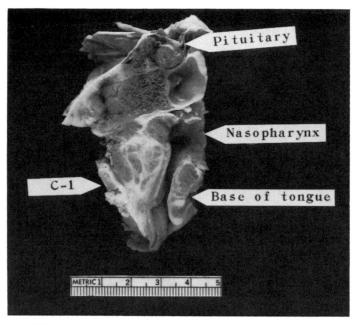

Fig. 23-15. Spheno-occipital chordoma removed at necropsy. Infiltration of bone with extension up behind the pituitary gland and down into the tissues behind the nasopharynx indicates the surgical inaccessibility of chordomas in this location. (Case contributed by Dr. P. T. Sloss, Grand Island, Nebraska.)

Treatment

Until recently, the treatment of chordoma was quite unsatisfactory. The tumor was only partially removed and the patient was afforded palliative benefit at best. The only cheerful aspects were that, owing to the slow growth of the tumor, a few patients obtained several years of freedom of symptoms after subtotal removal and some chordomas proved to be radiosensitive.

It has now been established that radical, complete removal of some sacrococcygeal tumors is feasible and should be attempted. The plane of excision must be well beyond the edge of the tumor to avoid recurrence due to implantation. For those tumors not amenable to complete removal and for inoperable recurrent lesions after surgical therapy, radiation should be employed.

As illustrated in Figure 23-15, spheno-occipital chordomas are so located as to preclude complete surgical removal. If radiation therapy fails and a chordoma in this location produces increased intracranial pressure, however, surgical intervention may be necessary.

Transnasal biopsy of the sphenoid sinus region may provide tissue for verification of the diagnosis of chordoma prior to institution of radiation therapy, since many spheno-occipital chordomas extend into this sinus.

Prognosis

Prior to adoption of the more radical surgical technique, even the patient with sacrococcygeal chordoma was doomed to eventual, though perhaps delayed, death from local extension of the tumor. The sacrococcygeal neoplasm often extended to block the genitourinary or gastrointestinal tract, and the spheno-occipital tumor produced lethal intracranial complications. Subtotal surgical removal sometimes produces gratifying remissions. A number of reports have lauded radiation therapy of chordomas, but it appears impossible to predict which tumors will respond.

Radical surgical techniques have produced prolonged survival and will no doubt afford permanent cure for some patients with less extensive sacrococcygeal chordoma. It must be remembered, however, that this tumor usually grows slowly and that long-term follow-up is necessary in the evaluation of any therapeutic regimen.

Bibliography

1935   Fletcher, E. M., Woltman, H. W., and Adson, A. W.: Sacrococcygeal Chordomas; A Clinical and Pathological Study. *Arch. Neurol. & Psychiat., 33:*283-299.

1935   Adson, A. W., Kernohan, J. W., and Woltman, H. W.: Cranial and Cervical Chordomas; A Clinical and Histologic Study. *Arch. Neurol. & Psychiat., 33:*247-261.

1935   Mabrey, R. E.: Chordoma: A Study of 150 Cases. *Am. J. Cancer, 25:*501-517.

1945   Givner, I.: Ophthalmologic Features of Intracranial Chordoma and Allied Tumors of the Clivus. *Arch. Ophth., 33:*397-402.

1952   Dahlin, D. C., and MacCarty, C. S.: Chordoma: A Study of Fifty-nine Cases. *Cancer, 5:*1170-1178.

1952   MacCarty, C. S., Waugh, J. M., Mayo, C. W., and Coventry, M. B.: The Surgical Treatment of Presacral Tumors: A Combined Problem. *Proc. Staff Meet., Mayo Clin., 27:*73-84.

1955   Utne, J. R., and Pugh, D. G.: The Roentgenologic Aspects of Chordoma. *Am. J. Roentgenol., 74:*593-608.

1957   Greenwald, C. M., Meaney, T. F., and Hughes, C. R.: Chordoma—Uncommon Destructive Lesion of Cerebrospinal Axis. *J.A.M.A., 163:*1240-1244.

1960   Forti, E., and Venturini, G.: Contributo alla Conoscenza delle Neoplasie Notocordali. *Riv. anat. pat. e Onc., 17:*317-396.

1961   MacCarty, C. S., Waugh, J. M., Coventry, M. B., and O'Sullivan, D. C.: Sacrococcygeal Chordomas. *Surg., Gynec., & Obst., 113:*551-554.

1964   Spjut, H. J., and Luse, S. A.: Chordoma: An Electron Microscopic Study. *Cancer, 17:*643-656.

1964   Kamrin, R. P., Potanos, J. N., and Pool, J. L.: An Evaluation of the Diagnosis and Treatment of Chordoma. *J. Neurol., Neurosurg., & Psychiat., 27:*157-165.

Chapter 24

Conditions That Commonly Simulate
Primary Tumors of Bone

ADEQUATE CONSIDERATION of all of the reactive, traumatic, infectious, metabolic, congenital, and other conditions of bone that may simulate benign or malignant neoplasms would require a volume larger than this one. My purpose in this chapter is to indicate the variety of problems that are encountered and to document briefly some of those most often seen in material sent to me for consultation from other pathologists. Pseudotumors of bone in hemophiliacs (Ghormley and Clegg, 1948), skeletal lesions of mastocytosis which may simulate carcinomatosis (Havard and Scott, 1959), and hydatid disease of bone which produces a severe problem not seen in the United States (Alldred and Nisbet, 1964) are among the conditions that will not be elaborated.

Metastatic Carcinoma

Metastatic deposits from carcinomas are by far the most common malignant tumors affecting the skeleton. Although the correct diagnosis is usually obvious when the clinical history is considered, it is often unsafe to assume that any given skeletal lesion or lesions are necessarily related to a proved carcinoma. The punched-out areas of destruction characteristic of myeloma, for example, may be mistaken for areas of lytic metastatic deposit. Metastatic carcinoma is especially likely to afford a diagnostic problem when only one skeletal lesion is found and no "primary" is known. A destructive process secondary to hypernephroma is particularly prone to simulate a primary lesion of bone, because this cancer has a tendency to produce a clinically solitary metastatic lesion and the primary tumor is in an obscure location. Carcinomas may invade bone by direct extension.

Metastatic carcinoma affects chiefly the older age groups. It is especially prone to involve the vertebral column, the pelvis, the ribs, the calvarium, and even the large bones of the limbs near the body. Metastasis of carcinoma distal to the levels of the knees and elbows, however, is uncommon.

Clinically the osseous lesions of metastatic carcinoma may closely simulate primary malignant tumor. Pain, with or without swelling, and symptoms resulting from pressure on neighboring structures or from pathologic fracture are the most prominent.

Roentgenologically, metastatic tumors usually produce irregular destruction of bone indicative of their malignant quality. Although most such lesions are osteolytic, many metastatic deposits from carcinoma of the prostate and some of those from other tumors are osteoblastic. Even malignant lymphomas sometimes evoke considerable sclerosis. Occasionally, especially in the pelvic bones, broadening of the osseous outline may result from periosteal elevation by the growing tumor and subperiosteal formation of new bone. The region of actual involvement by metastatic carcinoma is frequently more extensive than is seen roentgenographically.

Pathologically the lesions of metastatic carcinoma in bone do not present diagnostic characteristics from the gross standpoint. Lesions vary from those that are fibrotic owing to scirrhous reaction produced by the tumor to those that are extremely soft and mushy. The osteoblastic metastatic lesions so often seen from prostatic carcinoma are very dense and relatively characteristic. Histologically the average metastatic carcinoma to bone with its glandular or squamous elements is readily diagnosed. Even if these are absent the characteristic pattern of small islands of epithelial cells interspersed within a fibrous stroma are practically pathognomonic. Some highly anaplastic carcinomas with spindling nuclei closely simulate fibrosarcoma. In such instances, when one encounters a single metastatic lesion from a hidden primary, it may be extremely difficult to decide whether one is dealing with a primary malignant tumor. This is especially true of certain hypernephromas.

The *treatment* of patients with skeletal metastasis is becoming increasingly important. Certain carcinomas, especially those from the prostate and breast, are benefited by both medical and surgical hormonal therapy. Carcinoma metastatic from the thyroid may be held in abeyance for protracted periods by the use of radioactive iodine. Orthopedic surgical procedures in combination with

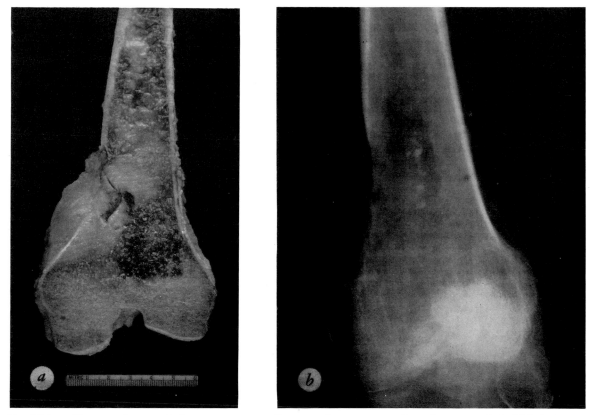

FIG. 24-1. *a.* Gross specimen and, *b,* roentgenogram of metastatic squamous cell carcinoma, grade 1. This lesion developed 10 years after below-knee amputation for a grade 1 squamous cell carcinoma of the foot. Popliteal lymph nodes were uninvolved and the route of this metastasis is obscure.

irradiation or other therapy are often of much value in the management of metastatic carcinoma to the skeleton. Amputation for solitary skeletal metastatic lesions must occasionally be considered. In the present series there is a case in which a solitary metastatic deposit developed in the distal part of the femur 8 years after removal of a hypernephroma, and amputation was followed by known survival for 11 additional years. Chemotherapeutic agents sometimes provide palliation.

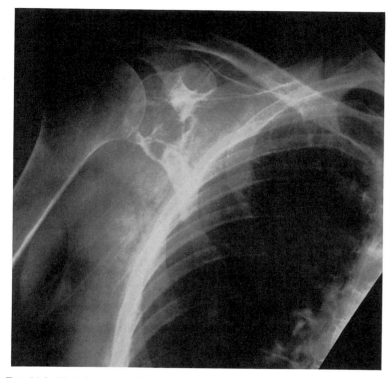

FIG. 24-2. Slightly expansile metastatic hypernephroma of neck of scapula. The renal tumor had been removed 6 years previously and for 18 months the patient had had shoulder pain. The scapular lesion was given radiation therapy, and when no other foci appeared, scapulectomy was performed and the patient was well more than 1 year later.

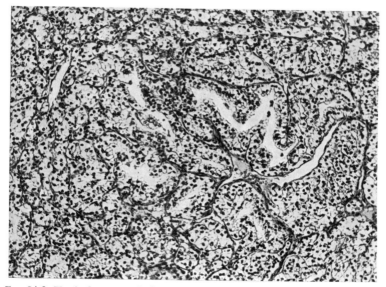

FIG. 24-3. Typical metastatic hypernephroma with clear cells in an organoid pattern ($\times$150).

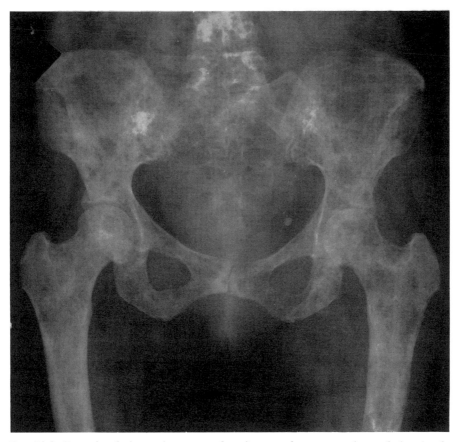

FIG. 24-4. Extensive lytic carcinomatous deposits secondary to a primary lesion in the breast. (Reproduced with permission from: Pugh, D. G.: *Roentgenologic Diagnosis of Diseases of Bones*. Baltimore, Williams & Wilkins, 1954.)

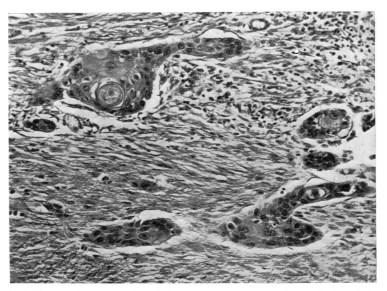

FIG. 24-5. Nests of cells of metastatic squamous cell carcinoma in the skeleton. Note the extensive fibrogenic reaction and the clusters of lymphocytes ($\times 150$).

CONDITIONS THAT SIMULATE PRIMARY TUMORS

Fibrous Dysplasia

Fibrous dysplasia is probably the result of an anomaly in the development of bone. It is characterized by the occurrence of one, a few, or numerous discrete skeletal defects. Yellow or brown patches of cutaneous pigmentation may accompany the bone lesions, especially in patients with a severe disseminated form of the disease. When, in addition to cutaneous pigmentation, such polyostotic disease is accompanied by signs of endocrine abnormality, especially precocious puberty in girls, the condition is commonly called "Albright's syndrome."

"Fibro-osseous dysplasia" is a term that is gaining acceptance for many of the defects of this type that involve the base of the skull and the jawbones. Dysplastic lesions at these sites often contain such an abundance of osseous trabeculae intermingled with the fibrous tissue that they are distinctly hard and may cast a dense shadow in the roentgenogram. Many, if not all, of the so-called osteofibromas and fibroosteomas in these locations are actually examples of fibro-osseous dysplasia.

Polyostotic fibrous dysplasia usually manifests itself early in life, as does also the monostotic form. The disease is relatively common, Pritchard being able to review 256 cases from the literature in 1951. Almost any bone in the body may be affected, and those lesions in the jawbones or at the base of the brain are especially likely to come to clinical and surgical attention.

Clinically, many of the lesions of fibrous dysplasia are completely asymptomatic and never discovered, as evidenced by the finding of occasional "silent" lesions in x-ray examination of the thorax. The dysplasia may produce defective growth and deformity and pain in any bone. The upper part of the femur is especially predilected. Those lesions that involve the bones of the face and skull usually produce signs and symptoms because of their size, such as focal swelling and exophthalmos. Deformity due to the mass is the usual problem presented by patients with lesions in the jaws. The lesions may become quiescent after puberty but this is by no means always the case.

Roentgenologically, the defects of fibrous dysplasia are usually well-defined zones of rarefaction. Expansion with thinning of the cortex is especially likely to occur in narrow bones such as the ribs. Those lesions with a large osseous component such as are commonly seen around the base of the skull and the maxilla are likely to be relatively radiopaque. This characteristic is accentuated if the lesion bulges into an air-containing sinus.

Grossly, examination reveals considerable variation in the lesions of fibrous dysplasia, but the average one is well defined and composed of dense fibrous tissue. Embedded in this fibrous tissue there are usually enough small osteoid trabeculae to impart a distinctly gritty quality. Slight to extensive cyst formation may be present, whereas those with marked ossification may resemble osteoma. Those lesions that arose from thin bones such as the maxilla may bulge into adjacent cavities or soft-tissue zones in a polypoid fashion.

Microscopically, the major feature is a proliferation of fibroblasts that produce dense collagenous matrix. Typically it contains more or less prominent trabeculae of osteoid or bone. These trabeculae have a completely meaningless arrangement as regards function. Metaplastic chondroid substance is sometimes present and on rare occasions it is so prominent that the question of a neoplasm of hyaline cartilage arises. Areas of degeneration may contain only relatively acellular fibrous tissue which is not diagnostic of fibrous dysplasia. Prominent regions of myxoid degeneration may obscure the basic lesion. Some are composed predominantly of osteoid and bone with only sparse fibroblastic elements separating the trabeculae. Sometimes, especially in lesions of the jaws and at the base of the brain, the osseous component is in the form of little spherical masses which are surrounded by the proliferating spindle cells in such a fashion that psammomatous meningioma is simulated. Mitotic figures may be found in the actively proliferating lesions of fibrous dysplasia. Benign giant cells and masses of lipophages are commonly associated with degenerative foci.

Treatment should be conservative. The lesions commonly stop growing at puberty. Therapy should be directed at restoring the normal configuration when the skull or jawbones are affected. In long bones, deformity secondary to the disease may require correction. Radiation therapy is probably of no value and, in a few recorded cases, sarcomatous transformation has followed its use. Fibrous dysplasia has little tendency to undergo spontaneous malignant change.

The *prognosis* in fibrous dysplasia is generally good. The deforming lesions of the jawbones or skull may sometimes recur, but ordinarily they respond favorably to additional conservative surgical therapy. Some of the large lesions in weight-bearing bones require curettage and bone grafting for the maintenance of function. Occasionally recurrence is a problem, but the long-term prognosis is usually good.

All 6 of the lesions of fibrous dysplasia that underwent malignant change in our total series had had irradiation as at least a part of their original therapy. Five of these were in the jaws.

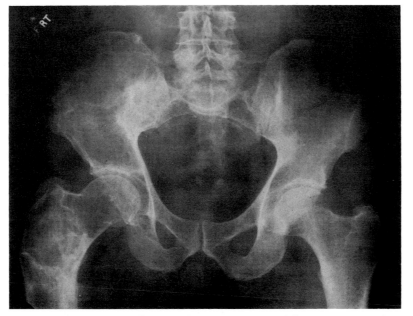

FIG. 24-6. Fibrous dysplasia involving right side of pelvis and upper part of femur. Roentgen therapy had been given 20 years previously. Although the roentgenogram does not suggest it, the sarcoma shown in Figure 24-11 has now complicated the femoral lesion. Increasing pain had been noted for 4 months.

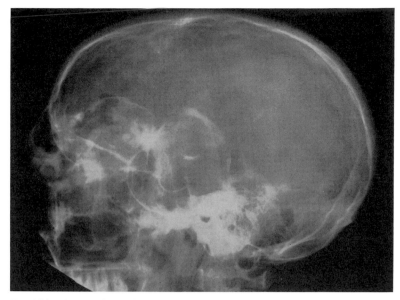

FIG. 24-7. Fibrous dysplasia causing pronounced distortion of base of skull and periorbital regions. Grossly this lesion was partially cystic.

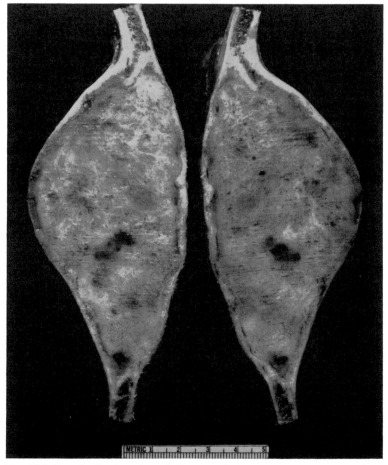

FIG. 24-8. Longitudinal section of rib expanded by fibrous dysplasia. (Reproduced with permission from: Zimmer, J. F., Dahlin, D. C., Pugh, D. G., and Clagett, O. T.: *J. Thoracic Surg., 31:*488-496, 1956.)

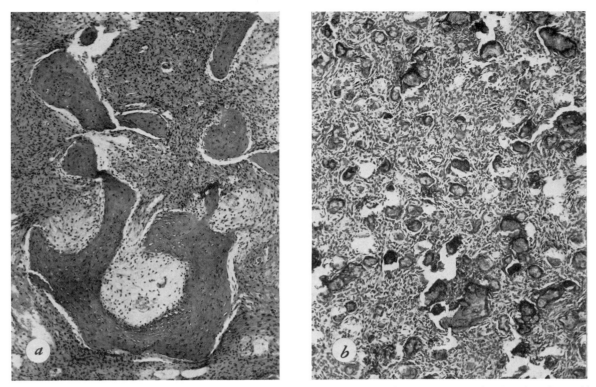

FIG. 24-9. *a*. Classic fibrous dysplasia with proliferating fibroblastic tissue and bizarre masses and trabeculae of osteoid tissue and bone (×75). *b*. Fibro-osseous dysplasia, in this instance producing spherical masses of osseous tissue. This pattern is often seen in lesions at the base of the skull and has been mistaken for meningioma (×100).

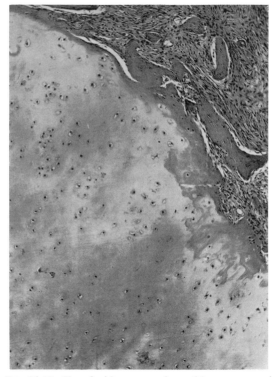

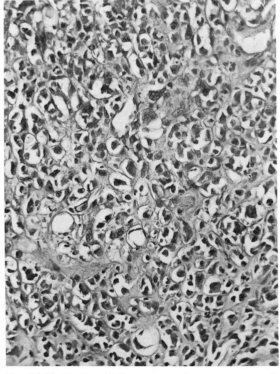

FIG. 24-10. Chondroid zones such as this may occur in lesions of fibrous dysplasia and, in rare instances, they dominate the histologic picture (×85).

FIG. 24-11. Postirradiation osteogenic sarcoma complicating femoral lesion of fibrous dysplasia shown in Figure 24-6 (×200).

CONDITIONS THAT SIMULATE PRIMARY TUMORS

Aneurysmal Bone Cyst

Aneurysmal bone cyst is one of the "variants" that has been justifiably excluded from the bona fide giant cell tumors. Features that make it logical to exclude this lesion from the neoplastic category include the observation that examples of it have regressed following incomplete removal. The cause of this strange process in bone is unknown.

In the present series, aneurysmal bone cyst has been somewhat less common than giant cell tumor of bone. No distinct sex predilection has been observed in reported cases. Nearly three fourths of the affected patients are less than 20 years of age, which is in striking contrast to the age distribution of true giant cell tumors, 90% of which occur in patients 20 years of age or older. Although aneurysmal bone cyst has been seen most commonly in the long bones, where it has a predilection for the metaphyseal region, almost any bone of the body may be affected.

Clinically, pain and swelling are the important features and they vary in duration from weeks to a few years. The lesion tends to increase in size until therapy is instituted. Vertebrae are relatively commonly involved (Cohen and co-workers, 1964), with the production of signs and symptoms owing to compression of the spinal cord and emerging nerves.

Roentgenographically, the lesion often has a characteristic appearance. A zone of rarefaction, which is usually well circumscribed and eccentric, is associated with an obvious soft-tissue extension of the process. In the classic case this soft-tissue extension is produced by bulging of the periosteum and a resultant layer of roentgenologically visible new bone which delimits the periphery of the tumor. The lesional area tends to show trabeculation. Fusiform expansion may be produced when small bones such as a rib or a fibula are affected.

Grossly, an aneurysmal bone cyst contains anastomosing cavernomatous spaces which ordinarily comprise the bulk of the lesion. The spaces are usually filled with unclotted blood, in which event blood may well up into, but does not spurt from, the tumor when it is unroofed. The egg-shell-thick layer of subperiosteal new bone which delimits the lesion is ordinarily readily discernible. Some of these lesions contain solid fleshy and friable or fibrous and granular zones which may comprise half of their bulk.

Microscopically, the essential feature is the presence of cavernomatous spaces, the walls of which lack the normal features of blood vessels. Thin strands of bone are often present in the fibrous tissue of these walls. An endothelial lining is unusual. Reconstruction of these cavernomatous spaces from curetted fragments may be extremely difficult. The solid portions of an aneurysmal bone cyst may be fibrous but they ordinarily contain a lacework of osteoid trabeculae similar to that observed in giant osteoid osteoma. Benign giant cells are often present in large numbers, thus accounting for the confusion of this lesion with genuine giant cell tumor. These solid zones with giant cells may resemble giant cell reparative granuloma of jawbones, which is likely a related lesion. The histopathology of aneurysmal bone cyst overlaps that of simple bone cyst, making differentiation difficult or impossible in some cases.

The most successful *treatment* has been surgical removal of the entire lesion or as much of it as possible. Occasionally, bone grafting of the resultant defect may be necessary. Recurrence sometimes develops. It may be difficult to determine when roentgenographic evidence of recurrence is sufficient to warrant additional treatment. Although irradiation has been advocated, especially for vertebral examples with compression of the spinal cord, three late postirradiation sarcomas have made us cautious about its use. These sarcomas developed at the sites of aneurysmal bone cysts of the tibia, the femur, and a vertebrae.

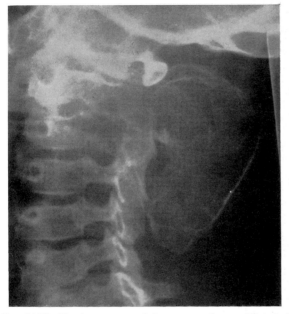

Fig. 24-12. Classic aneurysmal bone cyst of second cervical vertebra. (Reproduced with permission from: Dahlin, D. C., Besse, B. E., Jr., Pugh, D. G., and Ghormley, R. K.: *Radiology, 64*:56-65, 1955.)

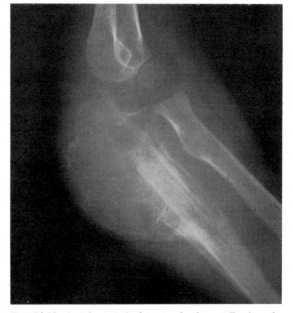

Fig. 24-13. Another typical example, here affecting the ulna. (Reproduced with permission from: Besse, B. E., Jr., Dahlin, D. C., Pugh, D. G., and Ghormley, R. K.: *Clin. Orthopaedics, 7*:93-102, 1956.)

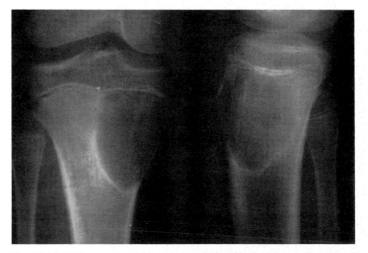

Fig. 24-14. This aneurysmal bone cyst of the tibia had not yet produced much expansion.

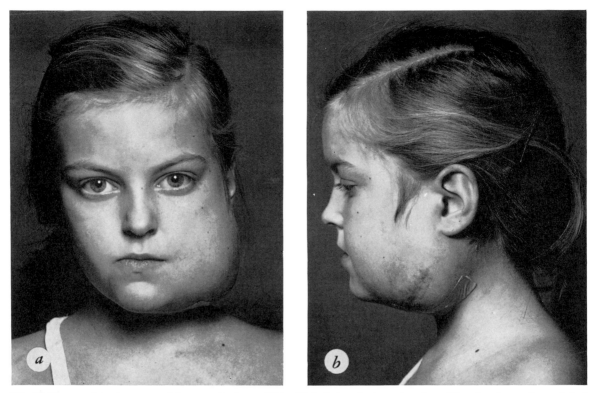

FIG. 24-15. *a* and *b*. Aneurysmal bone cyst of mandible. This lesion had produced swelling for 3 months and had recurred after incomplete removal. Wide excision with preservation of the mandible resulted in cure.

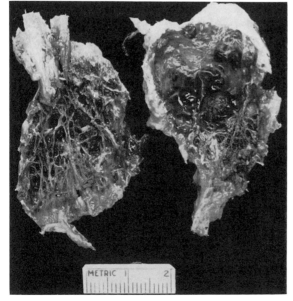

FIG. 24-16. Surfaces produced by sagittal section of aneurysmal bone cyst of upper portion of fibula. (Reproduced with permission from: Dahlin, D. C., Besse, B. E., Jr., Pugh, D. G., and Ghormley, R. K.: *Radiology, 64*:56-65, 1955.)

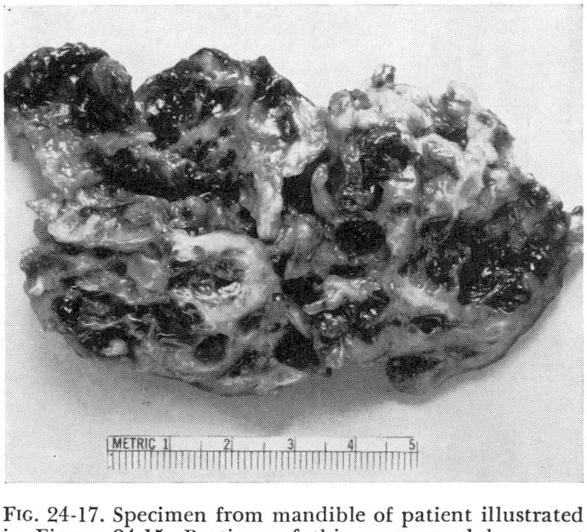

FIG. 24-17. Specimen from mandible of patient illustrated in Figure 24-15. Portions of this aneurysmal bone cyst exhibited the features of giant cell reparative granuloma.

CONDITIONS THAT SIMULATE PRIMARY TUMORS

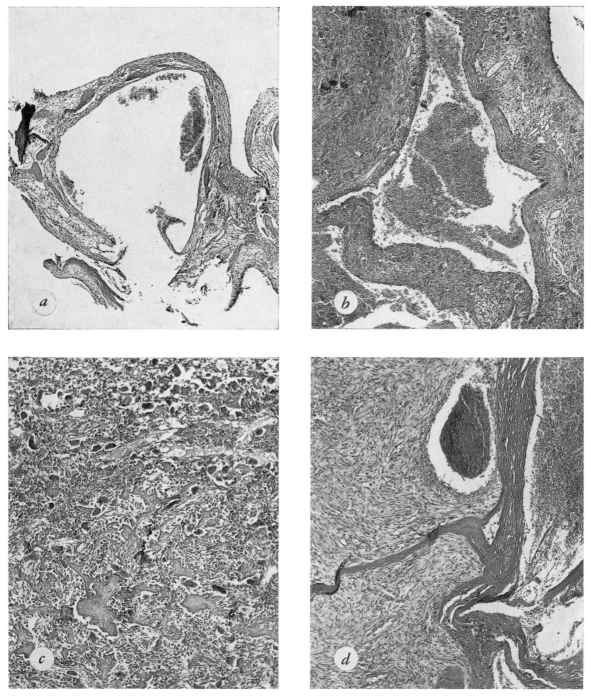

FIG. 24-18. *a*. Portion of the wall of a large cavernomatous space, showing that a smaller blood space is present in the wall (×40). *b*. Thicker and more cellular walls of blood spaces, here containing a few giant cells (×55). *c*. Solid portion of aneurysmal bone cyst, here containing osteoid trabeculae and numerous benign giant cells (×80). *d*. Solid fibrous area with cavernous space on right (×65). (Figure 24-18*b*, *c*, and *d* reproduced with permission from: Dahlin, D. C., Besse, B. E., Jr., Pugh, D. G., and Ghormley, R. K,: *Radiology, 64*:56-65, 1955.)

CONDITIONS THAT SIMULATE PRIMARY TUMORS

Heterotopic Ossification

Heterotopic ossification, often erroneously called myositis ossificans, may occur in muscle or other soft tissues. In its early or "florid" phase it may present such marked cellular activity that it may be mistaken for sarcoma. The lesions of this troublesome disease are rarely explored surgically, in their "florid" stage, so that they are not commonly encountered. The relative rarity of this disease, however, has delayed understanding of the peculiar tissue reaction associated with it.

Clinically, the patient may or may not have experienced significant recent trauma. Sometimes there is a history of unusual muscular exertion. A mass is present in most patients treated surgically. The mass commonly develops in as short a time as a week or two, and sometimes it recurs just as rapidly after surgical removal. This rate of development affords a diagnostic clue, since sarcomas rarely grow so fast.

Roentgenographically, in the earliest stages it may show no evidence of calcific substance. Usually, however, there is a more or less well-circumscribed, partially osseous tumor, which may give the false appearance of being attached to bone when viewed with only one projection. Some of the deeper-lying tumors may abut on the cortex of a bone and even be associated with some periosteal reaction. Ordinarily, however, stereoscopic studies reveal that the bone's cortex is not involved, a feature that aids materially in the differentiation from osteogenic sarcoma. With progression of the lesion, increased ossification develops until finally it is obvious roentgenologically that the process is benign.

Grossly, the tumor is well circumscribed except in the very early phases. It may be completely contained in the belly of a muscle, although an entirely similar process sometimes develops with no apparent relationship to a muscle. It is usually obvious that the lesion did not arise in bone. Ossification is characteristically most pronounced at the periphery of the mass. The central portion may contain small cysts.

Microscopically, active fibroblastic proliferation is the dominant feature and mitotic figures may be numerous. In all but the earliest lesions of this type, evidence that the fibroblasts are undergoing metaplasia to osteoblasts is present. These osteoblasts produce strands of new osteoid tissue that rapidly becomes well-formed osseous trabeculae. These are disposed in a somewhat parallel fashion that simulates the appearance of a callus. This "functional" arrangement of the osteoid and osseous trabecula, combined with the lack of true anaplasia in the proliferating cells, affords the histopathologist with the necessary diagnostic clues for the exclusion of sarcoma. Sometimes a chondroid phase is interposed between that of the proliferating fibroblasts and that of the osseous trabecula.

Treatment is usually unnecessary if one knows the correct diagnosis.

The *prognosis* is good whether the lesion is excised or amputation is performed because of an erroneous diagnosis. As indicated, sometimes the tumor recurs rather rapidly following excision, but such recurrences are, likewise, benign.

A few instances of malignant transformation of myositis ossificans have been recorded, but it is difficult to assess the authenticity of such cases. I believe that most of them represent erroneous interpretation of other processes. None were encountered in the Mayo Clinic material.

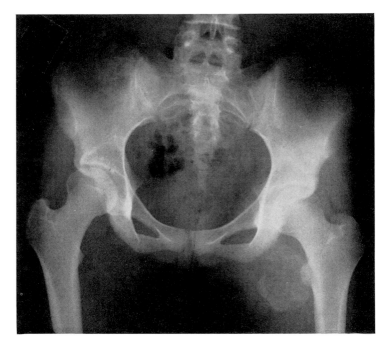

FIG. 24-19. Myositis ossificans. The patient had had local pain for 1 month. It began after strenuous gymnastics.

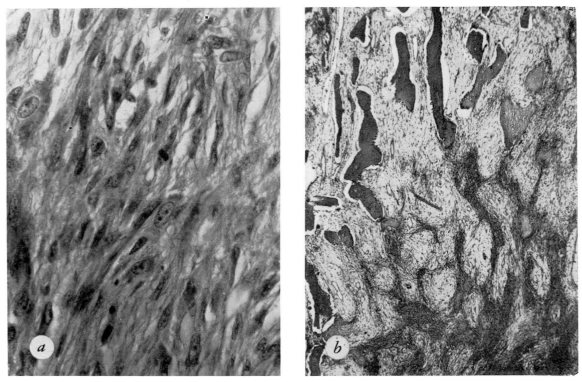

FIG. 24-20. *a.* Actively proliferating fibroblasts with mitotic figure in early lesion of myositis ossificans. Note that nuclei do not appear anaplastic ($\times$520). *b.* Here the fibroblasts have undergone metaplasia and are producing more or less parallel strands of bone ($\times$45).

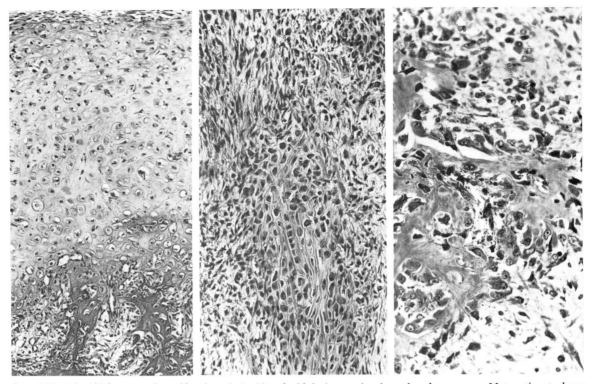

FIG. 24-21. "Florid" heterotopic ossification. *Left.* Chondroid foci may simulate chondrosarcoma. Maturation to bony trabeculae at bottom affords important evidence of their benign nature (×75). *Center.* Actively proliferating fibroblasts with a focus of osteoid tissue near center (×125). *Right.* More mature bony trabecula. The relatively large amount of cytoplasm favors the benign nature of the osteoblasts (×300).

Exuberant Callus

A healing fracture, in its early phases, exhibits marked cellular activity with abundant mitotic figures. At this stage, osteoid and chondroid material may not show the obvious functional arrangement of the reparative process, and the histologic appearance is ominous when studied out of context. Later, maturation of these substances will have resolved the problem. Baker, in 1946, emphasized that healing fractures are especially likely to simulate sarcoma in patients with fragilitas ossium. If the callus is the result of fatigue (march) fracture, which most commonly affects a metatarsal or the tibia, the underlying fracture may be roentgenographically obscure. This problem has been emphasized by Coley (1960) and by Linscheid and Coventry (1962). Traumatic avulsion of the periosteum can evoke the same type of healing reaction.

As in heterotopic ossification, nuclear evidences of malignancy are lacking. Again, the tendency for maturation of the proliferating elements into regularly arranged trabeculae is an important clue. In this type of reaction, the earliest signs of ossification appear adjacent to the bone, and the periphery of the lesion tends to be most cellular.

I am illustrating this problem because it is one commonly seen in material sent in for consultation from other pathologists. Even the proliferative subperiosteal new bone in Caffey's infantile cortical hyperostosis can pose a problem of this type to the histopathologist.

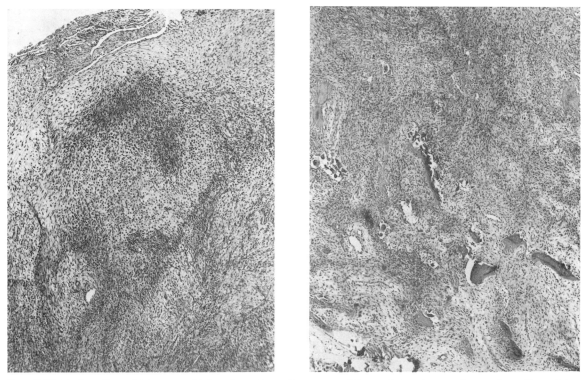

Fig. 24-22. Early callus which was mistaken for osteogenic sarcoma. These photomicrographs are from tissue taken from the lesion shown in Figure 24-23 below. The patient had injured his foot a month previously. *Left.* Periphery of reactive process. Maturation to bone is not evident and mitotic figures are numerous ($\times$35). *Right.* Near the metatarsal an orderly arrangement of bony trabecula is beginning to form ($\times$40).

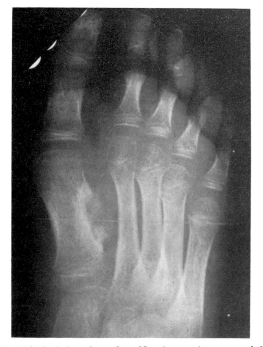

Fig. 24-23. Subperiosteal ossification as it appeared 1 month after injury. The histologic appearance is illustrated in Figure 24-22.

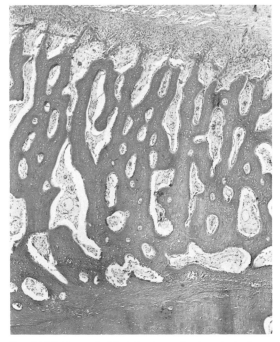

Fig. 24-24. Even at this late stage of subperiosteal new bone formation there is cellular activity just beneath the periosteum ($\times$40).

249

CONDITIONS THAT SIMULATE PRIMARY TUMORS

Simple Cyst

Simple or "unicameral" cyst of bone is of unknown cause but apparently results from a disturbance of growth at the epiphyseal line. It is relatively common and usually becomes manifest during the first 2 decades of life. In most cases it occurs in the upper part of the diaphysis of the humerus, the diaphysis of the femur, or the proximal part of the diaphysis of the tibia, in that order of frequency.

Clinically, the patient with a simple cyst of bone may have local pain, but in most cases the cyst comes to attention only after pathologic fracture has occurred. Occasionally there is swelling in the region.

Roentgenologically, there is often fusiform widening of the bone due to slight expansion in the cystic zone. The cortex is ordinarily eroded and thinned but it is intact unless pathologic fracture has occurred. Fine trabeculation through the lesion is sometimes seen, and a healed fracture may be evident as a partition through it. A simple cyst usually reaches maximal size before the patient has matured. Frequently, serial roentgenograms reveal that the epiphysis grows away from the region of the cyst so that it lies near the center of the shaft. A cyst not abutting on the epiphysis is referred to as a latent one.

Grossly, the cystic cavity may contain nothing, but is usually filled with a clear or yellowish-green fluid of low viscosity. The inner surface of the cyst wall frequently displays ridges separating depressed zones, and sometimes it is covered by a layer of fleshy tissue 1 cm or more in thickness. Not infrequently partial or complete septa are seen, the latter type making the cyst multicameral. Recent or old fractures produce modifications of this picture.

Histologically, the lining of the cyst may be merely a very thin layer of fibrous tissue. Thicker areas when present are composed of fibrogenic connective tissue which often contains numerous benign giant cells, hemosiderin pigment, a few chronic inflammatory cells, and lipophages. Because of their giant cell component some of these lesions have been erroneously classed with giant cell tumors. Individual septa, when present, resemble closely those seen in typical aneurysmal bone cyst. The histologic as well as the gross features may have been modified by fracture.

Treatment, when necessary, consists of curettage of the walls of the cyst with complete evacuation of its contents. Bone chips are ordinarily employed to fill the defect. It is difficult to determine the optimal time for treatment. Garceau and Gregory (1954) and others have noted a high recurrence rate if patients are less than 10 years of age, when the cyst is usually juxtaepiphyseal in location. The chance for permanent cure is good in patients that are more than 10 years of age, when the cyst ordinarily has been left behind by the growing epiphyseal line. Johnson and co-workers (1962) described four examples of the extremely rare sarcomatous change in simple cysts. None have been recognized in the Mayo Clinic material.

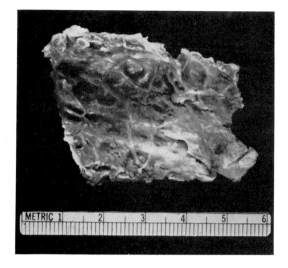

FIG. 24-25. *Above.* Inner surface of simple cyst of upper end of fibula. Note ridges separating depressed areas.

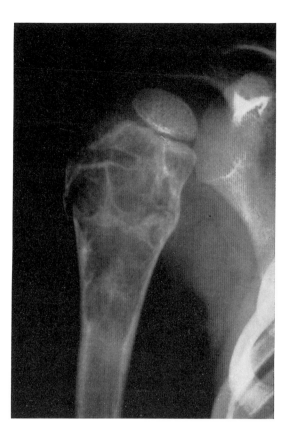

FIG. 24-26. *Above, right.* Classic appearance of simple cyst of upper portion of shaft of humerus. Fracture had occurred.

FIG. 24-27. *Right.* Lining of simple cyst. In this case there is a thick layer of fibrous tissue, along with fairly numerous benign giant cells ($\times 100$).

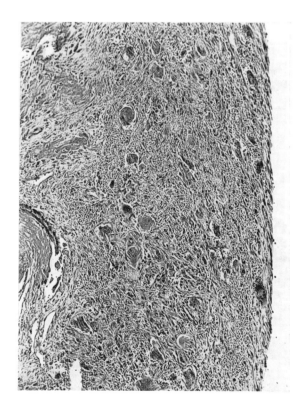

CONDITIONS THAT SIMULATE PRIMARY TUMORS

Epidermoid Cyst

Islands of squamous epithelium sometimes become embedded in bone and, with continued slow growth, a markedly expansile lesion may be produced. The majority of such cysts occur in the bones of the skull, Roth having collected more than 150 cases from the literature to 1964. In addition to causing expansion of the affected bone the cyst may protrude and displace adjacent soft tissue, including parts of the brain. Accordingly, some of them, especially if they are in roentgenologically obscure locations, may mimic the features of tumors arising in the brain. Sometimes an epidermoid cyst is dumbbell-shaped and protrudes beyond both the inner and outer tables of the skull.

Roth found records of more than 55 cysts of phalanges in the literature. Nearly all of these were in the hand. Except for squamous epithelium-lined cysts in the jaws, where they are common, and in the temporal bone, where they result from middle ear infection, epidermoid cysts are found in practically no bones other than the skull and distal phalanges. The evidence suggests that those in the skull are on a developmental basis and those in the phalanges probably on the basis of traumatic implantation of epidermis.

Numerous epidermoid cysts of the skull and only three of distal phalanges of the hand were encountered in my study of material from the files of the Mayo Clinic.

Roentgenologically, the rarefied defect in bone produced by an epidermoid cyst is typically very sharply defined and surrounded by a thin layer of sclerotic bone.

Grossly, epidermoid cysts are usually filled with a pearly white mass of inspissated, keratinized

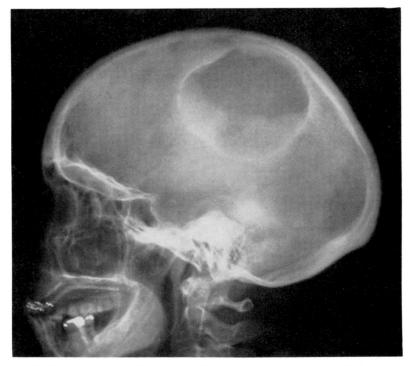

FIG. 24-28. Large epidermoid cyst of skull. It had produced a mass that bulged into the cranial cavity and outwardly as well.

252

squamous epithelium. The microscopic diagnosis depends upon demonstration of a squamous epithelial lining in at least some portion of the cyst wall.

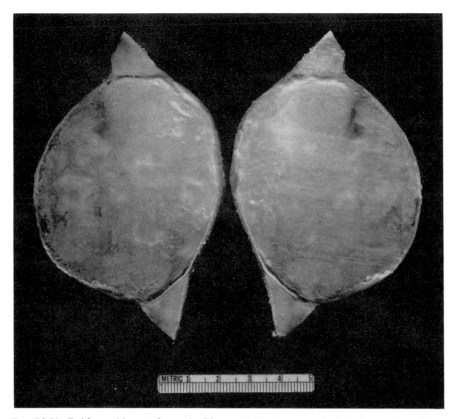

FIG. 24-29. Epidermoid cyst shown in Figure 24-28. It was excised in its entirety. Since the contents were very soft, the mass was frozen before it was cut for this picture. It bulges internally more than externally.

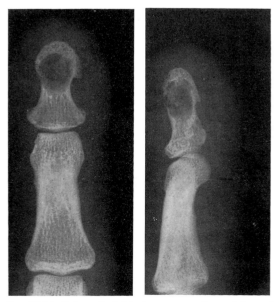

FIG. 24-30. *Left* and *right*. Anteroposterior and lateral views of epidermoid cyst of finger. (Contributed by Dr. J. W. Reagan, Cleveland, Ohio.)

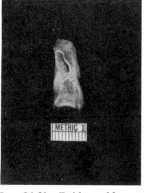

FIG. 24-31. Epidermoid cyst destroying part of terminal phalanx of finger.

CONDITIONS THAT SIMULATE PRIMARY TUMORS

"Cysts" Associated With Diseases of Joints

One must be suspicious that an osseous defect near a joint may be related to some primary synovial disease.

Severe degenerative joint disease is often accompanied by "cysts" in the juxta-articular bone. The pathogenesis of these more or less spherical zones of rarefaction is not clear. They are filled by a degenerative fibromyxoid material. They may be so extensive as to interfere with orthopedic surgical procedures designed to palliate the malfunction of the affected joint. When extensive they may produce the roentgenographic suggestion that neoplasm of bone is present.

Pigmented villonodular synovitis, especially when it affects the hip joint, sometimes results in similar "degenerative" cysts. Some of the cyst-like juxta-articular lesions in pigmented villonodular synovitis result from erosion of the proliferating masses of synovial tissue into the bone. Again, the process may be mistaken for primary disease of bone.

The inflammatory tissue of rheumatoid synovitis often produces rarefactive lesions of bone at the joints in the hands. Less commonly, significant defects adjacent to major joints or in the vertebrae are caused by invading granulomatous masses in rheumatoid disease.

Occasionally, specific infectious processes such as tuberculosis and brucellosis in joints invade and destroy juxta-articular bone.

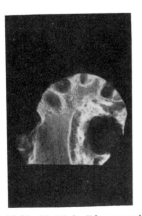

FIG. 24-32. Multiple "degenerative" cysts in femoral head of patient with pigmented villonodular synovitis. Cyst-like areas were filled with myxoid connective tissue. These cysts were just like those of degenerative arthritis.

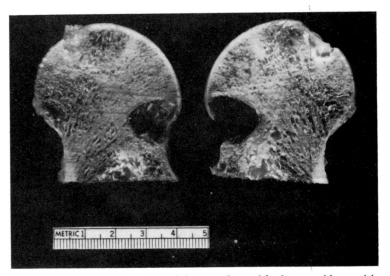

FIG. 24-33. Defect in femoral head from patient with rheumatoid synovitis. It was filled with granulomatous inflammatory tissue. (Reproduced with permission from: Hunder, G. G., Ward, L. E., and Ivins, J. C.: *Mayo Clin. Proc., 40*:766-770, 1965.)

Osteomyelitis

The alterations of bone that result from acute or chronic infection may produce roentgenographic changes that simulate those of bone tumors. Antimicrobial therapy sometimes attenuates the infection to such a degree that normal roentgenographic progression is distorted, thus increasing the likelihood of mistaking an infection of bone for a neoplasm.

Clinically, the febrile and septic course of acute osteomyelitis is sometimes obscured by therapy. Furthermore, some of the neoplasms, notably Ewing's sarcoma, produce fever and leukocytosis.

Roentgenologically, the earliest sign of osteomyelitis is irregular rarefaction, usually near the end of the shaft of a long bone. Periosteal elevation commonly occurs and one or more layers of subperiosteal new bone may be produced. Islands of dead bone which develop later are relatively radiopaque owing to the osteoporosis that occurs in the surrounding living bone. On occasion the roentgenographic shadow may simulate exactly that produced by a malignant bone tumor. Sometimes, specific chronic infections such as tuberculosis and brucellosis produce a discretely demarcated zone of bone destruction that resembles that produced by a slowly growing benign tumor of bone. At other times a large zone of sclerosis results from an indolent focus of infection in bone, and such a lesion can mimic the appearance of an osteoid osteoma in which the nidus is obscure.

Grossly, the granulation tissue present at the site of osteomyelitis may not be identifiable as non-neoplastic.

Microscopically, the differentiation from neoplasm is usually readily apparent. The granulation tissue characteristically contains numerous newly formed capillaries and an admixture of polymorphonuclear leukocytes, plasma cells, and lymphocytes in varying proportions. On some occasions, when almost a pure plasma cell reaction is evoked, the histologic pattern bears a resemblance to that of multiple myeloma. Ordinarily, however, the network of proliferating capillaries produces the unmistakable pattern one associates with reaction to infection.

The *treatment* of osteomyelitis varies with the organism responsible for the infection. Management of the condition is sometimes greatly facilitated by examination of fresh frozen sections at the time of operation. In certain specific mycotic infections, for instance, the diagnosis can be made or strongly suspected from the histologic appearance. Whenever the histologic pattern is that of a granulomatous type of inflammation, bacteriologic investigation can be appropriately directed. A wide variety of bacterial and mycotic infections can produce lesions in bone.

The possibility of malignant change in long-standing chronic osteomyelitis must be borne in mind. The usual malignant tumor is squamous cell carcinoma which develops from the regenerating skin at the edge of the cutaneous ulceration and invades the underlying already-diseased bone. An exacerbation of chronic symptoms or a flarcup in the quiescent stage of osteomyelitis should arouse suspicion of this complication. The carcinoma is usually well differentiated, but successful management depends on amputation.

More exotic tumors rarely complicate osteomyelitis as noted by Morris and Lucas (1964). Our total series includes one fibrosarcoma, one malignant lymphoma, and one rapidly lethal myeloma.

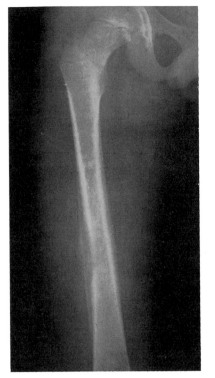

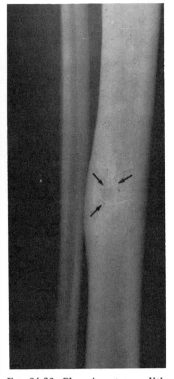

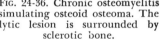

FIG. 24-34. An osteomyelitic lesion that roentgenologically simulates sarcoma. This, like the one shown in Figure 24-35, was caused by M. pyogenes and had destroyed bone and caused periosteal formation of new bone.

FIG. 24-35. Osteomyelitis of humerus simulating sarcoma. This occurred in a 9-year-old boy who had noted local pain for 1 month. The cultures from the lesion revealed M. pyogenes.

FIG. 24-36. Chronic osteomyelitis simulating osteoid osteoma. The lytic lesion is surrounded by sclerotic bone.

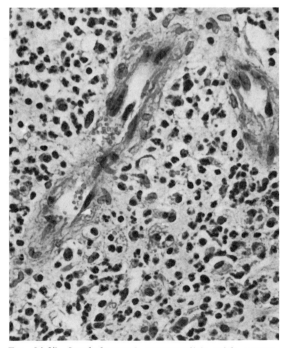

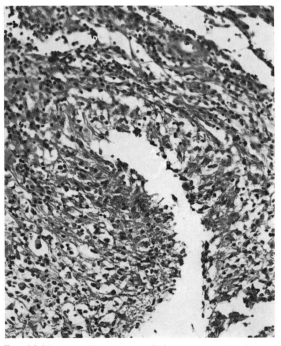

FIG. 24-37. Staphylococcal osteomyelitis with neutrophils, plasma cells, and capillary proliferation (×175).

FIG. 24-38. Brucellar osteomyelitis. The specific character of the infection is suggested by the clusters of epithelioid cells (×170).

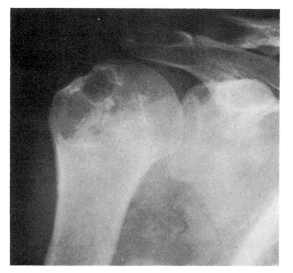

FIG. 24-39. Brucellar osteomyelitis simulating chondroblastoma of humerus.

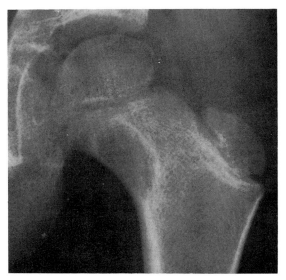

FIG. 24-40. Tuberculosis, producing a neoplasm-like rarefaction of the femoral neck.

Histiocytosis X (Reticuloendotheliosis)

This category includes a spectrum of conditions that range from the usually solitary and curable eosinophilic granuloma through the disseminated process that produces the Schüller-Christian syndrome to the fulminating, rapidly fatal variety known as Letterer-Siwe disease. Osseous lesions ordinarily dominate the pathologic picture of histiocytosis X, it being basically a disease of the reticuloendothelial system.

Diffuse malignant lymphomas have been mistaken for Letterer-Siwe disease. Letterer-Siwe syndrome usually affects very young children, whereas the Schüller-Christian syndrome and eosinophilic granuloma are seen most often in children and young adults. Practically any bone of the body may be affected, but there is a predilection for the skull.

A great variety of *symptoms* is produced. Ordinarily, patients with eosinophilic granuloma have a solitary painful focus and often a palpable or visible mass. The triad of the Schüller-Christian syndrome classically includes exophthalmos, often unilateral, diabetes insipidus, and rarefied defects of bones of the skull. A partial triad, however, has the same significance if other evidences of dissemination such as anemia, splenomegaly, fatigability, weight loss, and lymphadenopathy are present. Patients with histiocytosis X may complain of discharge from the ears owing to involvement of the temporal bones, loosening or falling-out of the teeth secondary to lesions of the jaw, and any of the symptoms that might be produced by focal destruction of bone. Any bone may be the site of a painful and sometimes expansile lesion. Vertebral involvement may result in collapse of a vertebral body with resultant neurologic symptoms. Cutaneous manifestations, lymphadenopathy, and splenomegaly are most common in the progressing, diffuse form of the disease. Pulmonary infiltration may become clinically important and, on rare occasions, it is the most significant evidence of the disease. Diffuse pulmonary lesions of histiocytosis X, on the other hand, may occur in the absence of osseous lesions; such patients are usually adults who are not seriously ill, may have episodes of spontaneous pneumothorax, and have an unpredictable but generally favorable clinical course.

Roentgenologically, the defects in bone are usually discretely defined. Periosteal reaction may be present when the cortex becomes eroded or when pathologic fracture has occurred. In the case of solitary lesions, such reaction combined with a poorly defined zone of rarefaction may produce a shadow like that of a malignant bone tumor. Multiple adjacent defects often become confluent. Lesions in the mandible are usually concentrated along the alveolar process. The teeth, in consequence, may appear to have no bony support, which indeed is the case. Moseley described the roentgenographic features in detail in 1962.

Grossly, the lesional tissue is soft. It may be gray, pink, or yellow.

The *microscopic appearance* is what links these three general conditions together. The salient and pathognomonic feature consists of foci of proliferating histiocytic cells. These histiocytes frequently have ill-defined cytoplasmic boundaries and characteristically contain an oval or indented nucleus. Multinucleated histiocytes may be seen. Although chromatin clumping and nucleoli are inconspicuous, mitotic figures are not uncommon. This has led to the confusion of histiocytosis X with malignant tumors, especially reticulum cell sarcoma on some occasions. Zones of necrosis are present in many of the lesions. The histiocytes may be swollen owing to cholesterol in their cytoplasm. Varying numbers of eosinophils, lymphocytes, and neutrophils are nearly always present.

The *treatment* of lesions seen in eosinophilic granuloma and the major ones in Schüller-Christian syndrome is roentgen therapy in moderate dosage. Steroids and other chemotherapeutic agents have been used successfully in the severe, disseminated forms of histiocytosis X.

Complete evaluation of patients who present with a defect characteristic of histiocytosis X is important in estimating *prognosis.* Those patients who have only one or a few lesions are usually cured by local irradiation. Patients with the Schüller-Christian type of disease have a poor long-term outlook, but prolonged palliation can be expected if therapy is administered judiciously. Enriquez, in a study of 116 patients with histiocytosis X at the Mayo Clinic (1966), found that those less than 3 years of age, those with more than 8 bones involved, those with hemorrhagic manifestations, and those with splenomegaly all had an ominous prognosis. Those who survived more than 3 years after the onset of symptoms had a good prognosis.

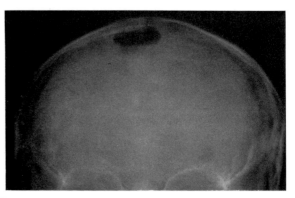

FIG. 24-41. *Right.* Skull defect produced by histiocytosis X. The skull is one of the commonest sites for lesions in this disease.

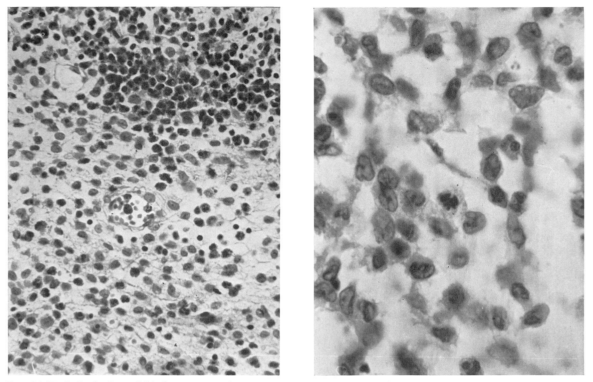

FIG. 24-42. *Left.* Lesion of histiocytosis X showing essential pale-staining histiocytes and darker eosinophils which commonly accompany the basic cells of the lesion ($\times$385). *Right.* Higher magnification to illustrate details of histiocytes. Note mitotic figure near center of field ($\times$1000).

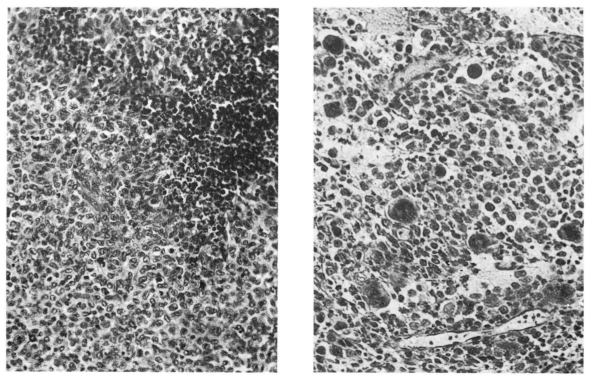

FIG. 24-43. *Left.* Characteristic cells of histiocytosis X dominate this field. Dark cells at upper right are eosinophils ($\times$245). *Right.* Multinucleated histiocytes such as those shown here are found in a minority of lesions ($\times$200).

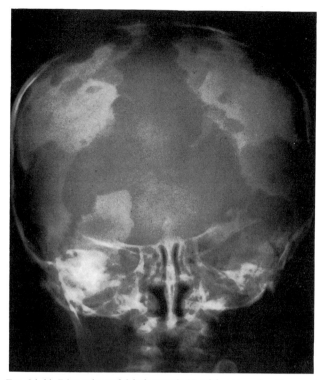

Fig. 24-44. Disseminated histiocytosis X with severe involvement of skull. This 3-year-old boy died the following year.

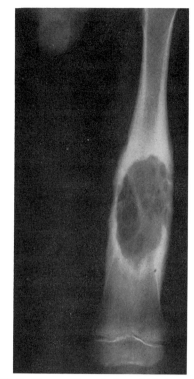

Fig. 24-45. Huge solitary lesion of histiocytosis X. Note marked sclerosis of adjacent bone.

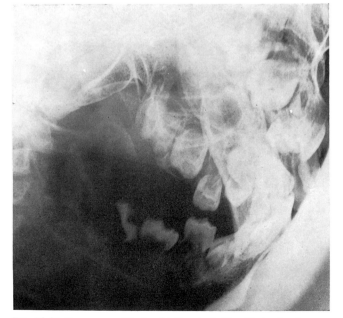

Fig. 24-46. Severe mandibular histiocytosis X with teeth about to exfoliate, which is a common complication.

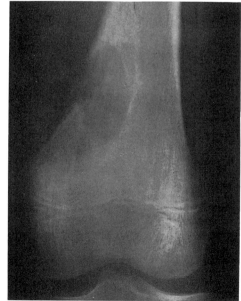

Fig. 24-47. Lytic lesion of histiocytosis X showing features suggestive of a malignant tumor.

Giant Cell Reparative Granuloma

This lesion is peculiar to the jawbones. It has been commonly confused with genuine benign giant cell tumor of bone. The concept that it is not a neoplasm but rather some peculiar reactive lesion is gaining acceptance. The lesion consists of proliferating fibroblasts and, often, zones in which metaplasia is resulting in the formation of orderly osseous trabeculae. A variable amount of vascularity and microcyst formation may be seen. The basically fibrogenic quality of the lesional tissue is the main feature that differentiates giant cell reparative granuloma from true giant cell tumor. Actually, true giant cell tumors are found so rarely, if ever, in the jawbones that one can practically exclude the possibility. The differentiation of these two lesions is important. Complete removal of giant cell reparative granuloma almost always effects cure, whereas true giant cell tumors recur in 50% of cases and 10% of them become malignant. Giant cell reparative granuloma commonly occurs in persons in the first decade or two of life as well as in older people.

There appears to be little difference between the lesions within bone that present the histologic characteristics of giant cell reparative granuloma and those that are basically soft-tissue tumors of the gums with little or no osseous involvement.

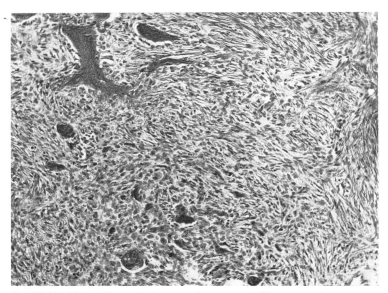

FIG. 24-48. Giant cell reparative granuloma of mandible. A few benign giant cells are present but the histologic picture is dominated by fibroblastic cells. Osseous metaplasia, which is almost always present, is seen at the upper left (×100).

261

CONDITIONS THAT SIMULATE PRIMARY TUMORS

Paget's Disease

Paget's disease is of unknown cause. It occurs in middle and old age. The pelvis, femur, skull, tibia, and vertebrae are common sites of involvement, although any bone may be affected. In early stages, resorption of bone is prominent. Later there is a mixture of destruction and repair of bone and, in the final stage, the reparative process is predominant and radiopacity is marked. A focal lesion of Paget's disease may simulate primary tumor of bone roentgenologically. With more diffuse involvement of the skeleton, differentiation of it from osteoblastic deposits on metastatic carcinoma may be a problem. Widening of the affected bone is helpful evidence that the sclerosing lesion is a manifestation of Paget's disease.

Sarcoma occasionally arises in Paget's disease to complicate the problem of roentgenologic diagnosis. The marked alteration of bone produced by Paget's disease sometimes obscures early signs of a superimposed malignant process.

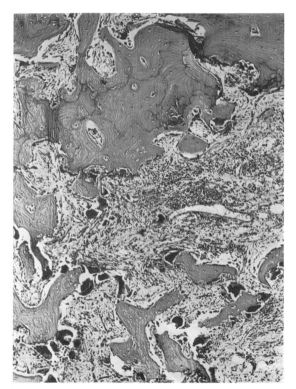

FIG. 24-49. Paget's disease with characteristic mosaic pattern in irregular osseous trabeculae. Osteoclasts are numerous and the marrow is replaced by vascular fibrous tissue ($\times 50$).

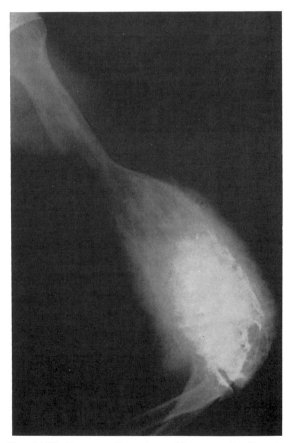

FIG. 24-50. Extreme distortion of humerus by Paget's disease. Such a lesion requires careful biopsy to exclude the presence of sarcoma.

Hyperparathyroidism

Hyperparathyroidism results from neoplasms or diffuse hyperplasia of the parathyroid glands. Ordinarily, diffuse demineralization of the skeleton occurs, but marked focal absorption sometimes produces a cyst-like appearance on the roentgenogram that can simulate that of a primary neoplasm of bone. In some instances the fibroblastic tissue that fills the defect is so exuberant that the contour of the bone bulges, thereby suggesting even more strongly that a neoplasm is present.

With widespread knowledge of the syndrome of hyperparathyroidism that prevails nowadays, the osseous lesions it produces are rarely subjected to biopsy. The diagnosis is best established by determinations of the serum calcium and phosphorus and by the finding of an increased amount of urinary calcium.

The lesion does not present pathognomonic histologic features. Where the osseous trabeculae are being resorbed, there is proliferating fibroblastic connective tissue usually so richly sprinkled with benign osteoclast-like giant cells that the diagnosis of giant cell tumor may be entertained. The basic fibrogenic quality of the lesion should, however, preclude the diagnosis of giant cell tumor because the latter lesion is not fibrogenic in its proliferating, diagnostic fields. Multifocal giant cell-rich fibroblastic islands partially separated by fairly well-formed trabeculae and the lack of typical features of other giant cell "variants" may alert the histopathologist to the possibility of a lesion's being the result of hyperparathyroidism.

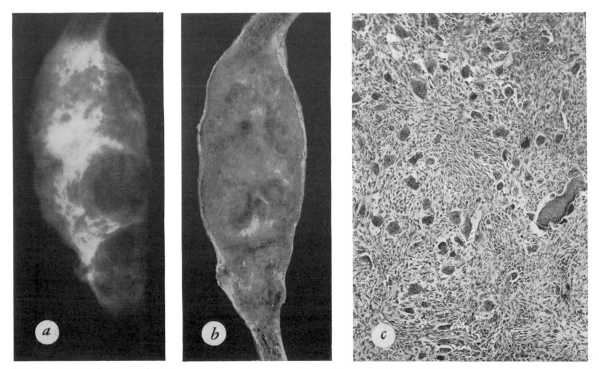

FIG. 24-51. *a* and *b*. Expanding "cystic" lesion of hyperparathyroidism involving a rib. Note that tumor is composed of fibrous tissue. *c*. Characteristic lesion of this disease. The fibrous tissue contains numerous giant cells of benign type. An almost completely resorbed osseous trabecula is seen at the extreme right (×100).

CONDITIONS THAT SIMULATE PRIMARY TUMORS

Synovial Chondromatosis and Para-Articular Chondromas

Cartilaginous metaplasia of synovium can give rise to one or innumerable cartilaginous bodies which may undergo partial calcification and ossification. In major joints this condition is monarticular and most often affects the knee. Numerous loose bodies or a conglomerate mass of osteocartilaginous tissue may develop. The diffuse process, with numerous cartilaginous nodules, may occur in bursae or tendon sheaths. Solitary chondromas are sometimes seen embedded in joint capsules, especially in the hands and feet; whether all of these are of synovial origin is debatable. Some of the chondromas of the hands and feet have convincing evidence of synovial derivation.

The *histologic* appearance of these proliferating cartilaginous tumors is what makes them important to the pathologist. In many instances, the nuclear abnormalities and numbers of multinucleated cells are so great that in the right context, as in the medulla of a major tubular bone, the diagnosis of chondrosarcoma would be strongly supported. Paradoxically, however, these cartilaginous masses are practically never malignant nor even premalignant.

The *prognosis* is good although the diffuse synovial lesions may recur since it is so difficult to remove every vestige of them. The solitary chondromas almost never recur after excision.

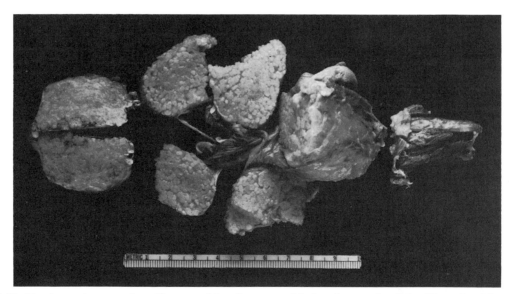

Fig. 24-52. Conglomerate mass of cartilage resulting from synovial chondromatosis of the iliopectineal bursa. This produced a significant intrapelvic mass. Although cytologically active, the diagnosis was established by finding metaplastic cartilage in encapsulating synovium. Excision of the mass has given a good clinical result now more than 6 years later. This is an extremely unusual location for this disease.

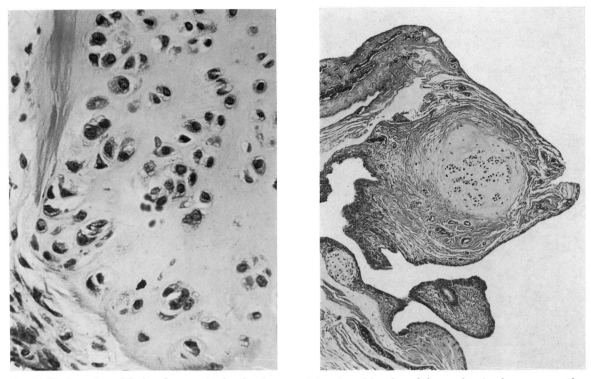

FIG. 24-53. *Left*. Synovial chondromatosis showing large nuclei and multinucleated forms that in the proper setting would constitute evidence suggesting malignancy ($\times$400). *Right*. Demonstration of origin from synovium such as shown here establishes the correct and benign diagnosis ($\times$50).

Bone Infarcts

Infarction of bone is common following decompression sickness, as in caisson workers, and in patients with sickle cell anemia. It is also being reported increasingly often as affecting part of the femoral head in the form of so-called idiopathic aseptic necrosis. Not so well known is that single or multiple osseous infarcts of unknown cause, although rarely seen, can occur in a variety of bones. These may be associated with local pain. In the early stages, according to Bullough and co-workers (1965), there may be no roentgenographic findings. Later, the lesion presents as an irregular area of density, sometimes with a cyst-like center. The density is the result of an ingrowth of new bone and impregnation of the necrotic zone with calcium salts. These infarcts may be mistaken for such things as calcifying cartilaginous neoplasms, cysts, and even osteoid osteoma with a surrounding halo of sclerotic bone. They differ histologically from the relatively common, asymptomatic "bone islands" seen roentgenographically. These latter lesions consist of a focus of bone that is merely much too dense for the region in question.

Furey and co-workers, in 1960, described two cases of the extremely rare complication of fibrosarcoma at the sites of bone infarcts.

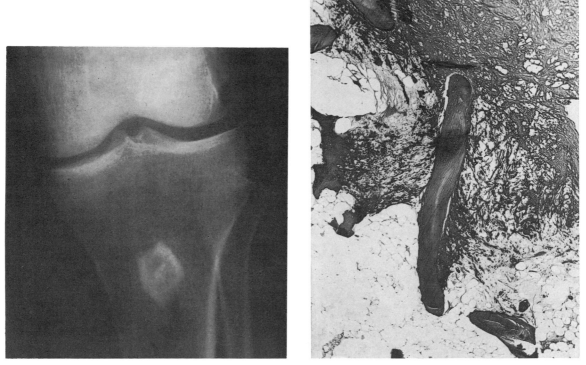

FIG. 24-54. *Left.* Bone infarct showing irregular radiodensity. *Right.* Necrotic osseous trabeculae with amorphous mineralization of the intervening degenerated marrow. This pattern is characteristic of an old infarct of bone (×30).

Bibliography

1946 Baker, S. L.: Hyperplastic Callus Simulating Sarcoma in Two Cases of Fragilitas Ossium. *J. Path. & Bact., 58:*609-623.

1948 Ghormley, R. K., and Clegg, R. S.: Bone and Joint Changes in Hemophilia With Report of Cases of So-Called Hemophilic Pseudotumor. *J. Bone & Joint Surg., 30A:*589-600.

1951 Pritchard, J. E.: Fibrous Dysplasia of the Bones. *Am. J. M. Sc., 222:*313-332.

1953 Lichtenstein, Louis: Histiocytosis X: Integration of Eosinophilic Granuloma of Bone, "Letterer-Siwe Disease," and "Schüller-Christian Disease" as Related Manifestations of a Single Nosologic Entity. *A.M.A. Arch. Path., 56:*84-102.

1953 Jaffe, H. L.: Giant-cell Reparative Granuloma, Traumatic Bone Cyst, and Fibrous (Fibro-osseous) Dysplasia of the Jawbones. *Oral Surg., 6:*159-175.

1954 Pugh, D. G.: *Roentgenologic Diagnosis of Diseases of Bones.* Baltimore, Williams & Wilkins.

1954 Garceau, G. J., and Gregory, C. F.: Solitary Unicameral Bone Cyst. *J. Bone & Joint Surg., 36A:*267-280.

1957 Eversole, S. L., Jr., Holman, G. H., and Robinson, R. A.: Hitherto Undescribed Characteristics of the Pathology of Infantile Cortical Hyperostosis (Caffey's Disease). *Bull. Johns Hopkins Hosp., 101:*80-99.

1957 Lichtenstein, L.: Aneurysmal Bone Cyst. Observations on Fifty Cases. *J. Bone & Joint Surg., 39A:*873-882.

1959 Havard, C. W. H., and Scott, R. B.: Urticaria Pigmentosa With Visceral and Skeletal Lesions. *Quart. J. Med., 24:*459-470.

1960 Wholey, M. H., and Pugh, D. G.: Localized Destructive Lesions in Rheumatoid Spondylitis. *Radiology, 74*:54-56.

1960 Coley, B. L.: *Neoplasms of Bone,* Ed. 2, New York City, Paul B. Hoeber, Inc., pp. 723-725.

1960 Furey, J. G., Ferrer-Torells, M., and Reagan, J. W.: Fibrosarcoma Arising at the Site of Bone Infarcts. A Report of 2 Cases. *J. Bone & Joint Surg., 42A*:802-810.

1961 Williams, A. W., Dunnington, W. G., and Berte, S. J.: Pulmonary Eosinophilic Granuloma: A Clinical and Pathologic Discussion. *Ann. Int. Med., 54*:30-45.

1962 Smith, J. H.. and Pugh, D. G.: Roentgenographic Aspects of Articular Pigmented Villonodular Synovitis. *Am. J. Roentgenol., 87*:1146-1156.

1962 Murphy, F. P., Dahlin, D. C., and Sullivan, C. R.: Articular Synovial Chondromatosis. *J. Bone & Joint Surg., 44A*:77-86.

1962 Linscheid, R. L., and Coventry, M. B.: Unrecognized Fractures of Long Bones Suggesting Primary Bone Tumors. *Proc. Staff Meet., Mayo Clin., 37*:599-606.

1962 Johnson, L. C., Vetter, H., and Putschar, W. G. J.: Sarcomas Arising in Bone Cysts. *Virchows Arch. path. Anat., 335*:428-451.

1962 Moseley, J. E.: Patterns of Bone Change in the Reticuloendothelioses. *J. Mt. Sinai Hosp., 29*:282-321.

1962 Lahey, M. E.: Prognosis in Reticuloendotheliosis in Children. *J. Pediat., 60*:664-671.

1964 Kim, S. K., and Barry, W. F., Jr.: Bone Island. *Am. J. Roentgenol., 92*:1301-1306.

1964 Roth, S. I.: Squamous Cysts Involving the Skull and Distal Phalanges. *J. Bone & Joint Surg., 46A*:1442-1450.

1964 Lichtenstein, L.: Histiocytosis X (Eosinophilic Granuloma of Bone, Letterer-Siwe Disease, and Schüller-Christian Disease). Further Observations of Pathological and Clinical Importance. *J. Bone & Joint Surg., 46A*:76-90.

1964 Alldred, A. J., and Nisbet, N. W.: Hydatid Disease of Bone in Australasia. *J. Bone & Joint Surg., 46B*:260-267.

1964 Cohen, D. M., Dahlin, D. C., and MacCarty, C. S.: Vertebral Giant-Cell Tumor and Variants. *Cancer, 17*:461-472.

1964 Morris, J. M., and Lucas, D. B.: Fibrosarcoma Within a Sinus Tract of Chronic Draining Osteomyelitis. Case Report and Review of Literature. *J. Bone & Joint Surg., 46A*:853-857.

1965 Johnson, L. L., and Kempson, R. L.: Epidermoid Carcinoma in Chronic Osteomyelitis: Diagnostic Problems and Management. *J. Bone & Joint Surg., 47A*:133-145.

1965 Hunder, G. G., Ward, L. E., and Ivins, J. C.: Rheumatoid Granulomatous Lesion Simulating Malignancy in the Head and Neck of the Femur. *Mayo Clin. Proc., 40*:766-770.

1965 Bullough, P. G., Kambolis, C. P., Marcove, R. C.. and Jaffe, H. L.: Bone Infarctions Not Associated With Caisson Disease. *J. Bone & Joint Surg., 47A*:477-491.

1966 Enriquez, P.: Unpublished data.

Chapter 25

Odontogenic Tumors

THE JAWBONES provide special tumors that derive from their dental structures. These lesions simulate neoplasms of osseous derivation. The following tabulation of these special tumors, short and somewhat simplified, should be useful to the general pathologist.

Ameloblastoma
Ameloblastic adenomatoid tumor
Ameloblastic fibroma
Ameloblastic odontoma
Complex odontoma
Compound odontoma
Myxoma (fibromyxoma)

Although dentinomas are included in many classifications, it seems likely that they are but variants of some of the above hamartoma-like tumors such as ameloblastic odontoma. Cementifying fibroma (periapical fibrous dysplasia) derives from the specialized bone around the dental roots and thus is not strictly odontogenic. Bulbous masses of densely ossified material surrounding dental roots are considered to be cementomas.

Cysts of the jaws are usually lined by squamous epithelium. Reference to the history and roentgenograms is necessary in determining whether they are related to unerupted teeth, to residual epithelial islands after dental extraction, or have some other genesis. These cysts and the "hemorrhagic" or "traumatic" cysts of the jaw, which have no lining, pose little diagnostic problem for the histopathologist.

Benign fibro-osseous lesions of the jaws are relatively common. They encompass such a wide spectrum as regards amount of osseous component that they defy strict classification. But pathologically they fit into the general category of fibrous (fibro-osseous) dysplasias. Benign, densely collagenous, fibroblastic tissue contains a variable amount of bone which typically arises as a metaplastic change in the former. Occasional lesions are large, expansile masses which may bulge into and distort the sinuses, and for which the term "fibrous osteoma" or "osteofibroma" is preferred by some. Most are centrally originating lesions that vary greatly in size and radiopacity. They may be incidental roentgenographic findings or produce pronounced distortion of the bone. A minority are a part of the polyostotic fibrous dysplasia complex. Even cherubism, with its fibrous expansion of the jaws of children that is characteristically familial, bilateral, and tends toward spontaneous resolution, is usually called fibrous dysplasia. The least conspicuous end of the spectrum is the periapical fibrous dysplasia mentioned above. All of these fibro-osseous lesions, although they may recur, are benign. Conservative surgical management is indicated. Unless exposed to radiation therapy they have practically no tendency to malignant change. Some osteogenic sarcomas of the jaws are so lacking in overt anaplasia that they pose a problem in differentiation from fibrous dysplasia.

Most of the primary malignant tumors of bone and some of the benign ones can occur in jawbones and must be considered in the differential diagnosis of defects in these bones. Metastatic carcinoma can simulate a primary tumor of the jaws. Giant cell reparative granulomas, considered in chapter 24, are a frequent cause of rarefaction of these bones.

Ameloblastoma

There are some 125 ameloblastomas in the Mayo Clinic's total series of oral lesions which includes 50 osteogenic sarcomas of the jaws. Ameloblastoma is the most common of the odontogenic tumors in our surgical series and yet it comprises only about 1% of the cysts and tumors seen in the area of the maxilla and mandible (Gorlin and co-workers, 1961). There is no notable sex predilection, and the tumor appears throughout adulthood and old age. It is distinctly rare in children. More than three-fourths arise in the mandible, most commonly in the molar-angle region. Slowly growing, the tumor is usually painless. Swelling, of more than 2 years' duration in two-thirds of the cases, is the usual symptom. The roentgenogram shows a cyst-like radiolucent expansion which may appear multilocular or unilocular and is simulated by a variety of lesions. The tumor often contains cysts and may be so predominantly cystic that squamous epithelium-lined cyst with incidental non-neoplastic ameloblastic elements in its wall becomes a differential consideration.

The proliferating epithelial elements belie their derivation from ameloblasts. The outer layer in the cellular islands is usually of cells of columnar type with nuclei tending to be away from the basement membrane. The cells often become stellate and loosely arranged in the centers of the islands. Although follicular and plexiform patterns are described, these merge in many tumors. A variable amount of non-neoplastic collagen may separate the epithelial islands. Sometimes, large zones of spindle-shaped epithelial cells are suggestive of sarcoma. Squamous metaplasia is relatively frequent and may be so marked as to suggest that the tumor is squamous cell carcinoma. Rare ameloblastomas contain cells that are granular; such cells may comprise the entire tumor. Some ameloblastomas are so vascular they have been called ameloblastohemangiomas. The histogenesis of melanoameloblastoma (melanotic progonoma, retinal anlage tumor) is obscure but this rare tumor of infancy is nearly always found in the jaws, especially the maxilla. By definition, ameloblastomas produce no recognizable mature dental substances. The extremely rare but distinctive calcifying epithelial odontogenic tumor described by Pindborg (1958) may be a variant of ameloblastoma; it behaves like one. It contains characteristic spherical calcific masses. Some of these peculiar ameloblastic tumors contain a substance that looks and stains like amyloid.

Treatment principles for ameloblastoma are still controversial, but it seems reasonable to adopt a relatively conservative attitude since metastasis practically never occurs. The tumor does have marked capacity to recur unless widely excised.

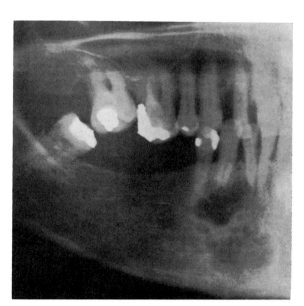

Fig. 25-1. Recurrent, multilocular ameloblastoma of the anterior part of the mandible.

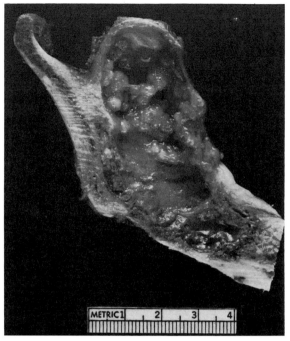

Fig. 25-2. Partially cystic ameloblastoma bulging from the region of the angle of the mandible.

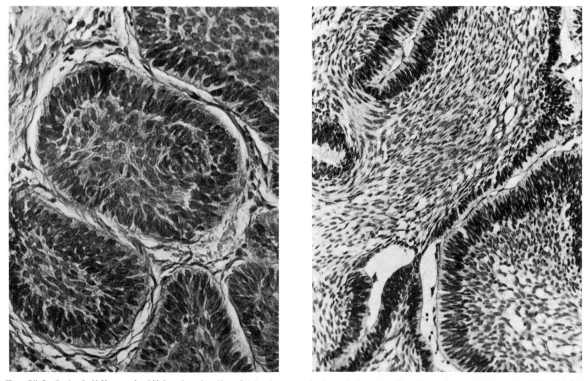

Fig. 25-3. *Left.* Solidly packed islands of cells which show typical peripheral palisading of ameloblasts ($\times$325). *Right.* In this tumor the cells of the centers of the anastomosing clusters show a prominent spindling quality ($\times$200).

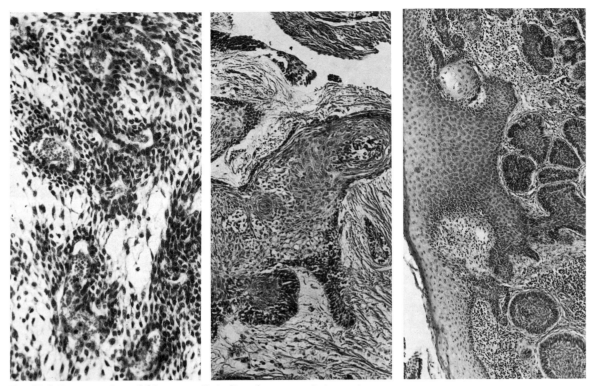

FIG. 25-4. Patterns of ameloblastomas. *Left.* Prominent vascularity such as seen here has prompted some to consider this lesion a hemangioameloblastoma (×200). *Center.* Squamous metaplasia, which is not an extremely unusual finding (×125). *Right.* Ameloblastoma eroding to and fusing with the gingival epithelium (×70).

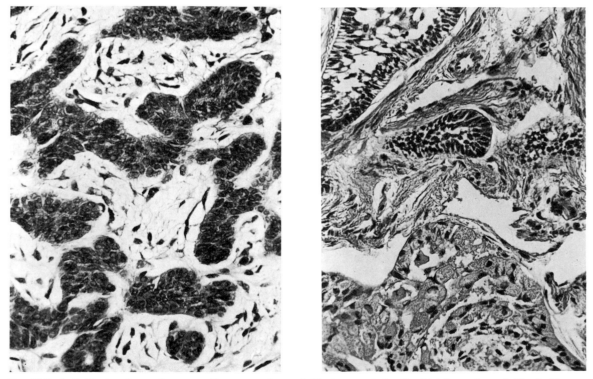

FIG. 25-5. *Left.* Trabecular pattern sometimes seen in ameloblastomas mimics the histology of ameloblastic fibroma somewhat. The characteristic fibrous component of the latter lesion is lacking (×250). *Right.* Granular cells such as these comprise part or all of an ameloblastoma in rare instances (×250).

Ameloblastic Adenomatoid Tumor

This tumor, also called adenoameloblastoma, should be distinguished from ameloblastoma because it responds to conservative surgical removal, having little tendency to recur. It is much less common than ameloblastoma. The Mayo Clinic files contain only eight recognized examples. Most of the some 40 reported tumors have been in patients aged 11 to 26; there has been a slight predominance in females. Two-thirds of the tumors have involved the maxilla, and nearly all of them have been located anterior to the first premolars. Tumefaction is the common symptom. Roentgenologically, the tumor produces a cyst-like zone which may display calcific material in a stippled pattern. The "cyst" often contains an unerupted tooth and resembles a dentigerous cyst. Grossly the lesion is often actually cystic, and the solid tissue may fill only a fraction of the cavity. The expanding process is well demarcated from surrounding tissue. Microscopically, the tumor is characterized by tubular, duct-like structures lined with columnar or cuboidal epithelium. The central spaces in some of these duct-like structures are empty, others are filled with acidophilic material, and still others are lined by a layer of pink hyaline material. Small calcified spherules or even larger mineralized masses may be found, sometimes within the tubular spaces. Masses of cells that produce whorl-like structures are found among the glandular-appearing elements. These epithelial cells sometimes resemble the stellate reticulum of ameloblastomas but they are usually distinctly spindle-shaped. These nests of cells lie outside the glandular component, which is in striking contrast to their location within the palisade of columnar cells in ameloblastoma. Although the cells are closely packed, they are regular in size and shape and do not appear anaplastic. The prognosis is excellent, local curettage being curative.

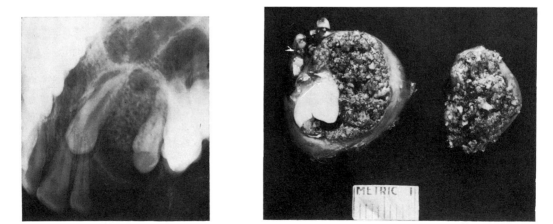

FIG. 25-6. *Left.* Ameloblastic adenomatoid tumor presenting as a cyst-like lesion containing the upper right premolar tooth. *Right.* Surgical specimen. Most of the premolar tooth was within the well-circumscribed tumor, but part of the root projected from it. (Reproduced with permission from: Stafne, E. C.: *Oral Surg., 1*:887-894, 1948.)

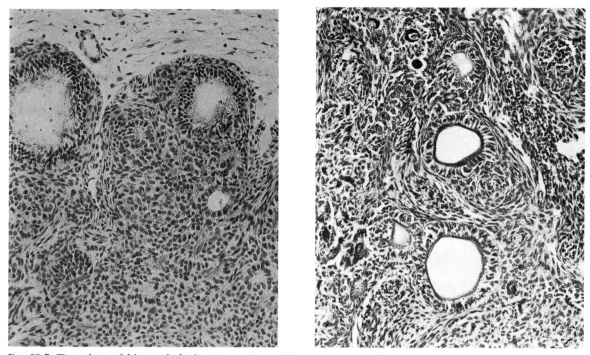

FIG. 25-7. Two views of histopathologic pattern of ameloblastic adenomatoid tumor. *Left.* Periphery of mass showing ductular structures of varying size and the slightly fusiform cells among them (×140). *Right.* Central portion of the tumor which has the same basic pattern. Small mineralized (darkly staining) masses are present (×140).

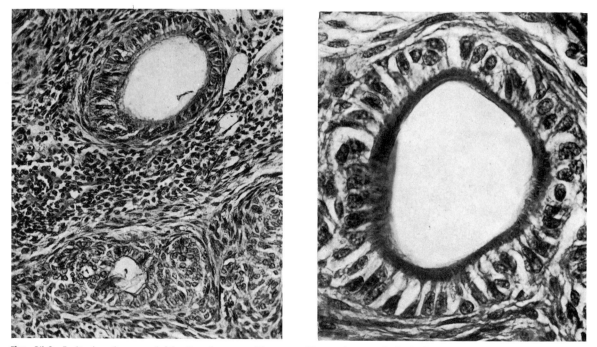

FIG. 25-8. *Left.* Another ameloblastic adenomatoid tumor illustrating marked similarity to the one above (×210). All tumors of this type are remarkably alike histologically. *Right.* Higher magnification emphasizes ameloblastic quality of cells lining tubular structures. This one has a thin hyalin-appearing lining. (This Figure and Figure 25-7 reproduced with permission from: Stafne, E. C.: *Oral Surg., 1*:887-894, 1948.)

ODONTOGENIC TUMORS

Ameloblastic Fibroma

This lesion, also called soft mixed odontoma, is rare. Six examples were found in our files. Proliferation of mesenchymal and epithelial odontogenic elements characterize this tumor. In contrast to ameloblastoma, in which the connective tissue is not part of the neoplastic process, ameloblastic fibroma contains an actively proliferating fibroblastic component. There is apparently no sex predilection. It is seen throughout childhood and adolescence but is rare in patients more than 21 years of age. The majority of these tumors affect the mandible, especially the bicuspid-molar region. Painless swelling is the rule and the lesion may be found incidentally on roentgenograms, where it produces a well-circumscribed cyst-like radiolucent zone. Occasionally an unerupted tooth is associated with the tumor. Grossly, the tissue is a soft fibrous mass. Histologically, the proliferating fibroblasts have plump nuclei that show little variation in size and shape. There are buds, cords, and islands of epithelial cells that are usually only a few cell-layers thick. Peripheral cells tend to become columnar as in ameloblastoma. If one studies many sections in an ameloblastic fibroma one may find evidence of hard dental structures such as dentin and enamel or preenamel. Hence this tumor overlaps histologically with ameloblastic odontoma, and both lesions probably should be regarded as hamartomas of a more primitive type than are the composite and compound odontomas.

Nearly all ameloblastic fibromas are easily cured by conservative surgical means, but a malignant counterpart in which fibrosarcoma arises in the stroma occurs. Two such cases were present in our series and several others have been documented.

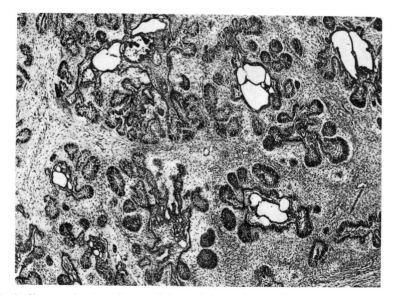

FIG. 25-9. Ameloblastic fibroma showing the ramifying and branching cords of ameloblastic cells and the associated fibroblastic proliferation (×48).

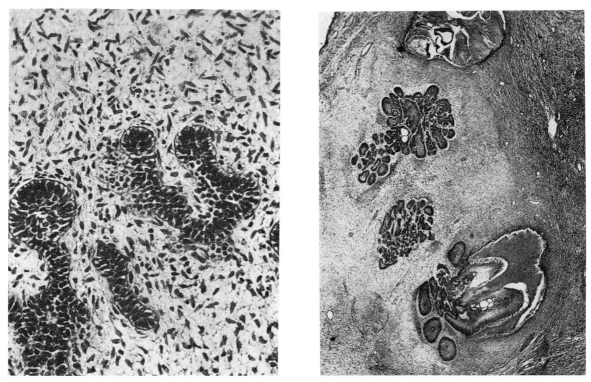

FIG. 25-10. *Left.* Higher magnification of ameloblastic fibroma to show the characteristics of the epithelial component and the plump uniform nuclei of the fibroblastic portion (×250). *Right.* Except for small foci of hard dental structure formation, the homogeneous masses shown here, this tumor was typical of ameloblastic fibroma throughout. Tumors like this emphasize the kinship of these various hamartoma-like tumors that reproduce dental structures or their precursors (×29).

Ameloblastic Odontoma

This tumor occupies a place between ameloblastic fibroma and the compound and composite odontomas. It contains foci of proliferating ameloblastic cells which introduce the hazard of mistaking the lesion for ameloblastoma. Dentin and enamel which are present in a poorly organized state differentiate it from ameloblastoma and indicate its basically hamartomatous nature. Parts of ameloblastic odontoma may resemble ameloblastic fibroma. Our files yielded only seven cases of this rare tumor which is usually found in children. Any part of either jaw may be affected but Gorlin and co-workers (1961) found a predilection for the premolar and molar areas. Delayed eruption or irregular position of teeth and swelling of the alveolar process may result from this tumor. The cyst-like zone in the roentgenogram may contain small or large radiopaque bodies. Nearly all of these well-cirmuscribed tumors are readily cured by conservative surgical means, but sarcomatous change in the connective tissue has been observed on very rare occasions.

275

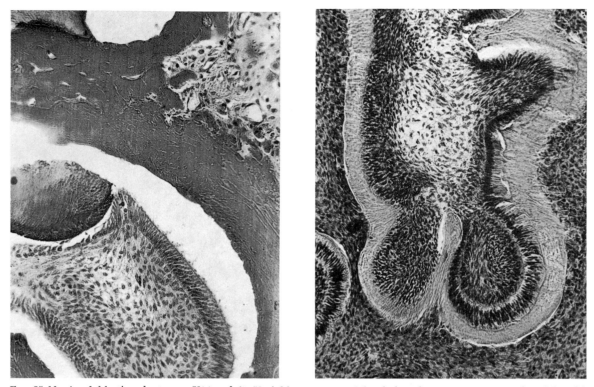

FIG. 25-11. Ameloblastic odontoma. *Upper left.* Variable amounts of hard dental structures are produced by this tumor. Dentin dominates this area but the dark mass at left center is early enamel matrix ($\times$250). *Upper right.* Here the ameloblastic proliferation is even more prominent ($\times$125). *Below.* Ameloblastic odontoma associated with unerupted molar tooth.

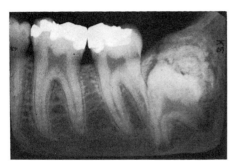

Complex Odontoma

This tumor lacks ameloblastic tissue, corresponding to a later stage of development of teeth than does ameloblastic odontoma. A disorderly mixture of hard dental elements characterize the lesion. It is considered to be somewhat more common in females and 6 of 11 cases affected this sex. It is found most often in older children and in young adults. It has a predilection for the molar portion of the lower jaw. The lesion is usually an incidental roentgenographic finding and is readily cured by simple removal.

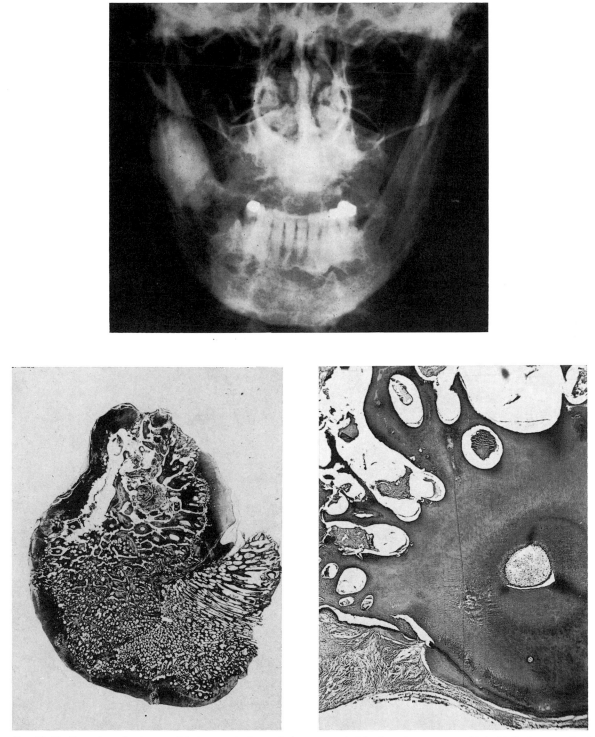

FIG. 25-12. Complex odontoma with its poorly formed, but recognizable dental structures. *Top.* Well-circumscribed and heavily mineralized tumor in ramus of mandible. *Lower left.* An entire complex odontoma (×3). *Lower right.* Higher magnification showing ramifying dentin in a background of fibrous tissue (×30).

Compound Odontomas

These tumors are composed of grossly recognizable teeth although they tend to be small and deformed. The number of teeth varies from three or four to many hundred. Complex and compound odontomas merge with one another, being arbitrarily separated on the basis of the degree of morphodifferentiation of the teeth. Both tumors are completely benign. Compound odontoma tends to occur in the incisor-cuspid region.

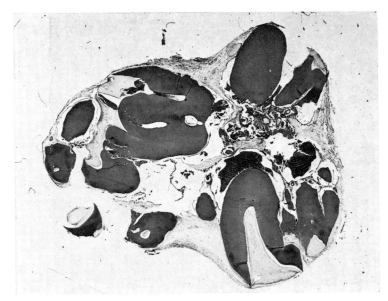

FIG. 25-13. Compound odontoma. Here the differentiation toward teeth is definite (×6). (Reproduced with permission from: Cina, M. T., Dahlin, D. C., and Gores, R. J.: *Proc. Staff Meet., Mayo Clinic, 36:*664-678, 1961.)

Myxoma (Fibromyxoma)

Myxomas of bone practically always occur in the jaws, which suggests that they are probably of odontogenic origin. This suggestion is supported by the resemblance of these tumors to the mesenchymal portion of the tooth germ. Some chondrosarcomas and even fibrosarcomas of the remainder of the skeleton show such prominent myxomatous alteration, probably a result of degeneration, that they have been classified erroneously among the myxomas and myxosarcomas. In our experience, myxoma of the jaws is approximately one-sixth as common as ameloblastoma. No sex predilection has been noted. Although almost any age may be affected, the majority are discovered during the second and third decades of life. The upper and lower jaws are about equally affected. This slowly growing lesion is usually painless but causes slowly progressive swelling, and sometimes severe facial deformity results. Roentgenographically the tumors may appear multilocular or unilocular. They cannot be distinguished from other cyst-like rarefying expansile lesions of the jaws. Grossly the tumor is soft, semitranslucent and may have a bosselated surface. Loose stellate cells dominate the histologic picture. They have long anastomosing cytoplasmic processes. The intercellular substance may be somewhat granular and basophilic. Some myxomas are hypocellular and obviously benign. Others contain relatively large and bizarre nuclei, suggest-

278

ing that they are more active, but follow-up studies indicate no correlation between cytologic abnormalities and ability of the tumor to recur. Sometimes zones within myxomas show considerable fibromatous quality but this does not appear to affect their clinical behavior.

The available evidence suggests that myxoma of the jaws has a capacity to recur similar to that of ameloblastoma, but it does not metastasize. The therapeutic goal should be total local removal of the lesion. Chondrosarcomas, osteogenic sarcomas and even fibrosarcomas with myxoid features can simulate myxoma and must be carefully differentiated from the latter.

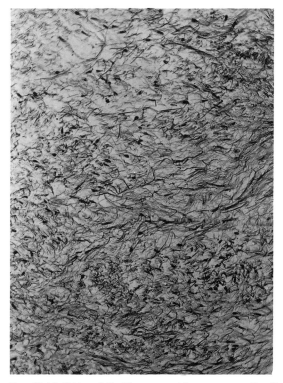

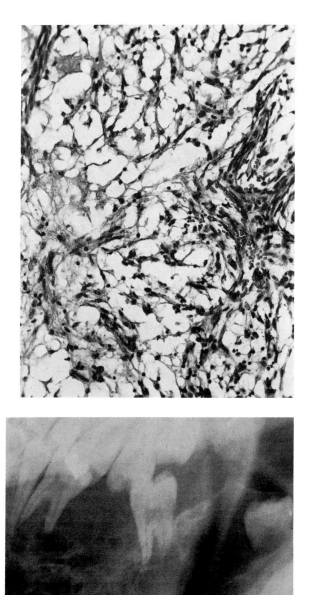

FIG. 25-14 *Upper left.* Myxoma with scanty, small cells and the characteristic, slightly fibrillar, and almost transparent matrix ($\times$140). *Upper right.* More cellular myxomas such as this have not been associated with a poorer prognosis in our material ($\times$200). *Right.* Expanding, "multicystic" myxoma which extended from the second bicuspid to the coronoid process of the right mandible.

Bibliography

1953   Berger, A., and Jaffe, H. L.: Fibrous (Fibro-osseous) Dysplasia of Jaw Bones. *J. Oral Surg.,* *11*:3-17.

1953   Jaffe, H. L.: Giant Cell Reparative Granuloma, Traumatic Bone Cyst, and Fibrous (Fibro-osseous) Dysplasia of the Jaw Bones. *Oral Surg., 6*:159-175.

1955   Small, I. A., and Waldron, C. A.: Ameloblastomas of the Jaws. *Oral Surg., 8*:281-297.

1958   Chaudhry, A. P., Spink, J. H., and Gorlin, R. J.: Periapical Fibrous 'Dysplasia (Cementoma). *J. Oral Surg., 16*:483-488.

1958   Pindborg, J. J.: A Calcifying Epithelial Odontogenic Tumor. *Cancer, 11*:838-843.

1958   Zimmerman, D. C., and Dahlin, D. C.: Myxomatous Tumors of the Jaws. *Oral Surg., 11*:1069-1080.

1959   Masson, J. K., McDonald, J. R., and Figi, F. A.: Adamantinoma of the Jaws. A Clinicopathologic Study of 101 Histologically Proved Cases. *Plast. & Reconstruct. Surg., 23*:510-525.

1960   Bernier, J. L.: *Tumors of the Odontogenic Apparatus and Jaws.* Atlas of Tumor Pathology, Section IV, Fascicle 10a, Armed Forces Institute of Pathology, Washington, D.C., National Research Council, pp. 9-107.

1961   Cash, C. D., Royer, Q. R., and Dahlin, D. C.: Metastatic Tumors of the Jaws. *Oral Surg., 14*:897-905.

1961   Cina, M. T., Dahlin, D. C., and Gores, R. J.: Odontogenic Mixed Tumors: A Review of the Mayo Clinic Series. *Proc. Staff Meet., Mayo Clin., 36*:664-678.

1961   Gorlin, R. J., Chaudhry, A. P., and Pindborg, J. J.: Odontogenic Tumors. Classification, Histopathology, and Clinical Behavior in Man and Domesticated Animals. *Cancer, 14*:73-101.

1962   Anderson, D. E., McClendon, J. L., and Cornelius, E. A.: Cherubism-Hereditary Fibrous Dysplasia of the Jaws. I. Genetic Considerations. II. Pathologic Considerations. *Oral Surg., 15* (Supplement 2): 5-16, 17-42.

1962   Cina, M. T., Dahlin, D. C., and Gores, R. J.: Ameloblastic Sarcoma. Report of Two Cases. *Oral Surg., 15*:696-700.

1963   Bhaskar, S. N.: Central Mucoepidermoid Tumors of the Mandible. Report of 2 Cases. *Cancer, 16*:721-726.

1963   Cina, M. T., Dahlin, D. C., and Gores, R. J.: Ameloblastic Adenomatoid Tumors. A Report of Four New Cases. *Am. J. Clin. Path.. 39*:59-65.

1963   Shafer, W. G., Hine, M. K., and Levy, B. M.: A *Textbook of Oral Pathology.* Ed. 2. Philadelphia, W. B. Saunders, pp. 200-236.

1964   Bhaskar, S. N.: Adenoameloblastoma: Its Histogenesis and Report of 15 New Cases. *J. Oral Surg., 22*:218-226.

1965   Pontius, E. E., Dziabis, M. D., and Foster, J. A.: Multicentric Melano-ameloblastoma of the Maxilla. *Cancer, 18*:381-387.

1965   Shear, M.: The Unity of Tumours of Odontogenic Epithelium. *Brit. J. Oral Surg., 2*:212-221.

1965   Tsukada, Y., de la Pava, S., and Pickren, J. W.: Granular Cell Ameloblastoma with Metastasis to the Lungs. Report of a Case and Review of the Literature. *Cancer, 18*:916-925.

1965   Vickers, R. A., Dahlin, D. C., and Gorlin, R. J.: Amyloid Containing Odontogenic Tumors. *Oral Surg., 20*:476-480.

Index

A

Adamantinoma of Jaws, 269, 270, 271
Adamantinoma of Long Bones, 8, 204
  age incidence, 205
  fibrous dysplasia in 206, 208, 210
  gross pathology, 207
  histopathology, 208
  incidence, 205
  localization, 205
  of jaw, 204, 269
  of Rathke's pouch, 204
  pathogenesis, 204
  physical findings, 206
  prognosis, 211
  roentgenologic features, 206
  sex incidence, 205
  symptoms, 206
  treatment, 210
Adenoameloblastoma, 272, 273
Age Distribution by Tumor Type, 9, 14, 15
Albrights, Syndrome, 238
Ameloblastic Adenomatoid Tumor, 272, 273
Ameloblastic Fibroma, 274, 275
Ameloblastic Odontoma, 275, 276
Ameloblastic Sarcoma, 274
Ameloblastoma, 269, 270, 271
Aneurysmal Bone Cyst, 242
  clinical features, 242
  gross pathology, 242
  histopathology, 242
  roentgenologic features, 242
  sarcoma in, 171, 217, 243
  treatment, 243
  "xanthic," 97
Angiosarcoma (*see* Hemangioendothelioma)

B

Benign Calcifying Giant Cell Tumor (*see* Benign Chondroblastoma)
Benign Chondroblastoma, 7, 38
  age incidence, 39
  gross pathology, 42
  histopathology, 42
  incidence, 39
  localization, 39
  physical findings, 40
  prognosis, 47
  roentgenologic features, 40
  sex incidence, 39
  symptoms, 40
  treatment, 47
Benign Giant Cell Tumor (*see* Giant Cell Tumor)
Benign Osteoblastoma (Giant Osteoid Osteoma), 8, 70
  age incidence, 71
  gross pathology, 74
  histopathology, 75
  incidence, 71
  localization, 71
  physical findings, 72
  prognosis, 77

  roentgenologic features, 72
  sex incidence, 71
  symptoms, 72
  treatment, 77
Brodie's Abscess (Chronic Osteomyelitis), 62, 256
"Brown" Tumor (Hyperparathyroidism). 263

C

Callus, Exuberant, 167, 248
Calcifying Epithelial Odontogenic Tumor, 269
Carcinoma, Metastatic (*see* Metastatic Carcinoma)
Cementoma, 268
Cherubism, 268
Chondroblastoma (*see* Benign Chondroblastoma)
Chondrogenic Tumors, 7, 18, 28, 38, 48, 138
Chondromyxoid Fibroma, 7, 48
  age incidence, 49
  gross pathology, 53
  histopathology, 53
  incidence, 49
  localization, 49
  physical findings, 50
  prognosis, 57
  roentgenologic features, 50
  sex incidence, 49
  symptoms, 50
  treatment, 57
Chondroma, 7, 28
  age incidence, 29
  gross pathology, 32
  histopathology, 33
  incidence, 29
  larynx, 28
  localization, 29
  multiple, 28, 31, 36, 37
  of soft tissue, 28, 264
  para-articular, 264
  periosteal, 28, 30, 33, 35
  physical findings, 30
  prognosis, 35
  roentgenologic features, 30
  sarcomas in, 36, 37
  sex incidence, 29
  symptoms, 30
  synovial, 28, 264
  treatment, 35
Chondromatosis, 28, 31, 36, 37
  synovial, 264
Chondrosarcoma, Mesenchymal, 138, 151
Chondrosarcoma, Primary, 7, 138
  age incidence, 139
  gross pathology, 144
  histopathology, 147
  incidence, 139
  localization, 139
  mesenchymal, 138, 151
  of soft tissues, 138
  physical findings, 141
  prognosis, 151
  roentgenologic features, 141

INDEX

sex incidence, 139
symptoms, 140
treatment, 150
Chondrosarcoma, Secondary, 7, 27, 36, 37, 138
  age incidence, 139
  gross pathology, 144
  histopathology, 147
  in chordoma, 228, 231
  in exostoses (osteochondromas), 27
  in multiple chondroma, 36, 37
  incidence, 139
  localization, 140
  physical findings, 141
  roentgenologic features, 141
  symptoms, 140
  treatment, 150
Chordoma, 8, 222
  age incidence, 223
  differential diagnosis, 228
  gross pathology, 227, 232
  histopathology, 228
  incidence, 223
  localization, 223
  physical findings, 224
  prognosis, 233
  roentgenologic features, 224
  sex incidence, 223
  symptoms, 224
  treatment, 232
Classification of Bone Tumors, 6, 11
Clinical Features, in Diagnosis, 4
Codman's Tumor (Benign Chondroblastoma), 38
Complex Odontoma, 276, 277
Compound Odontoma, 278
Cyst, Aneurysmal Bone, 242
Cyst, Epidermoid, 252
Cyst, "Hemorrhagic," 268
Cyst, of Jaws, 268
Cyst, Simple, 250
Cyst, "Traumatic," 268
Cysts Associated with Joint Disease, 254
  in osteoarthritis, 254
  in pigmented villonodular synovitis, 254
  in rheumatoid joint disease, 254

D

Degenerative Joint Disease, 254
Dentinoma, 268
Desmoplastic Fibroma, 8, 212, 219
Diagnosis, 3, 4, 5
  clinical features in, 4
  decalcification, 5
  gross pathology in, 3
  laboratory studies in, 4
  needle aspiration, 5
  rapid sections in, 4
  roentgenograms in, 3
  special stains in, 5
Diaphysial Aclasis (see Osteochondromas, Multiple)
"Disappearing" Bone Disease, 100, 101, 102, 104, 106

E

Ecchinococcosis of Bone, 234
Enchondroma, 28

Enchondromatosis (see Chondroma, Multiple)
Eosinophilic Granuloma, 257
Epidermoid Cyst of Bone, 252
Endothelioma (Ewing's Tumor), 186
Epiphyseal Chondromatous Giant Cell Tumors (see Benign Chondroblastoma)
Epulis (Giant Cell Reparative Granuloma), 261
Ewing's Tumor, 8, 186
  age incidence, 187
  gross pathology, 190
  histopathology, 191
  incidence, 187
  large cell variant, 186, 191, 193
  laboratory findings, 188
  localization, 187
  physical findings, 188
  prognosis, 194
  roentgenologic features, 188
  sex incidence, 187
  symptoms, 188
  treatment, 193
Exostosis (Osteochondroma), 18
  multiple, 18, 22, 27
  subungual, 18, 26
Extraosseous Cartilaginous Tumors, 28, 138, 264
Exuberant Callus, 167, 248, 249

F

Fibrogenic Tumors, 8, 90, 212
Fibroma, 8, 90
  age incidence, 91
  ameloblastic, 274, 275
  desmoplastic, 8, 212, 219
  gross pathology, 94
  histopathology, 95
  incidence, 91
  localization, 91
  periapical, 268
  physical findings, 92
  prognosis, 99
  roentgenologic features, 92
  sex incidence, 91
  symptoms, 92
  treatment, 99
  "xanthic," 97
Fibromatosis, 90
Fibromyxoma of Jaws, 278
Fibro-osseous Dysplasia, 58, 238, 268
Fibrosarcoma, 8, 212
  age incidence, 213
  gross pathology, 215
  histopathology, 216
  in chordoma, 228, 231
  incidence, 213
  in infarcts of bone, 212, 265
  localization, 213
  multicentric, 212
  myxoid, 218
  periosteal, 212
  physical findings, 214
  prognosis, 219
  roentgenologic features, 214
  secondary, 212
  sex incidence, 213
  symptoms, 214

treatment, 219
Fibrous Cortical Defect (Fibroma), 90
Fibrous Defect (Fibroma), 90
Fibrous Dysplasia, 238
    cherubism, 268
    clinical features, 238
    gross pathology, 238
    histopathology, 238
    in adamantinoma, 206, 208, 210
    polyostotic, 238
    prognosis, 239
    roentgenologic features, 238
    sarcoma in, 171, 239, 241
    treatment, 239
    "xanthic," 97
Fibrous Scars, 90, 93

G

Gardner's Syndrome, 58
Giant Cell "Epulis" (Giant Cell Reparative Granuloma), 261
Giant Cell Reparative Granuloma, 79, 261
Giant Cell Lesion, 78
Giant Cell Tumor, 8, 78
    age incidence, 79
    differential diagnosis, 78
    gross pathology, 82
    histopathology, 83
    incidence, 79
    in Paget's disease, 81
    localization, 79
    of jaw bones, 261
    metastasizing, 78, 87
    multicentric, 82
    physical findings, 80
    prognosis, 86
    roentgenologic features, 80
    sex incidence, 79
    symptoms, 80
    treatment, 86
    "xanthic," 97
Giant Cell Tumor, Malignant (see Malignant Giant Cell Tumor)
Giant Osteoid Osteoma (see Benign Osteoblastoma)
Glomus Tumors, 100
Gross Pathology in Diagnosis, 3

H

Hemangioendothelioma, 9, 100, 102, 104, 107, 108
    incidence, 101
    treatment, 109
Hemangioma, 9, 100
    age incidence, 101
    gross pathology, 104
    histopathology, 104
    incidence, 101
    localization, 101
    physical findings, 102
    prognosis, 109
    roentgenologic features, 102
    sex incidence, 101
    symptoms, 102
    treatment, 109
Hemangiomatosis, 100, 102
Hemangiopericytoma, 9, 100, 105

incidence, 101
localization, 101
Hemangiosarcoma (see Hemangioendothelioma)
Hematopoietic Tumors, 7, 116, 126
Hemophiliac Pseudotumors, 234
Heterotopic Ossification, 246
    clinical features, 246
    gross pathology, 246
    histopathology, 246, 247, 248
    malignancy in, 247
    prognosis, 246
    roentgenologic features, 246
    simulating sarcoma, 246
Histiocytosis X ("Reticuloendotheliosis"), 257
    clinical features, 257
    eosinophilic granuloma, 257
    gross pathology, 258
    histopathology, 258, 259
    Letterer-Siwe disease, 257
    prognosis, 258
    roentgenologic features, 258, 260
    Schüller-Christian syndrome, 257
    treatment, 258
Hodgkin's Lymphoma, 126, 129, 132, 134
Hydatid Disease of Bone, 234
Hyperparathyroidism, Simulating Neoplasm of Bone, 263

I

Incidence by Tumor Type, 11
Infantile Cortical Hyperostosis, 248
Infarcts of Bone, 265, 266

J

Juxtacortical Osteogenic Sarcoma (Parosteal Osteogenic Sarcoma), 176

L

Letterer-Siwe Disease, 257
Leukemia, 7, 126, 136, 193
Lipogenic Tumors, 9, 110
Lipoma, 9, 110
Liposarcoma, 9, 110, 112
Literature, General, 6, 16
Localization Data by Tumor Type, 12
Lymphangioma, 100
Lymphocytic Lymphoma, 126, 132

M

Maffucci's Syndrome, 28
Malignant Giant Cell Tumor, 8, 78, 86, 196
    age incidence, 197
    etiology, 196
    gross pathology, 200
    histopathology, 201
    incidence, 197
    localization, 197
    physical findings, 198
    prognosis, 203
    roentgenologic features, 198
    sex incidence, 197
    symptoms, 198
    treatment, 203
Malignant Lymphoma of Bone, 7, 126

INDEX

age incidence, 127
gross pathology, 131
histopathology, 132
incidence, 127
in osteomyelitis, 128, 130
localization, 127
physical findings, 128
prognosis, 136
roentgenologic features, 128
sex incidence, 127
symptoms, 128
treatment, 136
Massive Osteolysis, 100, 101, 102, 106
incidence, 101
Mastocytosis, 234
Melanoameloblastoma, 269
Mesenchymal Chondrosarcoma, 138, 151
histopathology, 153, 154
Metaphyseal Fibrous Defect (Fibroma), 90
Metastatic Carcinoma, 234, 269
clinical features, 234
pathology, 235
roentgenologic features, 234
treatment, 235
Multiple Chondroma, 28, 31, 36, 37
Multiple Myeloma (see Myeloma)
Multiple Osteochondromas, 18, 22, 27
Myeloma, 7, 116
age incidence, 117
amyloidosis in, 118, 121, 122, 124
extraskeletal, 116
gross pathology, 121
histopathology, 121
incidence, 117
in osteomyelitis, 121
laboratory findings, 118
localization, 117
physical findings, 118
prognosis, 124
renal changes, 116
roentgenologic features, 118
sex incidence, 117
"solitary," 116, 120, 124
symptoms, 118
treatment, 124
Myositis Ossificans (see Heterotopic Ossification)
Myxomatous Tumors, 7, 48, 145, 212, 278
myxoma of jaws, 278
myxosarcoma, 212, 218

N

Needle Aspiration in Diagnosis, 5
Neurilemmoma, 9, 114
Neurofibroma, 114
Neurofibromatosis (von Recklinghausen's), 114
Neurofibrosarcoma, 114
Neurogenic Tumors, 9, 114
Nonosteogenic Fibroma (Fibroma), 8, 90
Notochordal Tumors, 8, 222

O

Odontogenic Tumors, 268
ameloblastic adenomatoid tumor, 272, 273
ameloblastic fibroma, 274, 275
ameloblastic odontoma, 275, 276
ameloblastoma, 269, 270, 271

calcifying epithelial odontogenic tumor, 269
complex odontoma, 276, 277
compound odontoma, 278
myxoma (fibromyxoma), 278, 279
Ollier's Disease, 28, 31, 36, 37
Ossification, Heterotopic, 246
Ossifying Fibroma (see Benign Osteoblastoma)
Osteitis Deformans Simulating Neoplasm, 262
Osteoarthritis, 254
Osteoblastoma (see Benign Osteoblastoma)
Osteocartilaginous Exostosis (see Osteochondroma)
Osteochondroma, 7, 18
age incidence, 19
gross pathology, 23
histopathology, 24
incidence, 19
localization, 19
multiple, 18, 22, 27
physical findings, 20
prognosis, 25
roentgenologic features, 20
sarcoma in, 27
sex incidence, 19
symptoms, 20
treatment, 25
Osteoclastoma (see Giant Cell Tumor)
Osteofibroma, 268
Osteogenic Fibroma (see Benign Osteoblastoma)
Osteogenic Sarcoma, 7, 156
age incidence, 157, 158
biopsy diagnosis, 173
etiology, 27, 156
gross pathology, 163
histopathology, 167
in chordoma, 228, 231
incidence, 157
in Paget's disease, 156, 161, 172
juxtacortical, 176
localization, 157, 158
multicentric, 164
of jaws, 172, 173
of soft tissues, 156
parosteal, see Parosteal Osteogenic Sarcoma)
postirradiation, 156, 171
physical findings, 159
prognosis, 174
roentgenologic features, 159
sex incidence, 157, 158
symptoms, 159
treatment, 173
Osteogenic Tumors, 7, 58, 62, 70, 156, 176
Osteoid Osteoma, 8, 62
age incidence 63
gross pathology, 66
histopathology, 67
incidence, 63
localization, 63
physical findings, 64
prognosis, 69
roentgenologic features, 64
sex incidence, 63
symptoms, 64
treatment, 69
Osteoma, 58
fibrous, 268
of paranasal sinuses, 58, 59

parosteal, 58, 60, 61
Osteomyelitis, 254
  carcinoma in, 255
  clinical features, 255
  fibrosarcoma in, 255
  gross pathology, 255
  histopathology, 255, 256
  malignant lymphoma in, 128, 130, 255
  myeloma in, 121, 255
  roentgenologic features, 255, 256, 257
  treatment, 255
Osteosarcoma (*see* Osteogenic Sarcoma)

P

Paget's Disease, Simulating Neoplasm, 262
  giant cell tumor in, 81
  sarcoma in, 172
Para-Articular Chondromas, 264
Parathyroid Osteopathy, 263
Parosteal Osteogenic Sarcoma, 8, 176
  age incidence, 177
  differential diagnosis, 178, 180, 182
  gross pathology, 179
  histopathology, 182
  incidence, 177
  localization, 177
  physical findings, 178
  prognosis, 185
  roentgenologic features, 178
  sex incidence, 177
  symptoms, 178
  treatment, 185
Parosteal Osteoma, 58, 60, 61
Periosteal Chondroma, 28, 30, 33, 35
Periosteal Desmoid, 90
"Periosteal" Fibrosarcoma, 212
Periosteal Hemangioma, 103
"Phantom" Bone Disease, 100, 101, 102, 104, 106
Pigmented Villonodular Synovitis, 254
Plasma Cell Leukemia, 118

Plasma Cell Myeloma, 116
Postirradiation Sarcoma of Bone, 171, 196, 212

R

Rapid Sections in Diagnosis, 4
Recklinghausen's Neurofibromatosis, 114
Reticuloendotheliosis (Histiocystosis X), 257
Reticulum Cell Sarcoma (*see* Malignant Lymphoma of Bone)
Rheumatoid Synovitis, 254
Roentgenograms in Diagnosis, 3

S

Schüller-Christian Syndrome, 257
Simple ("Unicameral") Cyst of Bone, 250
  clinical features, 250
  pathology of, 250
  roentgenologic features, 250
  treatment, 250
  "xanthic," 97
Skeletal Distribution by Tumor Type, 9, 12, 13
"Solitary" Myeloma, 116, 120
  prognosis, 124
Special Stains in Diagnosis, 5
Subperiosteal Giant Cell Tumor (Aneurysmal Bone Cyst), 242
Subungual Exostoses, 18, 26
Synovial Chondromatosis, 28, 264

T

Tori, 58
Tumors of Unknown Origin, 8, 78, 186, 196, 204
Tumors of Vascular Origin, 9, 100

U

Unclassified Tumors, 9
"Unicameral" Cyst of Bone (Simple Cyst), 250

V

Vascular Tumors, 9, 100

X

"Xanthoma" ("Xanthofibroma"), 90, 97